The Essential Guide to
Trauma Sensitive Yoga

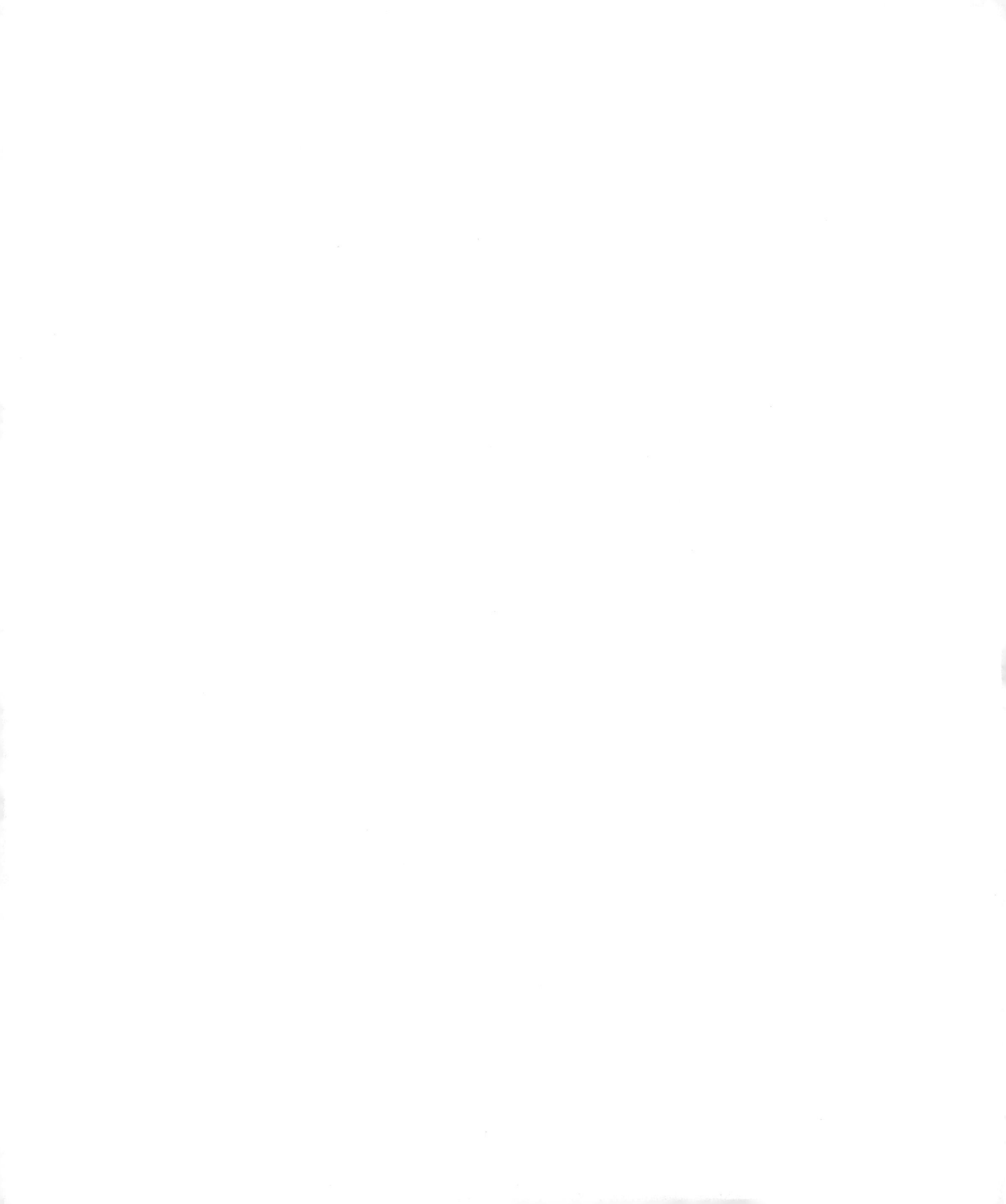

The Essential Guide to

TRAUMA SENSITIVE YOGA

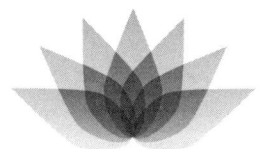

How to Create Safer Spaces for All

LARA LAND

Foreword by Michelle Cassandra Johnson

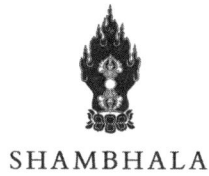

SHAMBHALA

SHAMBHALA PUBLICATIONS, INC.
2129 13th Street
Boulder, Colorado 80302
www.shambhala.com

Cover art: Cat Grishaver
Cover design: Cat Grishaver
Interior design: Steve Dyer

9 8 7 6 5 4 3 2 1

FIRST EDITION
Printed in the United States of America

Shambhala Publications makes every effort
to print on acid-free, recycled paper.
Shambhala Publications is distributed worldwide by
Penguin Random House, Inc., and its subsidiaries.

LIBRARY OF CONGRESS CATALOGING-IN-PUBLICATION DATA
Names: Land, Lara, author.
Title: The essential guide to trauma sensitive yoga: how to create
safer spaces for all / Lara Land.
Description: First edition. | Boulder, Colorado:
Shambhala Publications Inc., [2023]
Identifiers: LCCN 2022030143 | ISBN 9781611809886 (trade paperback)
Subjects: LCSH: Psychic trauma—Alternative treatment. | Yoga—
Therapeutic use. | Yoga—Study and teaching.
Classification: LCC BC552.T7 L37 2023 | DDC 616.89/165—dc23/eng/20220816
LC record available at https://lccn.loc.gov/2022030143

CONTENTS

FOREWORD

I REMEMBER ARRIVING A FEW MINUTES LATE TO THE OPENING activities for the Yoga Service Council Conference in May 2018. I was in a whirlwind of a time in my life preparing to move back to North Carolina from Portland, Oregon, after having been in Portland for a little less than a year. I was stressed, grieving the loss of my father and grandmother, and I felt groundless in many ways. I went into the room where the opening of the conference was being held and sat in the back. I didn't feel very social, and I really didn't know many folks in attendance at the conference. I sat and watched folks on the stage chant, invite us in, and share guidelines and agreements for our time together.

Someone on stage encouraged us to say hello to folks and to build community. This is what yoga is about: union and coming into community. Even though I knew this was the meaning of yoga, the thought of building community at that point in my life triggered a response in my nervous system. I knew I would have to summon a vast amount of energy to make new connections while tending my grieving, broken, and unsettled heart. I wanted to turn inward and instead was invited to turn outward. Yoga asks us to do both and to see the relationship between our internal experience and how we show up in the world.

I returned to that same room for the second day of the conference. This time I didn't sit in the back; I sat in the third row next to someone I had not yet met. The conference presenters invited us to share names and a little about ourselves with the person next to us. I turned to the person next to me, and her name was Lara. She had a lot of energy and seemed eager to connect. We chatted, and I learned some about her story of yoga and service. I shared some about my own story of yoga and justice. After that moment of connection, I knew Lara was someone I wouldn't forget. There was something about her energy that let me know she was truly committed to yoga as a pathway for service and healing. For me, yoga is a reclamation of our wholeness and humanity. Yoga has the potential to support us individually and collectively in healing our trauma. It was clear to me that her vision and experience of yoga mirrored my own.

Throughout the years, I continued to follow what Lara was doing and deepened my practice and devotion to yoga as a way of living. When Lara reached out to me to write the foreword for *The Essential Guide to Trauma Sensitive Yoga: How to Create Safer Spaces for All*, I didn't have to take long to think about the request. I had not yet read *The Essential Guide to Trauma Sensitive Yoga*, and I trusted the offering that Lara was contributing to the practice and long lineage of yoga was going to be a unique and significant one.

Lara and Three and a Half Acres Yoga's work is shifting the landscape of yoga, specifically trauma-informed yoga. Lara invites yoga teachers, facilitators, and practitioners of yoga to notice the trauma that lives inside their nervous systems because of the horrors that happen on a daily basis—racism, transphobia, ableism, sexual violence, the carceral system, classism, and other toxic systems rooted in dominance. Lara takes what she has learned from her lived experience and in the numerous trainings in which she has participated, her experiences teaching in various communities and starting a nonprofit, and her intuition about the world and what is needed at this time and asks yoga teachers, facilitators, and practitioners to consider what it might be like to slow down, return to a state of homeostasis, practice mindfulness techniques, and practice the various limbs of the eight limb path of yoga to heal our trauma.

The Essential Guide to Trauma Sensitive Yoga: How to Create Safer Spaces for All is a comprehensive guide to better understand trauma and how trauma lives in the body—both the individual body and our collective. This resource offers countless practices focused on how to come back into the body, be that through pranayama (breathwork), movement, or meditation. It shares detailed information about what to look for if you are seeking a trauma-informed yoga teacher or class and breaks down what yoga teachers need to study, practice, and be knowledgeable about to offer a trauma-informed class. During this time when so many are turning toward yoga and contemplative practices for their recovery from prolonged isolation due to COVID-19, losses due to systems of oppression, and nervous system dysregulation due to so much uncertainty, Lara's book is a vital and critical resource for yoga teachers and practitioners. The divine spark that I saw in Lara when I first met her will continue to shine through this offering and beyond.

MICHELLE CASSANDRA JOHNSON

INTRODUCTION

In March 2008, I returned to the United States with nowhere to live and not sure of what I would be able to do professionally. I had spent the better part of my Saturn Return year—an astrology-indicated time of transitional growth—studying and volunteering in India and Rwanda. I had given up my longtime Brooklyn apartment and was largely disconnected from my former New York yoga community. The stock market had crashed, which meant most of my private yoga clients, who made up the bulk of my teaching income, were not renewing their contracts.

Being away from my chosen career path for so long had me feeling like a runner held back before a big race: filled with ideas and energy and ready to share my recent experiences. I created Bring Back the Light, a workshop on karma, yoga, and service that I planned to pitch to religious organizations, schools, and businesses. I thought I was going to transform the way the world (or at least the New York tri-state area) thought about yoga, especially the way it implemented charity. No one could stop me, not even my mother, who reminded me that no one was spending money on yoga during a deep economic recession.

I rented a studio apartment on 127th Street in Harlem. I had heard great things about Harlem and was eager to get to know the community as I settled into my new home. Instead, I promptly got an offer to teach daily yoga at 6:30 a.m. in Greenpoint, Brooklyn—an hour away.

With no savings and no job alternatives, I said yes to the long, disjointed commute. After ten months, as I trudged (yet again) across the Pulaski Bridge at 6 a.m., my red rain boots filled with knee-deep snow, I knew that it was time for a change. It was time for me to open my own studio in the Harlem neighborhood I had grown to love.

In 2011, I opened Land Yoga on the ground floor of a condominium in the heart of the busy Frederick Douglass Boulevard (Eighth Avenue) corridor. A cluster of businesses had opened, and I felt that I was a part of a community-building moment. I made it a priority to reach as many people as possible, especially complete beginners. My team of teachers, wellness practitioners, college interns, and I, offered classes, workshops, massage, acupuncture, Reiki, pre- and postnatal offerings, children's parties, art shows, demonstrations, and cooking classes. We even brought yoga to local parks, schools, street fairs, and festivals. I dreamed about doing in Harlem what I had done in Rwanda: bringing yoga to folks who had been through intense trauma to support their health and healing. I wanted to do it smartly and sustainably, avoiding the mistakes I had witnessed from others in the nonprofit world. It was an idea that I kept brewing as I made Land Yoga strong enough to take on an additional enterprise.

Drawn from my time in Rwanda, my scope of "trauma" included people who had experienced abuse, had limited resources, and were marginalized within our communities. I hadn't yet come to understand the traumatic stress of daily life as a Black American in our country due to living with structural racism, microaggressions, othering, and exoticism. My experience of living and forming my yoga studio in Harlem opened my eyes to and led me to further research these types of traumas. I'm deeply indebted to my BIPOC friends and mentors in the community who trusted me enough to share their experiences and showed patience and compassion for me in these early days of my learning how best to address the community's needs.

THREE AND A HALF ACRES YOGA

Then, in 2014, Eric Garner and Michael Brown were murdered by police (in New York City and Ferguson, Missouri, respectively). The senselessness of their deaths circled and circled inside of me. I felt that I had to do something—however small, with the skills I had—to make a positive difference. I mapped my thoughts and entrepreneurial vision and soon had the initial structure for Three and a Half Acres Yoga, a nonprofit designed to broaden access to yoga and breathing and mindfulness techniques, focusing on communities that have experienced trauma.

The name Three and a Half Acres Yoga is derived from a quote from my Ashtanga teacher Sharath Jois, who made the connection for me between clean air and mental health. He taught that a person needs three and a half acres of tree-filled land to breathe properly and that without the access to this generous amount of clean fresh air, clear thinking is not possible. With my nonprofit, I aspired to create the benefits of this acreage through relaxation, lung expansion, and increased breath capacity through yoga.

Our classes and trainings support practitioners and teachers alike in recognizing their power to generate positive change. We offer stress reduction for those dealing with the trauma associated with these high-profile deaths and ongoing social injustices. The techniques we use assist practitioners in finding their vision and activating their voices. In addition, this work trains others in how to de-escalate contentious situations.

We formed partnerships with organizations such as Harlem United, the Food Bank of New York, and Children's Aid Society. I created a separate arm of the organization to bring yoga to the New York Police Department. I traveled all over Harlem and upper Manhattan to visit precincts at roll calls, which are held at the start of officers' shifts and when they get their daily briefing. The first time I went I was shaky as I explained the benefits of yoga and urged them to join our free classes for cops. Over time, my voice grew confident, my pitches got better, and officers started coming to class.

Trauma sensitive yoga for police is a sensitive, controversial offering; many people feel no police reform is possible and that our free offerings are misdirected. Our feeling counters that: yoga is revolutionary. It teaches the habit of pausing before action, giving that one extra second to slow things down. We become less directed by our "reptilian brain" and more aware of conscious choice. This habit has the potential to disrupt reactionary responses, and we hope to get our yoga classes into the Police Academy to plant the seeds of awareness from day one of training.

Our targeted work has had a positive response. Officers have become regulars at our yoga classes with a few enthusiasts wrangling coworkers to join them. We have also been able to do some powerful work with the NYPD Law Enforcement Explorers program, which brings local youth and officers together to practice yoga side by side and connect with one another. I was honored for leading these efforts by former Mayor Bill de Blasio on National Night Out, a campaign to promote better partnerships between community and police. Our work with the NYPD Law Enforcement Explorers program was also featured on NY1, our local cable news network.

However, now that the NYPD has its own health and wellness department, we have suspended most of these classes and are focusing on broadening access to yoga for survivors of trauma in five major categories: housing and food insecurity, domestic violence, LGBTQIA+, recovery, and justice issues such as integration after incarceration and immigration. We are also looking at how to actively support folks affected by climate crisis disasters as that need becomes more and more urgent.

Our program teachers are trained in yoga trauma sensitivity and in best practices for avoiding trauma triggers in yoga class, as well as how to interpret yoga teaching in a way that is empowering for the practitioner. This means the practice is rooted in reinforcing autonomy and nurturing the practitioner's ability to tune in to their inner knowledge about what is best for them. The cost of training is covered by volunteer commitment. When the volunteer commitment is complete, we hire the volunteers we most believe in and they become teachers, mentors, and trainers.

Our work has had an impact on the lives of yoga teachers and their students, including those who have faced a wide variety of trauma as the result of drugs, abuse, age, discrimination, and housing insecurity. We have found that our method of teaching is effective for all, regardless of the origin of trauma, because it is born of adaptability.

THE TRAUMATIC EVENT THAT SHOOK THE WORLD

As I set out to write this book in the winter of 2019, I could not have predicted the way our methods would be tested by the new traumatic event each one of us was about to face: the arrival of COVID-19 in early 2020. Living through a pandemic is traumatic. It has changed many of us, all at once and within the briefest of periods, from outgoing, social beings to homebodies afraid to be near strangers. In New York City, I witnessed previously polite neighbors sneer when folks came too close, scurry to the edges of apartment lobbies with their heads down as if hiding, and rush each other at the grocery store for toilet paper and disinfectant.

Survival instincts are embedded in each one of us, in our DNA. They can "flip our lids," turning us into selfish and single-minded lunatics, especially when scarcity or perceived scarcity enters the mix. Collective intelligence, collaboration, and altruism are also embedded in our genetic code for survival. We know this because it feels good to do good. In fact, the Dalai Lama himself often speaks about a kind of wise selfishness: "If you help others with sincere motivation and sincere concern, that will bring you more fortune, more friends, more smiles, and more success."[1] He also reminds us we will have more helpers available when our time comes for needing assistance.

The writer and activist Adrienne Maree Brown asks so eloquently in her seminal *Emergent Strategy: Shaping Change, Changing Worlds*, "Do you understand that your quality of life and your survival are tied to how authentic and generous the connections are between you and the people and place you live with and in?"[2] The human challenge is that it is hard to know how much we are connected to one another when we are in a stress response because of the way it narrows our vision. As the Buddhist minister and author Lama Rod Owens recently reminded me in an episode of the podcast *Ten Percent Happier*, we have to practice the kind of meditation that awakens us to our connectivity when things are not difficult. When times become difficult, that knowledge is instilled in us, and we are ready to lean in though our nervous systems want to lead us elsewhere. "When a crisis happens," he said, "actually what happens is I just fall into my practice."[3]

Even with all my yoga and meditation training, when the pandemic hit I felt fear and mistrust of others arise within my body. Stepping outside my door was enough to make my heart rate go up. Grocery stores felt like minefields. Nothing and no one felt safe to the point that when I finally did start meeting friends again (outside and at a social distance), I didn't know how to be with them. I remember running into my friend Kristin on the street one day. We stood across from each other, faces half-covered by our masks, trying to connect, but our bodies kept doing a strange shuffle and our words came out trite and superficial. It was hard to know where to start our conversation. There was both so much to say and the feeling it had already been said. We needed a kind of silent, emotional communion, with the nuances of touch and facial expressions. With those methods unavailable, we just flapped around like fish out of water before scurrying off.

I know my experience was not unique. Fear can envelop us in an instant and stay with us long after the trigger has departed. We will all be working through the triggers and aftermath of COVID-19 for some time in our own unique ways.

Many people were shocked during the pandemic by how we handled or were unable to handle low-level challenges—myself included. This is because of how stressed to capacity our systems were. When already so stretched, the smallest burden can overwhelm the system. Have you heard the Chinese proverb "If you want to know what water is, don't ask a fish"? It seems that we didn't know how stressful the environment we were swimming in was until COVID-19 hit. Since 2020, many Americans (and people worldwide) have woken up to the buzzing stress they and their fellow citizens are facing as the result of structural and systemic racism, environmental stress and species loss, economic insecurity, few and poor social safety nets, an individualistic perfectionist culture, and a sea of social media designed to breed competition and isolation. We are living at a time and in a society that encourages a pace of life so traumatic to all our systems. The practices of trauma-informed yoga help revise that narrative and slow it to a more humane speed.

When a person is already dealing with institutional or other traumas, a new traumatic incident triggers the body into a traumatic response. Another person may respond to the same event without trauma. Another may even experience post-traumatic growth, a positive psychological change that can come for some from their struggles. All responses to trauma are correct ones: they all exhibit the genius of the mind-body system that protects us from harm we cannot bear. Our body responds with its unique internal intelligence, drawn from personal history living in each of our cells.

We are living in an era of enormous trauma with a likelihood of more traumatic incidents to come. We are going to need some help to get through it. One of the best things we can do is prepare, to understand and regulate our systems. If you are feeling stressed, practice yoga. If you are feeling good, practice yoga, too. The fruits of the practice, the ability to calm yourself and recognize when you are becoming dysregulated, will help you now and later.

Promoting Inner Guidance in Group Yoga

Though a handful of books explain trauma-informed yoga teaching for the individual, this is the first book that outlines the tough job of teaching the individual in a group setting. My message to teachers is to get to know the individual student and why they are there. Guide each student on their personal journey and help them awaken their own inner guidance and launch a self-led voyage. My hope is that this book will help you do that while serving as a resource to the practitioner, providing guidance on everything from what to look for in a teacher to what to focus on in each pose and how to create a devoted home practice. I hope it inspires both teacher and student to rethink the role of yoga, the yoga teacher, and the relationship between teacher and student in yoga spaces everywhere.

Note to Readers

The nature of this book requires that I discuss, sometimes in detail, traumatic incidences and responses. Witnessing or hearing about trauma can be triggering. As you read, check in with your nervous system, taking breaks to regulate yourself through grounding, shaking out, immersing in nature, journaling, calling a friend, watching a show, or seeking out any other resource that supports your nature. Take your time.

Defining Trauma

Trauma is traditionally regarded as a psychological and medical disorder of the mind. The practice of modern medicine and psychology, while giving lip service to a connection between mind and body, greatly underestimates the deep relationship that they have in the healing of trauma. The welding unity of body and mind that, throughout time, has formed the philosophical and practical underpinnings of most of the world's traditional healing systems is sadly lacking in our modern understanding and treatment of trauma.

—DR. PETER A. LEVINE,
Waking the Tiger

NAMING THINGS MATTERS. IT GIVES THOSE THINGS WEIGHT and provides a way for us to communicate and legitimize what we know is happening to us. Yet so often science is slow to identify the experiences we have long recognized anecdotally. Clinical diagnoses are not fixed things. They change as science advances, representation increases in the field, and scientists are pushed to expand the framework of their research to include a larger variety of experiences. For this reason, we can expect new definitions of trauma to come into our consciousness as more and more marginalized people take power and their experiences are brought into the light.

We often think of trauma as a single instance, such as a violent attack, but there are many kinds of trauma, even some that get passed down through generations. The *Diagnostic and Statistical Manual of Mental Disorders* (DSM-5) published by the American Psychiatric Association defines post-traumatic stress disorder (PTSD) as "exposure to actual or threatened death, serious injury, or sexual violence." It explains that exposure may include direct experience, being a witness, learning about an event that happened to a loved one, or repeated contact with details surrounding a traumatic event, as is often the case with nurses, therapists, and police.

PTSD is the most recognized result of trauma, but there are many other trauma- and stressor-related disorders. The DSM-5 lists reactive attachment disorder, disinhibited social engagement disorder, acute stress disorder, adjustment disorders and other specified trauma- and stressor-related disorders, and unspecified trauma- and stressor-related disorders. Nowhere, however, in DSM-5 is race-based traumatic stress injury (RBTSI) listed, detailed brilliantly by Dr. Gail Parker in her book *Restorative Yoga for Ethnic and Race-Based Stress and Trauma*.

To give further context to the complexity and social factors behind the DSM-5 definition, sexual violence as a potential PTSD trigger was only recently added. We may want to ask ourselves what other traumas are absent from the clinical definition of PTSD and how that affects the more than forty-one million Americans who receive counseling each year.

"Trust science" has become the mantra of the Progressive Left and a plea for those who have fallen prey to conspiracy theories, and yet we must also acknowledge that the science we love and trust lives within, not beyond, the influences of culture, stereotypes, and racism. The scientific and medical communities are only just starting to recognize the ways systematic oppression creates trauma. They are also just beginning to understand the ways trauma is biologically inherited (through epigenetics)[1] and perpetuated as we (often without realizing it) preemptively protect ourselves against harms our ancestors faced that are no longer relevant to us today.

Just as scientific trauma diagnoses are evolving, so is the scientific validation of yoga practice as a preventative and healing modality. Two decades ago, my Indian teachers taught me that yoga was a science, but it is only in recent years that yoga has been given scientific credibility in the West. These days you can find yoga instruction in schools, therapy sessions, and doctors' prescriptions (though it is rarely covered by health insurance companies). Scientific research shows yoga practice reduces blood pressure, aids in the management of type 2 diabetes, reduces the body's stress response, and increases our tolerance to pain. But at its heart, yoga is still experiential. When folks ask me, "What are the benefits of yoga?" I always suggest they practice and then tell me. Through regular practice, yogis have experienced the ways that yoga addresses and heals all kinds of trauma, regulates our systems, and teaches us to be self-aware, resilient, and cognizant of choice.

RECOGNIZING TRAUMA

Trauma-informed yoga teachers are not clinicians. You do not need to determine the specific type of stress a student has or diagnose PTSD or other forms of post-traumatic stress to bring relief. Nor is it important to cite yoga studies and prescribe yoga poses as though they are pills. What is important is becoming aware of all the ways trauma can show up in your classroom and to be responsive to students' needs by offering yoga the way it was intended to be shared: with respect, adaptability, compassion, and choice.

Gail Parker writes in the preface of *Restorative Yoga for Ethnic and Race-Based Stress and Trauma* that "until now, ethnic and race-based traumatic stress has been a neglected area of inquiry in most trauma-informed therapeutic modalities, including trauma-informed yoga. Yet many of us working in the field of stress reduction and trauma recovery, and those of us living the reality, recognize it as a real and unique source of emotional injury."[2] My experience shows me that this is true.

- If a person feels unable to live freely, or experiences threat or repression throughout the day or the threat of future repression, that causes trauma.
- If a person is exposed to images and stories of folks like them that suggest they should be fearful and limit their expression and impact on the world to stay "safe," that is traumatizing.
- Being silenced is traumatizing.
- If a person works in a job where accidents occur or where folks are often intimidated or arrested, this is traumatizing, as is arrest and imprisonment.
- If a parent or caregiver is lost, especially early in life, due to death or abandonment, or if they came and went unexpectedly, this can create trauma.
- Not getting needs met, or a perpetual lack of resources, produces trauma.
- Accidents and natural disasters may cause trauma.
- Climate change is traumatic.

- Sickness of self or a loved one may cause trauma as can surgery and other invasive medical events.
- Birthing a child can be trauma inducing. (It was pretty traumatic for me!)
- Ecological grief around species loss and our heightened anxiety over the future loom large over many people on the planet, creating trauma.

You don't have to go to a war zone to see the effects of trauma. It's in our communities, in our homes, and in us. The adverse childhood experiences (ACE) study by Kaiser Permanente (1995–1997) drew lots of attention by showing that negative childhood experiences are far more common than anyone expected. We now know that two out of three children experience at least one adverse event in childhood, and those who do are much more likely to experience a second traumatic instance. We must consider that trauma is in every room we enter, sometimes just beneath the surface. It's alive and present in every shared space, yoga class, and community.

Healing Ourselves First

"Hurt people hurt people," the saying goes. Part of my purpose for sharing trauma-informed yoga practices has been to disrupt that cycle. We disrupt not just by offering to aid others but also by recognizing the pain within us and working to soften it through self-compassion. In taking a look at ourselves and the ways we have hardened and defended ourselves against pain, we naturally grow to understand others and have compassion for their circumstances as well. This, in turn, helps them on their path to health and well-being, which is also the path for our own healing.

So much of the work we do to become trauma-informed yoga teachers is about healing ourselves. Dr. Kristin Neff is an author and pioneer in the field of self-compassion. Her research helps us understand how doing our inner work positively affects others. For instance, she writes in her book *Fierce Self-Compassion*, "Self-compassionate people tend to have more compassionate goals in their close relationships, meaning they tend to provide a lot of emotional support to others they are close to. . . . They're more accepting of the flaws and shortcomings of others, and better at perspective-taking or considering outside viewpoints."[3]

As we recognize and soften toward the pain in ourselves, we broaden our awareness of all the places trauma lives in others: the hidden nooks and crannies, the obvious spaces that we haven't been able to see. This is an important first step. The next step is to recognize that though traumatic events affect us all, they affect us in different ways depending on a multitude of factors, including our previous experiences, culture, community, resources, and biology.

THE POWER OF PREVIOUS EXPERIENCES

For many reasons, a person who has experienced trauma once is more likely to be faced with trauma again. Though we can't say that having previous experience with trauma means they will have a worse future trauma, we can say that retraumatization is a real concern. If a person has just recovered or is working on recovering from a trauma and experiences another one, this new experience can compound and negatively affect recovery. Ideas of the world as dangerous can be reinforced. In fact, the world the individual is living in may be unsafe.

Marcy Tropin, a teacher at my yoga studio, Land Yoga, and the author of *Yin Yoga Master Class: A Memoir*, survived ongoing childhood abuse. When later in life she found herself being arrested in her home on false accusations, a second traumatic event, it brought back the intense horror of her previous entrapment. How could her life post–child abuse have led to that arrest? Marcy shared with me how the trauma from that event affects her life. "The PTSD manifestations of anger, depression, anxiety, and ADD [attention deficit disorder] are like dirty windows that muddy perception of events in daily life," she said. From research we know trauma can make it hard to form healthy positive relationships and to trust others. It can sometimes escalate conflicts. "The biggest problem with my childhood abuse," Marcy explained, "was I was never diagnosed with PTSD. Once I was arrested and my shrink said, 'You have PTSD,' I thought, *Okay, now I know what I am working with!* In any situation I have, I ask myself if I'm reacting to the actual situation that's happening or if it is the PTSD that is in front of it."

People who have been through multiple traumas experience more emotional dysregulation, disassociation, and trouble learning new knowledge and retaining memories. The adverse long-term health consequences include increased risk of heart disease, cancer, and even reduced life expectancy. In Marcy's case, she has found a way to offset

Teacher Spotlight: Samantha Lucas

Samantha (she/her) and I met in Mysore, India, in 2008. Samantha is open and real in a way that is unusual and refreshing. She always has an interesting take on things and a sweetness and humor that I was drawn to from the time we met. After she had a devastating motorcycle accident, I visited her in the hospital and witnessed her great courage and unbreakable commitment to her yoga practice. Samantha has a wealth of embodied knowledge and life experience, and it's an honor for me to have her story and perspective included in this book.

∼

I discovered Ashtanga yoga and from day one, I thought, *This is it for me*. It got me out of a deep depression. I've struggled with depression my entire adult life. I was doing really well and then in 2016, I was in a motorcycle accident and I lost my right leg below the knee. I remember in the hospital bed thinking, *How am I going to practice? Will I ever practice?* When you have such a catastrophic injury,

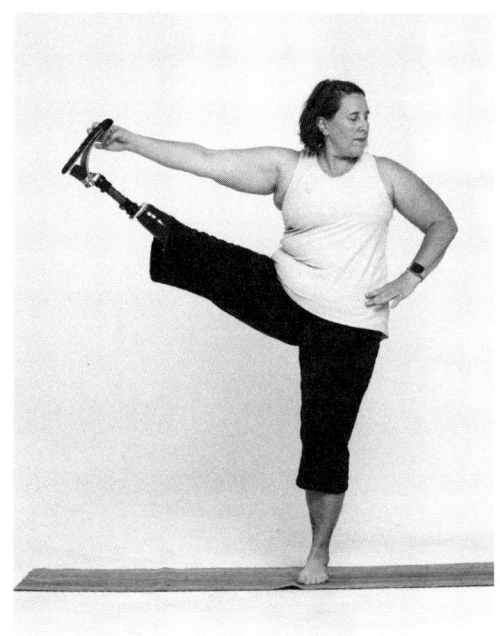

you just don't know. I started doing pranayama in the morning before nurses came to draw blood. Then I started doing Surya Namaskar in bed, mainly breathing. And then I started doing the seated postures in bed on just my left side, because I could do that. It's a long recovery process when you have an amputation, especially a traumatic one. It takes a long time to figure stuff out. I remember still being in the hospital, in the physical therapy room, and I thought, *Let me see if I can do Downward Dog.* I pushed up into it on one leg and I realized, *Okay, I'm alright. I can do this.* There was a long time where all I could do was get to the mat and do some Sun Salutations. The accident changed how I approached Ashtanga yoga. I adjusted as I needed to. And the best thing that I discovered was, your practice is there, whether you're doing one Sun Salutation or whatever your practice. It doesn't matter how much you do or what. The quality of your mind and your breath within what you're doing becomes your practice.

∼

Sam credits the fact that she had been practicing regularly for years before her motorcycle accident with how quickly she was able to access its benefits after the trauma. "Prana started flowing with the first Sun Salutation," she said. "It took some more time for my body to catch up, but in just a few days I was already emotionally where I was before the accident. It's very powerful. It's within you, and it solves a lot of things. My practice is probably a lot deeper than a lot of people doing advanced postures—maybe not physically but emotionally and pranically."

Sam experienced several childhood traumas that she has identified as leading to physical blocks in her yoga practice. She was molested by her brother, who claimed that it didn't count because they were not biologically related. She was then retraumatized by her parents' reaction, which was to act like it never happened.

∽

I was supergood at powering through and pushing it all down. Not dealing with it. I was emotionally shut off from that [childhood] trauma. Then having the accident, that kind of rewound time. I thought I had worked through all that stuff, and then you have another trauma and then you realize, no, it's still all right there. All you can do is keep practicing. I feel like yoga opens your eyes to whatever the struggle is, so you get better at being able to identify what's happening. That it's okay. Maybe yoga calms you enough to acknowledge that the feeling you are feeling right now is not the end of the world.

Getting to the mat when you're in physical pain is really hard. I was told putting your legs up the wall helps you heal faster, and I realized that my pain was relieved by a longer closing (inversion sequence). So I forced myself to stay there a lot longer. Jeff, my husband, would always show up at 7 a.m., when the hospital opened. He would instantly know if I hadn't gotten my yoga practice in on that day, because if not, I'd be struggling with everything. I learned very early on that I had to do something to keep my emotions calm. The emotional pain without practice was far greater than the physical pain with practice. Every time I've stopped practicing for whatever reason, I think, *You are only hurting yourself by not practicing.*

these adverse impacts through yoga practice, walking her dog, therapy, and knowledge of the way PTSD works. Becoming aware of and using coping skills that work for you is called *resourcing*, and it is very important to the healing process.

THE POWER OF BEING BELIEVED

A key component of healing trauma is a survivor being believed or feeling they would be believed if they shared their experience of trauma. When a person's trauma is not validated, they may have trouble not only healing but also recognizing their own trauma. Even when a trauma is recognized, some cultures may be more likely to downplay the condition and approach it as solvable via force of will and fortitude, hiding it from others and missing the crucial assistance of qualified professionals. Even when a trauma survivor receives support from professionals, understanding their trauma through the lens of the culture may influence how they experience it and certainly how they describe their trauma. For example, the individual might focus on describing physical symptoms and omit or downplay emotional upheaval.

Many cultures have stigmas attached to trauma that make it difficult for a person suffering to seek help even if they do recognize the trauma. They may feel at risk of alienating themselves or being judged, or they may have internalized the stigmas around trauma or the cause of their trauma. Many trauma survivors navigate deep shame because of internalized societal messaging—*I should have been able to avoid this, get away from it sooner, recover from it faster*. Because of this societal-induced shame, they may try to suppress symptoms of traumatization via drug and alcohol abuse or hide from friends and family using work and other excuses to avoid those who know them best. The tragedy of this is that authentic relationships play an essential role in trauma healing. Being without them, by contrast, can cause additional harm.

Seeking medical care for trauma can be fraught. If an individual is living somewhere where the dominant culture is not their own and they have experienced discrimination in medical settings, they may be averse to seeking help, which will negatively affect recovery. Even without first-hand experience of discrimination in these settings, knowledge of implicit biases may influence a person's decision to get help. Sadly, treatment is also likely to be affected by implicit bias, as clinicians' biases have been proven to influence both diagnosis and treatment.[4]

The Power of Community

Another factor that influences a trauma's impact is the survivor's community. Community is defined as a feeling of fellowship with others as a result of sharing common attitudes, interests, and goals. In short, community is our real-world social network. In multiple studies, social support is a key indicator of how an individual will progress through trauma. An individual's ability to seek and sustain support is strengthened in two ways: (1) if the community of a traumatized individual recognizes trauma as having serious and scientifically proven effects on the brain and body, and (2) if the community and the individual share the same definition of trauma.

A community can enforce or override cultural norms or pressures. If the community embraces all the types and definitions of trauma, encourages reaching out for support, and celebrates the healing process, an individual whose family or ancestral culture doesn't may find themselves better able to heal. That the individual doesn't feel loneliness,[5] a common companion to trauma and another trigger of adverse health effects, on top of the trauma is a big factor toward recovery.

As individuals, we may have one core community but we inhabit many. We have our neighborhood communities, religious communities, and work communities, as well as other circles drawn around partners and children. As yoga teachers we create community, or sangha, around the practice. We have our yoga studios, our online spaces, our yoga friendships, and companion yoga activities such as book clubs or getting tea and coffee with fellow practitioners. The conscious creation of a safe and supportive community is a way for us to have a profound impact on our students. By offering a space, even if it is virtual, and making it as supportive, educated, and trauma sensitive as possible, you are creating sangha.

Sangha, spiritual community, is one of the three jewels in Buddhism, and many believe it is even the most important. When survivors can rely on a sangha for support, the burden of recovery is alleviated. In a spiritual community, practitioners lean on each other for both support and growth. The meditation and mindfulness teacher Larry Yang speaks on sangha in his book *Awakening Together*: "Our needs are not solely an individual matter, even though we might feel them personally. It is the practice of sangha to naturally take care of others with grace and ease—to share our joys and sorrows together in communion with the full range of our collective experience."[6] No one is alone. We are all interdependent.

Teacher Spotlight: Pratiba Premkumar

Pratiba (she/her) came to yoga after a running injury led her to seek exercise that would be gentle on her joints. As she gradually experienced the powerful effects of the breath-mind-body connection through yoga, she came to realize it was a practice that was more than simply exercise. Pratiba completed her trauma-informed training through Three and a Half Acres Yoga in 2019. Shortly after her training, she began teaching a weekly yoga class for the Urban Resource Institute for women transitioning out of domestic violence situations.

I got into a series of bad relationships, and it got worse when I met this one guy who love-bombed me. I started drinking a lot, relying on my drinking just to escape. Eventually that relationship ended. You would think after the relationship ended, I would have stopped drinking as much, but I started drinking more. It was a way to deal with my PTSD, so it got really bad the year after that. I was taking yoga classes during this time, and I felt horrible about myself. I went to this one studio where the teacher was always so nice to me that I always made sure, even if I had drunk way too much the night before and could barely get up, that I went to her twice-weekly classes. I was walking around with so much shame weighing down on me constantly, day-to-day. Just going to yoga class and the kindness helped me heal in its own way. And eventually I made the decision to stop drinking.

A few months later I saw a posting on the wall for teacher training, and I took that. Then yoga became less about exercise and more about the whole yoga philosophy. One of the course assignments was to choose one of the eight limbs of yoga and discuss how it applies to your life. I chose tapas—passion, sticking to something—and how I used it to stop drinking. If you want to change something, just stick to that commitment, stoke that fire. Fire is transformative.

The teacher who was nice to me inspired me to get into trauma-informed yoga. Being with people, showing a little kindness to people who are going through something, even if it's the tiniest little thing, can be beneficial. Trauma-informed yoga is different than Vinyasa. It's more about mindfulness and an approach of gentleness. That's what I like about it.

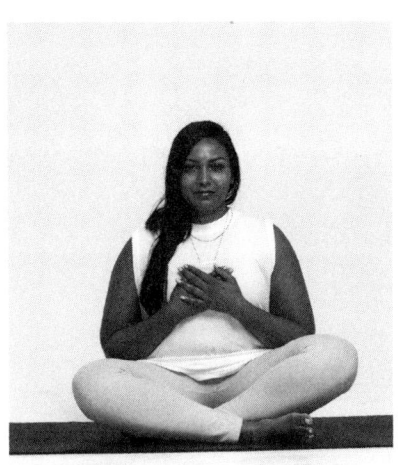

BEING A SUPPORTIVE RESOURCE
FOR YOUR STUDENTS

Pratiba was able to find a healthy yoga situation, but not everyone has access to the same resources. Not everyone has access to a mental health professional who specializes in trauma or the insurance or co-pay to cover visits, let alone the time to take off work or find and pay for the childcare needed during mental health appointments. Sometimes lack of resources means lack of access to information about trauma or money for necessary medication.

Yoga is a resource that can also come with accessibility issues,[7] and trauma sensitivity is one of them. By taking the time to make your yoga offerings trauma sensitive, you are making them more accessible and providing a valuable resource. It takes nothing away from those of your students who have been spared trauma to make your classes trauma sensitive, and it gives much needed security and protection to those who have. You can further that contribution by having additional resources prepared for your students such as names of trauma-sensitive health-care professionals, literature on trauma, and information on support groups.

Some of your students will need more than yoga to heal from trauma. Knowing the limits of your knowledge and expertise, and being able and eager to refer out, is key to limiting harm to yourself and your students. Below are some other modalities that might benefit your students. A basic understanding of complementary modalities will help you guide them. Be mindful when referring out that you are not diagnosing and that your student does not feel rejected or get a sense that they are some-how more broken than you can handle. Keep the conversation open about your own limitations in knowledge and expertise.

Complementary Therapies for Trauma Survivors

Instead of overpromising on the benefits of yoga, the time has come for yoga teachers to build a supportive referral network for students who need more than yoga. Teachers can forge relationships with clinicians in the categories below by attending networking groups through BNI (Business Network International) or your local Chamber of Commerce. When referring, it's preferable to know the therapist and have a sense for how they work. If possible, consider asking for a sample treatment ses-sion so you understand their methods. Before referring out, know if the clinician is taking new clients, if they accept insurance, and if they work virtually as well as in person.

Psychotherapy

Psychotherapy is what is commonly known as talk therapy. The patient talks about their life and their trauma, and the doctor works with the patient through the healing process by talking and listening. Weekly sessions can be limited to a few or continue for years, with the individual alone or including family members. Sometimes medication is prescribed in combination with therapy.

Cognitive Behavioral Therapy

A cognitive behavioral therapist focuses on helping the patient recognize negative behaviors and mental patterns in their life and replace them with positive ones. In cognitive behavioral therapy (CBT), the emphasis is on reprogramming the brain by practicing alternative thought patterns. The patient will often work on building their tolerance to potentially triggering stimuli by using this method.

Eye Movement Desensitization and Reprocessing

Mental health professionals with certification in eye movement desensitization and reprocessing (EMDR) facilitate the client's remembering of traumatic events while directing them to focus on external stimulus. This is usually experienced as lateral eye movements, although hand tapping and audio stimulation may also be used. Through these movements, new learning pathways are established in the brain, which often results in rapid and long-lasting healing.

Group Therapy

Group therapy typically involves one or more psychologists and five to fifteen patients who have a similar issue in need of support. Participants are often surprised by how much they benefit from being in a group. When sharing, the others act as a sounding board and in some cases may even help with problem-solving. As a listener, participants may find it comforting that others are also struggling and they are not alone.

Somatic Therapy or Somatic Experiencing Therapy

Somatic therapy or somatic experiencing therapy incorporates the mind, body, and spirit into healing work, specifically focusing on how the physical body holds tension. Somatic therapists help their patients release pent-up tensions as a way to release their trauma and to recognize and work with bodily sensations as a way to process experiences and live trauma-free.

BIOLOGICAL FACTORS OF TRAUMA

How a person is affected by trauma is contingent on social and cultural factors and with the structure and workings of the individual's brain and body chemistry. Each of us is unique, and therefore, each of us will have our own experience dealing with trauma. The discovery of the brain's neuroplasticity was a neuroscientific breakthrough; now we know the structure of the brain changes depending on how we use it. Nurturing patterns of brain functioning that support recovery will make those patterns stronger and eventually turn those positive patterns into habits. This is part of the work of trauma-informed yoga. Still, it's important to note that not all brains recover in the same way. Not all brains come back from traumatic events to their pre-trauma state. Not all brains were at the same developmental stage when the trauma was introduced to them. The mind-body has no "correct" response to trauma. Each response is the individual mind-body system's intelligent way of protecting the survivor, and it must be honored.

Your Brain on Trauma

So what happens to the brain on trauma? One of the most obvious things that happens is the amygdala becomes activated. The amygdala, the almond-shaped structure located within the temporal lobe of the brain, is part of the limbic system, the middle section of the brain known as the emotional center. Structures within the limbic system send and receive signals to and from the hypothalamus (the automatic reptilian part of our brain) and the prefrontal cortex (the thinking/rationalizing part of our brain). The amygdala's primary role is to alert us to danger.

When the amygdala signals, the hypothalamus hears it loud and clear. The hypothalamus is the part of the brain that regulates the body's breath, heart rate, temperature, and other autonomic processes. At the first signal of danger from the amygdala, the sympathetic nervous system becomes engaged and sets off a series of physiological responses. Adrenaline is secreted and circulated. This increases our heart rate, which quickly pushes blood into vital organs. The lungs open and breath becomes more rapid. Cortisol and epinephrine cause sugars and fats to be released from the liver, flooding the blood, sending energy to the large muscles of the body. Your body's sympathetic nervous system has kicked into gear, which means you are aroused and ready to respond to the crisis.

At the same time the amygdala is firing, the prefrontal cortex—the part of the brain that assesses, calculates, and plans—is doing the opposite; it's slowing or shutting down. (We don't need long-term planning in a moment of crisis.) Other nonessential bodily processes—such as reproduction, digestion, and functions related to growth, among others—slow or stop as well. All systems are working together now to attend to the crisis that triggered the stress response.

Consider this from the perspective within a person who's been traumatized. In this individual, the stress response continues to signal long after the incident has passed. The amygdala remains hyperactive, keeping the body in a state of panic. In this hyperactive state, the brain perceives nearly everything in the environment as dangerous, signaling the body to react as if it is in immediate danger and continuing to send out all those stress hormones. As trauma specialist and Somatic Experiencing developer Dr. Peter Levine explains in his trauma resource staple *Waking the Tiger*, "When arousal continues (because discharging it is too threatening), we find ourselves in a no-win situation. We feel compelled to find a source of threat, but the compulsion is internally generated and even if an external source of threat is identified, the compulsive hypervigilant stance will continue because the internal arousal is the threat." Trauma results, Levine writes, when "the neo-cortex overrides the instinctual responses that would initiate the completion of this cycle."[8] Long-term planning and other functions unimportant to the perceived threat continue to remain shut down or repressed, and the system fluctuates between hypo- and hyperarousal (flight, fight, freeze) states indefinitely.

Imagine trying to navigate the world while this radical fluctuation is flooding your automatic systems. How do you know which of the warning signals your body is sending are valid, to distinguish between real and imagined threat? How do you regulate emotions or understand expectations? It is challenging to get comfortable because triggering and dysregulation can happen unexpectedly. To cope, perhaps you begin to retreat inward. This might mean avoiding any places that could be triggering, such as spaces that are dark, hard to exit, new, or at all resemble the place of the inciting trauma. You may not want to go out during certain hours or be anywhere you can't leave quickly.

Your body may pull inward into a more protective stance. Certain muscular holding patterns are similar to a fetal position. Perhaps your chest curls to protect the heart, bringing the arms in with it. Your head may dip down, tucking the chin. Your brain is telling your body that it is unsafe and should protect itself. However, your body's positioning also sends signals back to the brain. By remaining in protective positioning, it tells the brain that there is danger, unconsciously escalating the situation.

The prefrontal cortex remains offline, and a lingering fogginess makes it difficult to think clearly and make good decisions. You try to concentrate, but you simply can't. Days and eventually weeks go by and you have not responded to important requests. Other people think you're lazy or even perhaps rude. You misread social cues and respond inappropriately to those around you. You begin to feel you can rely on neither your instincts nor your reasoning for good decision-making, and this makes you even more afraid. You have nothing to hold on to.

Sometimes the combination of the triggered amygdala and the lethargic prefrontal cortex results in the opposite response: radical inhibition. In this case, the survivor employs actions and behaviors that may seem adolescent, like they are acting out, which is a sign of the diminished functioning of the problem-solving and socially regulating part of their brains. (In fact, the prefrontal cortex isn't fully formed until our midtwenties—a good case for restricting activities with long-term consequences until then!) Sometimes trauma survivors tend to break social norms by oversharing, disrupting, and dismissing boundaries. This can also be due to the brain's compulsion to relive the traumatic incident, until they can play the whole thing out with an ending where they are able to escape or triumph, or due to a survivor feeling deep hurt and shame, manifesting in violence against themselves.

In these cases, the survivor may appear to stretch endlessly outward, even recreating events similar to those that caused the initial trauma. They may also be unconsciously looking for some sensory feedback indicating a boundary but feeling little or nothing in the way of an edge. Instead of having a fear-based survival mechanism that uses inhibition to protect against risk of future pain, the body simply does not register pain. They are tuned out, numb, disassociated from the experiences they are living. In these cases, when asked to comment on a particular part of the yoga experience, students will tell you they feel nothing.

Trauma's Long Arc

Brain fog, jitters, overreactions to the slightest stimuli, and increased aggression are just a few of the impacts of trauma. Interpersonal relationships can suffer as the person impacted by trauma has trouble focusing on others or is actively trying to avoid others to hide what they are going through. Due to hypervigilance, the inability to sleep or sleep deeply is common and further diminishes brain function at horrifying levels. According to Dr. Matthew Walker, the author of *Why We Sleep*, "There is no major psychiatric condition in which sleep is normal. This is true of depression, anxiety, post-traumatic stress disorder (PTSD), schizophrenia, and bipolar disorder (once known as manic depression)."[9]

Studies show that yoga helps folks sleep, and some yoga teachers have taken note of that. My dear friend Pamela Stokes, the founder of Yoga2Sleep and a certified yoga therapist, started her company after experiencing how her own challenges with insomnia and secondary post-traumatic stress (PTS) could be alleviated with yoga. In her *Yoga Journal* article "How One Yoga Teacher Found Strength After Her Husband's War Injury," Pamela talks about returning to her practice after near burnout taking care of her husband. "Finding my flow," Pamela writes, "down-regulated my central nervous system and empowered me to explore additional forms of self-care. By focusing on myself and surrendering to awareness, I found more compassion for myself. As a result, I was able to create the space necessary to be a more present and loving caregiver."[10]

Avoidance is a common coping mechanism that pushes away the feelings that come with processing the traumatic experience. To avoid those feelings, the trauma survivor may choose to stay in a state of hyperactivity and distraction, use alcohol or drugs, or adopt any number of habits including downplaying what happened and engaging in high-risk behaviors.

Having some understanding of and sensitivity to humankind's universal trauma response makes you better able to accommodate a student who may need a position near or viewing the door instead of automatically assuming they want to be able to exit your class early for superficial reasons. It helps to clarify behavior that seems abnormal and to curb the instinct to jump to judgment when people don't meet ideas of social norms. It reveals why your students may have a hard time remembering movement sequences or poses from week to week.

The way a being reacts to trauma is normal, protective, necessary, and lifesaving, until it's not. As the psychoneurobiology researcher Dr. Robert Sapolsky makes a compelling case for in his book *Why Zebras*

It's typical for a trauma survivor to create circumstances similar to the inciting incident in an unconscious effort to reenact the event. Reliving a traumatic event and trying to work out the response to it differently both in physical reality and in the mind is a very common rabbit hole for trauma survivors to fall into, often resulting in increased trauma and agitation.

As yoga teachers, it's important we know all of this is going on when designing our classes. It helps us recognize why a seemingly simple request such as having our student sit in silence for a few minutes is not always an inviting proposition. Some talking or activity is usually needed to mute the past experience and can be an anchor for developing deeper concentration down the line. Knowing and integrating this fact alone can make your class much more trauma sensitive.

Don't Get Ulcers, our response to threat is biologically important. That we can't turn it off after the threat has passed is what is damaging. Over time, the extended response to past trauma may cause more injury to the already harmed individual.[11] It may keep them from jobs, travel, forming and engaging in deep interpersonal relationships, and many other fulfilling life experiences, as well as harm their health. Even so, it's hard to say when the time is right for the individual to stop protecting themselves. As yoga teachers, we don't know what experiences they go back to after we see them in class and what protections they need to survive inside their bodies. We don't know if the flood of memory would come back with a fury if they were to relax in a safe-as-possible environment, such as our class. Are they ready for that? As trauma-informed yoga teachers, our approach must be extraordinarily slow and nonstriving, with the student always leading the way.

Exercise: Broadening Awareness

Consider again the bulleted list on page 11 of what experiences can lead to trauma. Is this the first time you have read such a detailed and expansive definition of trauma? How does this impact you as a yoga teacher and human? Write down the ways this alters your view of others in your life, family, social networks, and community.

Core Concepts

- The definition of trauma is constant, but its scope is always evolving.
- Trauma may not be obvious, but it is present in every shared space.
- A person's response to trauma is determined by factors other than the trauma itself, such as previous experience, being believed, community, resources, biology.
- Traumatization happens when the mind-body system is overwhelmed and cannot regulate itself post trauma. Signs of this are hypervigilance, avoidance, brain fog, dissociation, oversharing, and self-harm.
- A prolonged stress response can lead to serious health consequences, though it may also serve as a necessary protection to the survivor.
- It is up to the survivor to decide if they want to let go of their defenses and at what pace.
- As a yoga teacher, don't overpromise healing. Offer referrals for clinicians who can support your students with modalities in addition to yoga.

Exercise: Looking at Past Traumas

Take some time to consider and journal on past traumas you and your ancestors have experienced and how that history has an impact on how you navigate the world.

For instance, what comes to mind when I think of my family history is my grandparents' escapes from Nazi Germany. I recognize how they needed to carry and rely on essential survival techniques during this time such as staying in close relationship with others like them for support and insider information, working longer than required hours once in the US, and getting quiet about much of their past, including their first language, for quick assimilation. These practices have been passed down not only through the family lineage, pushing us toward perfectionism even when new threats have not existed, but also through a coded agreement to be successful—but not so much that we stand out. I can feel into my paternal grandparents' personal stories of hard work and eventual success in their new country. I can trace the line through the generations to my quirky but previously invisible-to-myself ways of understanding the world, opportunities, and others. And I can mourn the ways my tendencies toward perfectionism, born of their struggle, have in the past harmed my relationships, both with myself and others. All known and unknown histories live within each of us and influence our moment-to-moment behavior without permission, unless we own up to it and explore it.

Softening the Trauma Response through Yoga

> At its root yoga is a practical, structured, scientific framework and embodiment practice that aims at curing our personal and social ills.
>
> —SUSANNA BARKATAKI,
> *Embrace Yoga's Roots*

WHAT IS YOGA? ACCORDING TO DR. SHYAM RANGANATHAN'S study of Patanjali's Yoga Sutras, yoga is "taking responsibility for your mental life, which is basically philosophy (YS I.2–3). Three practical ideals that structure the philosophical practice of yoga are devotion to lordliness (*īśvara praṇidhāna*); unconservativism, or pushing one's boundaries (*tapas*); and self-governance or self-control (*svādhyāya*) (YS II.1)."[1] Together, Barkataki's and Ranganathan's interpretations align with my view of trauma-informed yoga and its purpose.

To achieve yoga or work toward yoga, we use a variety of practices from the Yoga Sutras, Hatha Yoga Pradipika, and other texts that include mindful movement, breathwork, self-discipline, deep study and contemplation, ethics, and concentration. Together these practices work to heal trauma by addressing the whole person. Unlike talk therapies, which often address only one part of what it is to be a living human being, often cognition or cerebral activity, yoga aims to advance the whole self. It does so in two channels: **top-down regulation**, which involves observing the fluctuations, sensations, thoughts, and emotions of the mind-body system from a witnessing perspective; and **bottom-up regulation**, which uses breathwork, movement, and touch. When the practices of yoga honor the intention of the tradition and the unique architecture of the individual, the results are profound and transformative. As the expert trauma researcher Dr. Bessel van der Kolk writes in his best-selling work

The Body Keeps the Score, "The act of telling the story doesn't necessarily alter the automatic physical and hormonal responses of bodies that remain hypervigilant, prepared to be assaulted or violated at any time. For real change to take place, the body needs to learn that danger has passed and to live in the reality of the present."[2]

In the West, yoga postures, or asanas, are the most recognized components of the yoga system of practice. Indeed, asanas are crucial to trauma healing. When we take a new posture, many signals are sent to the brain, and these signals change the state of the body and the mind. The breathing, awareness, intention, concentration, and self-study occurring while in the shape or asana, however, are what lead to transformation. By varying the position of the body and the awareness and intention we give to that position, we can achieve different results. Many of these results, such as capacity to stay engaged when aroused, counter the negative impacts of traumatization.

You will never convince the mind to let go of trauma through thinking alone, but if you involve the body, the mind will change. Every unprocessed life experience is stored in the body in some way. Most of us deny or are disconnected from how profound an impact our mental and emotional lives have on the body until the body makes it known. Our back goes out, our stomach cramps, our jaw aches, we can't move our neck—only when these alarms sound do we start investigating what's been going on in our lives and how our bodies are bearing it. Where trauma is involved, this tightening of the body is likely its best defense and may be a defense it still needs. Asanas that are introduced without trauma sensitivity in mind can leave a person defenseless, overwhelming the nervous system, and cause additional harm. Instead, trauma sensitive yoga presents options that allow for the slow and safe opening and releasing of tensions, emotions, and memories. Even this release can be too swift; trauma sensitive yoga teaches the student how to notice when they need to pump the breaks to stay in control. Though some practitioners find the initial release of practice intense, they also report through regular practice emotional releases become much smaller and more manageable.

START BY GROUNDING

It's typical for folks to report a feeling of leaving their body after a trauma. The trauma is too much to handle, so the body's wisdom creates an escape via disassociation, the experience of watching one's life as if it's happening to someone else. This is nothing short of ingenious in moments of trauma but can have negative consequences after the fact: not being present with friends, difficulty experiencing the full richness of life, dangerous risk-taking, and trouble retaining memories. Yoga practices can help students stay in the present, as they feel ready, fully embedding their life experiences. As a teacher, you will be inviting your students to ground in the present moment by consciously bringing awareness to the body and into the sensations that arise through the senses. You will teach them to watch for when the mind wanders and coax it back to the sensory information available in the here and now. As their ability to ground themselves grows stronger in yoga practice, so will it in life off the mat.

Grounding practices are used by therapists to help their clients when experiencing panic attacks, disassociation, and other nervous system dysregulation. They involve directing the five senses into experiences of the present moment, and they are especially effective in response to flashbacks. A grounding practice often begins by placing the feet firmly on the ground. Some grounding exercises focus exclusively on the feet, experimenting with how they feel as they connect with the floor.

An extension of the ground is any stable surface the body interacts with, especially surfaces that bear the practitioner's weight, such as the floor, wall, or chair, all of which are well suited to a yoga space. Sitting in a chair or lying on the floor, with or without support props, is the basis for grounding practices. Squatting is also a form of grounding. It connects us to the earth and keeps us low, engaged, and alert. I suggest using these types of grounding practices at the beginning of class.

Try it now. Take a moment now to notice your position. If you are seated, bring your feet in contact with the ground or the surface below them, such as the footrest if you are in a wheelchair. Now turn your attention to the feeling of your feet making contact. Even in cases of paralysis, many people express they can experience sensations in those parts of the body through directed attention and enhance them via visualization.[3] If you are in a chair and your feet don't touch the floor, place blocks or a stack of books under them to create contact with a grounding surface.

Without moving anything, can you allow your feet to take more support from that surface? Is there a way of letting go of extra tension? You can try this same exercise with the seat of your body in a chair or your whole body lying on the ground, if that position is available. What happens when you accept support and stop trying to hold yourself up?

Teacher Spotlight: Timothy Lewis

I first met Tim (he/him) on New Year's Eve 2017 when he walked into my yoga studio, Land Yoga, for our annual candlelit yoga event. He was eager to learn and share knowledge in a way that made him stand out. After class he signed up for a two-month membership to the studio and started coming regularly to early morning classes, as he is a schoolteacher. He often shared book recommendations or asked about a chanting or pranayama technique. (Tim really gets self-study!) He participated in the Three and a Half Acres trauma-informed yoga teacher training to learn pose adaptations and trauma sensitivity. He's used that knowledge most notably with his mother, something we've often highlighted within the nonprofit organization.

I don't remember the first time I heard the word *yoga*. I come from a traditional Black Baptist family. So, when there was talk of a spiritual practice, it was just hands-off, you don't talk about that. The first time I was introduced to the idea of yoga, it was through the lens of stretching. From the very first yoga practice I gained a greater awareness of my body than I ever had before. I grew up as an athlete, but understanding the mechanics of the body and being honestly curious about it only came through yoga. As I became more open to yoga, I also felt a huge resistance. All the excuses not to practice would pile up. And then all of those layers started to shift. I have had to break through the barrier of being the only Black person in a yoga space, but I kind of thrive on being uncomfortable. I become curious. I'm generally attracted to things that go against the grain.

My journey as a yoga teacher is so interesting. I needed something to keep me going in the teaching profession. I was feeling such burnout, isolation, frustration, and I didn't know how to navigate it. In that two hundred–hour (yoga teacher training), one of the first sort of exercises that we did, I remember crying like crazy. It opened up things in a way that became a tool for self-study and curiosity. Then I started to learn more about philosophy and that opened up a whole other thing. There's the training aspect of it, the reading and studying materials and practicing for yourself and getting tools, and then finding unique ways to do that in the classroom. I've always been of the mindset that you can't teach what you don't know, and practice is a

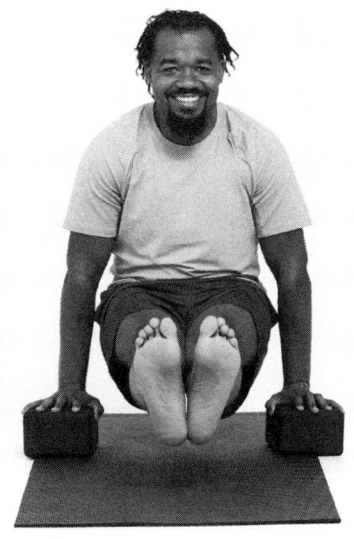

critical part of one's learned experience. The opportunity to do trauma-informed yoga teacher training felt essential. If you work in New York City with young people, the question is not "Is there trauma?" but rather "What degree of trauma are we dealing with?"

Then my mom was hospitalized with COVID-19 in March 2020, when literally there was nothing but unknowns. We would talk on the phone, and I would say, "I don't want you to talk. Just listen to me. I want you to just focus on the breath, just pay attention to *I am breathing in and I am breathing out* and just count to ten." Then I'd say, "Every time that you lose track, just remind yourself, *I am breathing in. I am breathing out*." That was one of the first times that I spoke to her about the power of the breath and how it calms the nervous system, helping her ease the panic that rose when preparing to walk with the oxygen tube in her nose, for example.

After she got home, yoga was an easier sell because she already had let her guard down and was open to yoga as an idea that did not conflict with religion. Because we've been doing yoga for so long now, I've started to talk to her a bit about gratitude. I wasn't introduced to that growing up. We always start with just kind of settling in, grounding, and focusing on the breath. Recently I've tried to incorporate more poses for upper-body strength. I recognize a lot of change in her. I see that she's more active. Her diet is changing. She's paying attention to her health. She is more curious, and she's getting out and doing things. And I would say that we are closer. The conversations that we have are definitely richer.

Grounding is the first step in becoming present. To become present means to have a full sensory awareness of the present moment. It's a superpower anyone can use and that can be made stronger through encouragement and practice.

TRISTANA: UNION OF AWARENESS

The word *yoga* itself suggests presence. It comes from the Sanskrit root *yuk*, meaning "union," and is often defined as the union of ourselves with the present moment. Though some define the union as one with a greater energy force or an idealized version of self, perhaps both those aspects of divine connection and highest self are here in the present moment.

When the present moment is safe, here-and-now awareness holds trauma survivors in refuge. Though past memories can be devastating and the future anxiety-ridden, the now may present a pocket of safety to relax into. In trauma sensitive yoga we offer presencing work with the caveat that the student can choose to go away, disengage, self-distract at any time and that that choice is okay. They can always come back to intentional yoking yoga practice when they feel ready or continue to shift back and forth, pendulating between concentration and purposeful distraction as they choose.

The presencing practice I teach is a three-pointed awareness called Tristana, which comes from the Ashtanga tradition. The three points are steadying one's eye gaze on one spot (*drishti*), listening to a sounded (*ujjayi*) breath as one makes it, and feeling the body in posture as one complete shape in space (what some might call embodiment).

Each part of the Tristana has many benefits. Drishti keeps the eyes steady on one spot. Doing so reduces visual stimulation and helps pull attention inward. It also grounds the practitioner in the present moment. For someone who has been through a trauma, this may be challenging at first as their body is telling them to be hypervigilant, searching the space for threat. Over time, softening the gaze on one spot and resisting shifting the eyes can override the hypervigilance and calm the body. Another benefit to the practitioner is knowing others in the class are also being encouraged not to look around. It can help them feel a sense of anonymity and reduce shyness around moving their body in new ways.

The second point of focus, listening to the sound of one's breath, reins in our sense of hearing and has similar benefits in reducing hypervigilance and turning attention inward. The sound of the ujjayi breathing appeals to most people. It's compared to the ocean or a white noise machine, sounds that are universally relaxing. As the practitioner listens more deeply to their sounded breath, they may find their inner mental dialogue falls away. This brings great peace to those who are tormented by negative thoughts.

The third part, cultivating full body awareness, has similar benefits to the other elements of the Tristana. The practice is an anchor, helping the practitioner to ground into the present moment and reduce external and internal stimuli. It also awakens body awareness, something which is often muted post trauma. I also find the practice of capturing a feeling of the whole body reduces the teacher's and student's inclination to "fix" postures. This can assist tremendously in encouraging self-acceptance.

Practicing the three-pointed Tristana helps the student remain in the

Postures, breathwork, and even word choice can be triggers for trauma survivors, if not offered gently and with the option to opt out. Trauma-surviving students are regularly alienated in yoga classes led by teachers who don't know how to give supportive options. Students are left feeling that they "can't do yoga," so they quit a practice that, if taught sensitively, could have helped them. Or they stay with a point of concentration that is too triggering, causing deep emotional harm. These outcomes can easily be averted by consistently providing a few anchoring options to your students.

present moment via its wholeness of sensory awareness. It also provides a way for an individual to shift focus (within the Tristana) if one of the three options (breath, gaze, or body awareness) is too triggering. David Treleaven, the author of *Trauma-Sensitive Mindfulness*, offers many ways to pump the brakes in his trauma-sensitive mindfulness training. He writes, "To support their window of tolerance,[4] survivors must learn they can shift their focus away from traumatic stimuli during mindfulness practice."[5] If too much attention on breath is triggering, the practitioner can focus on what they see or feel. They can still completely engage in the practice and avoid feeling like they're "bad practitioners."

Sometimes a break from focused practice is necessary. You should reassure your students that this is always an option. They may want to shake out, take a walk, or just simply take a break from intense concentration. Students can be invited to return to practice when they are ready.

Not everyone's present moment is comfortable, but many people can find a feeling of ease when the mind isn't caught in past regret or future anxiety. Teachers guide students to look for what's happening in the here and now—the support of the ground or chair below, the sound of the breath or the teacher's voice, or a small unmoving spot on the ground up ahead—and focus on the sensations present when one's focus is guided in those directions.

AWAKENING SENSATION, AWAKENING CONNECTION

Part of the dissociation that happens in response to trauma is a lack of sensation in the body. This highly intelligent way of escaping from pain can linger as a defense mechanism post trauma. Yoga provides an opportunity (when the individual is ready) to wake up that sensation again. In trauma sensitive yoga, we do this by slowly and intentionally bringing the mind's attention into different parts of the body. For many students, the simple act of asking the mind to become aware of the different parts of the body will lead to those parts waking up. At the beginning, folks may feel nothing, but over time most people begin to notice small sensations as the mind-body connection strengthens.

Awakening sensation is a tool everyone can employ to make use of the vast information our body is giving us at any moment. Contemporary life emphasizes the thought process and mental reactions, which are distinctly removed from the body. Sadly, a dulling of bodily sensation or our consciousness of those sensations is all too common.

Once parts of our body are enlivened again with sensation, they can become more responsive to the mind's instructions. We begin testing this using simple movements linked with breath, such as lifting up the arms (with the inhale) and bringing them down (with the exhale). As these movements get more refined and more closely match inhalations and exhalations, we can start focusing on subtler movements and smaller parts of the body. This seemingly simple act of the body doing what we tell it to has stunning implications. More awareness and sensation in our body, and the ability to move it as desired, can lead to more autonomy and more self-confidence, key benefits of trauma sensitive yoga.

Many yoga poses aim to release tension, a comfort trauma survivors in particular can benefit from. When we relax the muscles of the body, signals are sent to the brain telling it that it too is in a relaxed state. In yoga we deepen this response by using full, slow breathing, which also resets the nervous system, stimulating the parasympathetic (rest and digest) functions to come online.

This slow, diaphragmatic breathing, Ujjayi Pranayama, is proven to increase vagal tone, an essential component of healing trauma. The vagus nerve is a cranial nerve that runs from the brain, down the body, and through the gut, interacting with most of the body's organs. When it is well "toned," the body can process emotions more subtly and can relax faster after experiencing stress. Dr. Elizabeth Cohen, a Land Yoga practitioner, clinical psychologist, and author of *Light on the Other Side of Divorce*, shared with me that she uses ujjayi breathing frequently outside of yoga class. "I use it before I walk into my kids' room to regulate my nervous system and before I interact with them as their moods (as teens) are so unpredictable. I use it before I give a talk to 'cleanse' myself and prepare for the transition, and I use it when I need to connect with a hard client and feel my spine again."

Other practices found in yoga—meditation, movement, massage, socializing, and chanting—are also known to increase vagal tone. This is a great argument for incorporating these exercises into your teaching in a trauma-sensitive way. We will look more deeply into some of these practices in the following chapters. For now, here are some brief guidelines:

Meditation: Meditations are focused on the present moment and guided. Avoid creative visualization, affirmations, and long silences.

Massage: Bring in massage by offering the opportunity for students to engage in simple self-touch such as kneading shoulder and arm muscles. Placing one's own hands on the heart and belly is also self-regulating but can trigger release, so be mindful. When seeking a restful pose, some students prefer to cup their eyes with their palms or bring their hands to the back of the neck and forehead instead.

Socializing: Socializing can be integrated into class via beginning- and end-of-class check-ins, as well as through the creation of group agreements and by finding moments of laughter in class, an underused tool for connecting us all.

Offering time for sharing can enrich the yoga experience but should only be done by a skilled teacher who knows how to hold the boundaries and the energy of the space. Sometimes what one student shares can be a release for them and yet trigger another student. Ask students to issue a warning before jumping into one of those shares and get permission from the group to tell their story. It's a delicate balance; it takes a strong leader to keep the space safe for everyone.

The same is true when incorporating **chanting** into class. The Three and a Half Acres Yoga teacher Nikki Walker (profile on page 38) is a master at introducing sound vibration into her classes. She always gives the option for students to hum, chant silently, make up their own words, or opt out. Releasing stress through sound vibration can be intense and emotional, so as with each step in a trauma-informed yoga setting, it's important to go slowly. Start short and simple, and resist the urge to add or intensify the practice as you might in other yoga settings.

Teacher Profile: Nikki Walker

Nikki (she/her) was introduced to Three and a Half Acres Yoga by Karen Archer, a former board member. They are both voice-over actors, and Karen knew Nikki was also a certified yoga instructor. Nikki enrolled in the Three and a Half Acres Yoga trauma-informed teacher training in 2018. From the get-go the team could tell she was a star. Nikki was an eager volunteer and became a favorite of many of our partners. Her excellence was the catalyst for creating the new position of senior teacher within the organization. In addition to senior teacher, Nikki is now a teacher trainer and a junior board member.

~

In 2017 I was diagnosed with MS and my world was turned upside down. My body was not the same as it had been yesterday. My left side became weaker, and I thought, *What is this?* That summer, my (Kundalini) yoga teacher sent me an email offering me a scholarship for teacher training. My first response was, "I don't think I can

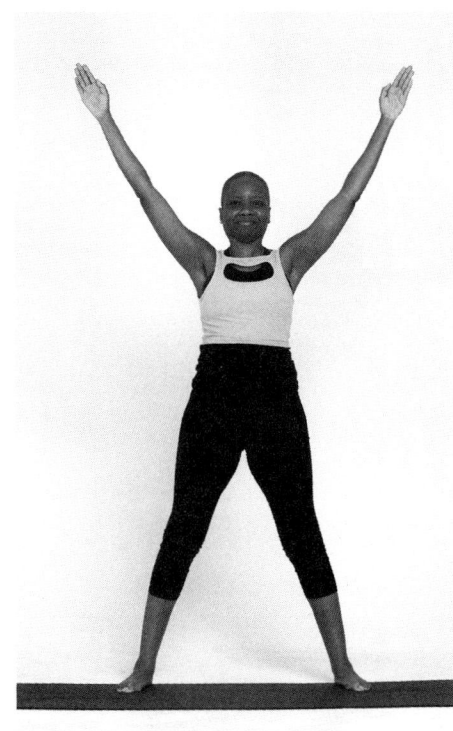

teach anyone because something's wrong with my body." And you know what she said? She said, "No, you should teach *because* of what you're going through with your body. It's going to teach you a lot. Become a teacher. Be a teacher." I accepted the scholarship.

Yoga helped me to come to terms, to deal, and to transform myself. I keep moving forward. No, I'm not moving like I used to when I was in my twenties and thirties and earlier forties, but I'm able to do it for a longer time. I'm actually getting stronger.

Yoga has taught me that living with MS can be a wild and beautiful adventure. You're constantly living in a new body every day. It's easier to breathe through and stretch through the uncertain times. I have the ability to release all of my fears. Yoga reminds me to accept my body and myself exactly as I am. The body is a divine gift. I might as well enjoy the hell out of it. Life is too short.

Breath really is our medicine. Not saying anything against medicine—medicine, we love you. But breath helps us heal. It helps us to release resentment, to release heartbreak, and to invite the new. To invite love, to invite release, to invite life. It's divine. It's our best food.

Some things I teach that are different are holding your arms up in a V shape for victory. Sometimes I try to do it for sixty seconds, which you wouldn't think is hard, but for a lot of people that's really challenging. Ultimately it's very calming, especially when you bring a mantra in. You can whisper the mantra or just think the mantra if you are uncomfortable saying the words.

I also bring laughter to my classes—bringing our belly, our navel, our heart into laughing out loud. It moves everything and makes the class lighter, which makes it more accessible. And I incorporate student's suggestions into class. Every person you meet is a teacher. The best teachers in my life were my nieces when they were four, five, and six years old!

RELAXATION AS SELF-CARE

Caring for myself is not self-indulgence, it is self-preservation, and that is an act of political warfare.

—AUDRE LORDE

The state and position of our muscles have a notable impact on our brain. Even if life circumstances have not changed, the simple act of releasing tensions in the body will create more peace. Just like smiling makes someone feel happier, lengthening the spine and expanding the chest makes someone feel more open, confident, and aware.

Some activists suggest that relaxing at a time of so much injustice and oppression could make us lazy and inactive. This is true only if we mistake relaxation for tuning out. Yoga asks the opposite of us. Yoga asks that we consciously cultivate awareness and practice the inner calm that results from focusing on and doing our duties in life with a quality of service. This means releasing our actions into the world without entangling ourselves in the results. By doing so, we are able to remain in service longer, without burnout and without passing on our traumas to others. The call to take this kind of action goes as far back as the Bhagavad Gita, "Your right is to action alone; Never to its fruits at any time. Never should the fruits of action be your motive; Never let there be attachment to inaction in you."[6]

If well cared for, a calm nervous system has a unique ability to awaken to awareness of injustice and to work against injustices long term without burnout. This doesn't mean, however, there aren't times for anger or that we should deny reality in order to float in an ignorant state of calm. This is the opposite of the awakening to which yoga asks us to be present. Anger does not indicate that one is a lesser yogi. In the yoga process, feelings are never to be stuffed down; instead, they are to be acknowledged and explored. The call to "stay calm" and "be positive" in the face of injustice is a gross misunderstanding of what yoga texts like Patanjali's Yoga Sutras teach. It has been used to silence important voices and has caused deep harm and further trauma to those already facing the trauma of daily systematic oppression. In fact, as Michelle Cassandra Johnson states in her book *Skill in Action*, "Feeling the pain, individually and, more importantly, collectively allows for us to grieve, to acknowledge and truth tell, and to aspire to be better than the legacy that white supremacy has left us."[7]

When viewed through a historical context, we see that yoga was never meant to be separate from social and political activism. Yogis' call to recognize oneness is as much about working to realize a world in which we are all seen and treated as one in our personal relations, actions, and social networks as it is coming to recognize that we are all made of the same matter: stardust and pure awareness.

FINDING ONE'S TRUE VOICE

In my decades of teaching yoga, I have witnessed again and again how the practice of yoga changes the temporary or present emotional state and long-term traits in people who commit themselves to it. As the muscles relax, defenses that had been impeding expansion—physical and mental, creative and emotional—begin to disappear. After an extended period of regular practice, it's not unusual for a person to experience a sense of waking up, sometimes coupled with a feeling of loss at the time spent "sleeping" in their life. They see things anew.

As the chest cavity and lungs are opened through the practice, the breath deepens and has room to expand. Vocal resonance has more depth and becomes more attuned, subtle in its ability to match the individual's inner intent. (We practiced many yoga techniques in my acting training as an undergraduate at Boston University, and they were always included in courses about finding one's true voice.) As Kristin Linklater, the vocal coach and author of *Freeing the Natural Voice*, said, "If the work to free the voice has been deeply absorbed, the person will be naturally freer; the person and the voice will be unified."[8]

Being able to speak up, speak out, give the world an accurate account of our inner truth is a boldly satisfying accomplishment, sometimes shockingly so. I've seen students suddenly begin to say what they mean without holding back or apologizing meekly. One of my students rarely spoke when I met her, and when she did, her voice was barely audible. In two years of practice, she had a complete vocal rebirth. It was deeply exciting to experience together, and this renaissance led to her exposing sexual harassment she was experiencing in the workplace. The practice of yoga was also a main support for her after she spoke up, an act that drastically changed her life situation. She was removed from her job, and she filed a lawsuit that became the center of her life. When her life was in upheaval, the consistency of the yoga movements, community, and principles was a source of stability.

When our experience has the freedom to be expressed via the breath and sound vibration, it is no longer trapped in the body. Trauma is released. Those who experience trauma are often inhibited from expressing their needs and desires or are forced to repress those wishes after they go unmet or result in opposing responses. Expression can be a form of healing.

Breath and Increased Conscious Awareness

Yoga makes conscious and ultimately alters what were previously unconscious and autonomic nervous system processes of the body, most notably the breath. This is another way it is such a powerful healing modality for trauma.

We bring awareness of breath to every posture and every moment that we are in yoga practice. We work on having an even breath pace and sound, for both inhales and exhales and from breath to breath, whether we are engaged in an easy or difficult posture. We practice staying in awareness and therefore noticing when the breath pace increases or the breaths become shorter. With mindfulness we are able to watch the experience of stress on the body and make choices around it. Simply by enacting this awareness, the body responds by slowing down. We can consciously slow it down by deepening our breathing when that option is available to us. When breath pace is decreased, the parasympathetic nervous system is activated, telling our body to relax and increase heart rate variability. As we practice slowing down in the face of challenges on the mat, this neural pattern becomes stronger in all aspects of life.

Neural pathways that fire a lot get stronger and fire faster. These become our go-to responses, and other patterns begin to weaken. Over time and through yoga practice we can make a parasympathetic nervous response a dominant response to stress: we can train ourselves to relax when triggered. Processes that seemed automatic, like breath and the release of stress hormones, become more in our control. Remember that prefrontal cortex discernment part of our brain going offline in crisis? If the body isn't signaling a crisis, we hold on to that functioning. We have more agency when challenged, and we retain clarity of thought, leading the way to better decisions. As one might imagine, this can have life-changing and lifesaving effects. This is the gift of a trauma-informed yoga practice and one that anyone can learn and use.

As we slow down, we realize we are not our thoughts. Though the mind may fire rapidly with stories of self-criticism and doubt, we are, from a place of calm, able to watch those thoughts arise and pass. We learn this as awareness builds within each posture and we begin to hear all the thoughts that fire off when we ask our body to do something even mildly uncomfortable, such as be still for five breaths. Angry, limiting self-talk may amplify; self-criticism gains rapid speed; or frustration may be turned at the teacher or other students. Sometimes, instead, the mind will distract us with reminders of things we have to do, imaginings of better times ahead, or revisiting something we did or said earlier. No matter the thought, the challenge is to remain in present-moment awareness as much as possible. When we do this, we see how rapidly the thoughts pass, making way for new, sometimes contradictory ones. This knowledge leads to deeper understanding about our mind and how fleeting and unreliable our thoughts can be. It changes our relationship to our thoughts and calls us to look for something deeper when seeking enduring truth.

Off the mat this translates to better decision-making and more responsive, less reactive behavior. Students of yoga become better at waiting after a particularly distressing thought (instead of reacting) to see how they feel after a breath or two. Knowing the breath can powerfully slow things down and change one's perspective, this tool is now available at any time.

BUILDING CONFIDENCE, SHEDDING STORIES

Anxious thinking, loss of confidence, doubt, and shame are common and can be crippling after trauma. Survivors are often plagued with thoughts about themselves as being bad or lacking. These ideas are connected to an awareness of how society sees trauma survivors and a response to the Medusa complex, a post-trauma effect where survivors can't turn away from it in their mind's eye, often circling around and around the experience looking for ways they could have done better.

As survivors come to understand that those thoughts are just stories they are telling themselves, not fact, the stories lose their power and make way for new beliefs around courage and fortitude. This process begins as they get space and perspective around their thinking, and its power grows as they expand their ability to decipher and make better decisions around signals within their body. It gains even more speed as they begin to do things with their body and mind that they had previously considered beyond their potential, such as staying in a posture though their mind is racing or balancing on one foot as their quads are firing. Yoga shows us that we can do hard things without harming ourselves or losing compounded stamina. We may even gain strength through our efforts.

The way that yoga aids a trauma survivor in self-understanding and rebuilds the foundation for trusting personal instincts cannot be overstated. Once the nervous system is slowed down and much of the stress is released from the body, students begin to become conscious of their thoughts and start disentangling the misleading stories their minds are telling them. They begin to get more trustworthy information from the mind-body system. When the body is calm and the amygdala's fire alarm is not going off as constantly or unreasonably, they can begin to focus on the times when it does fire and explore what is triggering that arousal. Then using a relaxed, articulate system of inquiry, they can make insightful choices around if and how to react. Survivors begin to trust themselves again. They can make sense of what to let pass and what to dig into.

Establishing Boundaries

A reestablished connection to self-confidence is a deep desire of most trauma survivors, and it is at the heart of trauma sensitive yoga techniques. There is only one way to promote this as a teacher: by getting out of the way of the student. Your job is to stay curious about their experience and make way for them to have or not have any sensations, asking questions that open their curiosity rather than lead them to where you believe they need to go. This is the only way they will be able to come to uncorrupted self-knowledge on their own. Any sense that you have a preference for their experience or that they should please you would

Teacher Spotlight: Elsie Scimecca

Elsie (she/her) was a graduating member of Three and a Half Acres' first Washington, DC, cohort, which also became our first online training class after its dates coincided with COVID-19 lockdowns. She's been a leader and a trouper when it comes to transforming our programs and trainings to the digital platform. Her classes are accessible, inviting, and visually appealing, making the journey to calm, peaceful connection through the screen an easy one.

~

I'm seventy-three years old. I've been doing yoga for twelve years. My daughter runs a yoga studio, and she's a wonderful teacher. I had started some running to get in shape and I kept getting injured. My daughter said, "Mom, you have to come do some yoga and balance out." So I started. I liked it more and more as I did it, and I ended up doing more and more yoga and less and less running. After a few years, my daughter said, "You were my longest-lasting beginner student. You really know what it's like for them. I think you'd be a good teacher for beginners." So, I have primarily taught beginners.

I've been in pretty good health, and I credit yoga with some of that. My mother had pretty bad osteoporosis when she got older, but I have had very good, stable bone density test results. I grew up with a lot of allergies and asthma. I do feel like the focus on a slow, steady, deep breath has been a benefit for me in yoga. I am very grateful for yoga and what it's done for me. It's changed my body and my quality of life in terms of what I can do. I can keep up with my grandchildren. Plus they're super-impressed if I can do a headstand or backbend. They just can't believe that Grandma can do that!

I worked in schools for a number of years, and I worked with a lot of kids that had experienced trauma. Also, some of my older sisters have physical challenges that they're facing, so I felt like it'd be really cool if I could teach postures that involved chairs. My oldest sister is in assisted living now, which really got me interested in teaching trauma-informed yoga at the facility. I brought her to my beginner's class a few times, and I could see how helpful that was to her. I don't know what I would do if I couldn't do yoga anymore, so I'm glad to know trauma-informed yoga and all its modifications. I can probably continue it in one way or another until very old age.

I looked at some different styles of chair-yoga offerings and they don't have the same benefit of the core from Ashtanga. Adapting the postures of Ashtanga to the chair while keeping as much of the original intent is really a good thing. I feel like you should never sell students short; you should always be giving them the options of moving deeper into the poses and not feel that because they're in a shelter or an assisted living facility that they must have a totally modified system. Maybe they can do more, and maybe they will over time. Older students who might have significant physical issues, who maybe cannot raise their arms above their head, will enjoy small changes that are so pleasing to them—and to me. And even if they don't, they can just enjoy the practice and enjoy being able to move and breathe and meditate in a group while they're practicing yoga.

destroy this highly sensitive step back into self-confidence and crucial reclaiming of autonomy.

Only when a student can trust the information they are receiving from their own mind-body system can they reestablish and trust new, healthy boundaries. Boundaries are the lines we put up around us to set a distinction between our body, thoughts, energy, and emotions and those of others. They are the rules that guide us around what we can and cannot do or feel for another human being, and they are based on how going past them makes us feel. As Jivana Heyman writes in *Yoga Revolution*, "Boundaries are the best form of self-care. They allow us to focus on what the body and mind need to flourish, rather than what other people think we need or what other people need from us."[9]

Recognition and observance of boundaries can be aided by the right teacher. A great teacher encourages their students to show up for themselves and celebrates their self-trust even and especially when that leads to the student opting out of a practice or not pushing themselves. They show their students compassion and consistency and bear witness to their profound journey, helping them to remember how far they've come. The teacher reinforces the students' innate abilities, reminding them that the answers to all their questions are inside. The teacher never claims to be a healer, leader, or guru but instead stands beside students looking out with them at where they are going, reminding them how far they have come.

A teacher can help a student recognize, trust, and appreciate their boundaries. These can be around how deep they want to stretch, how much they want to open/release, and how closely they want to interact with the teacher and others in the practice space. Boundaries are a beautiful and necessary part of a healthy life. Many modern, non-trauma-trained yoga teachers think their job is to push through boundaries and create openings. This is not the work of a trauma-trained yoga teacher. Trauma fractures boundaries. Trauma-informed yoga is a tool for reestablishing healthy ones.

The teacher can assist in boundary setting by vocalizing when they see a student confused about trying to assert a boundary or unsure if they are safe or right to do so. They can say, "I see you are coming up against _____. What do you want to do?" They can help them navigate toward the trusted signals they've been developing and reading in their body and making the right decisions for themselves. They can reinforce safety and remind students that yoga isn't about being as open and flexible as possible but uniting with self and the moment. That comes from being in balance, from holding strength and flexibility in equal esteem, and by celebrating the boundaries and limits our body is asking of us.

The power dynamic between trauma survivors and yoga teachers is important because those who have been affected by trauma tend toward codependency, lack of self-esteem, and loss of self-knowledge. They can have a hard time finding healthy boundaries and can become easily attached to those who seem able to save them. This dynamic is very fraught, and yoga practitioners are confronted with this danger again and again when they come to yoga to heal and are violated by teachers who use the opportunity to abuse their power. If yoga environments are to be made as safe as possible, teachers must be accountable. Even better, all teachers should have trauma-sensitivity training and actively eradicate hierarchical ideology in the yoga classroom by asking students what they want to do instead of demanding to be followed.

BUILDING A LIFE THAT IS SATISFYING AND FUN

Along the way, as self-awareness, confidence, and boundaries are blossoming, students begin to notice something else: yoga is fun. It provides an opportunity to relax, take chances, grow, and play. Practiced alone and in community, yoga offers a lot of choice in the way one can experience it. It can and often does start to influence a person's whole life, from

Recently, the meditation coach Oneika Mays shared with me a story about a woman she was teaching meditation to on Rikers Island. They had been working together in one-on-one sessions for some time, and the woman seemed to really enjoy and benefit from the meditation instruction. Then one day she decided she didn't want to come to meditation anymore. Instead of being offended or disappointed, Oneika relayed that she felt happy. She saw that in jail, a place where individuals have very little in the way of choice, this woman had found an opportunity to make a choice for herself—setting a boundary—and Oneika celebrated that. "I believe that liberation and agency are in the choosing," Oneika says.

what they eat to the way they perform habitual tasks. One begins to feel how different foods affect us and make choices around those feelings. Patterns of overdoing or overtrying, as well as other habits, show up in practice, and we see them reflected in life off the mat. At the same time, yoga philosophy, such as the *yamas* and *niyamas*, and more curiosity around the other (non-asana) parts of yoga start to become of interest. These guidelines offer a road map for a life built on ethics and living one's values, a path many find deeply satisfying. Finding like-minded friends who also live strong ethics and provide spiritual support is another natural outcome.

Yoga shows practitioners how to determine and use appropriate amounts of effort toward meeting goals. It awakens them to times they are doing tasks more as a distraction rather than for better outcomes. Most of us need to learn to do less and allow for more flow. In this way, yoga creates an ease in life revealing when to push forward and when to let go. It can feel, when practiced with proper use of energy and effort, like a kind of rest and recharge that can be otherwise challenging to find for trauma survivors, who tend to be hypervigilant and unable to relax.

COMPLEXITY, IMPERMANENCE, AND RESILIENCE

Finally, yoga awakens in practitioners the ability to see the complexity in things. As we explore sensations and emotions and begin to notice all the parts these feelings are made of, we notice how they move and morph in the body, often becoming something surprising and new. After months of regular yoga practice, an area in our body that feels as hard as a rock is suddenly as fluid as water. Upon investigation we realize things may not be as simple as we had thought, and we start shedding binary labels such as stiff or flexible, damaged or healed. The relationship with complexity grows as students traverse the complicated questions of nonstriving, nonharm, honesty, boundaries, and devotion prescribed in the Yoga Sutras.

Yoga helps us understand and accept the fact that we live in a body—and in a world—that is impermanent and constantly changing. Within this knowledge lies the freedom to embrace the self as it grows and changes, to resist the inclination to try to return to some imagined pre-trauma self and instead to meet each moment with wonder and an acknowledgment of its newness and potential. As the great meditation teacher Joseph Goldstein writes in *Mindfulness: A Practical Guide to Awakening*, "A deep reflection on this great truth of impermanence enlarges the context of our own experience and loosens the bonds of craving and attachment. It is the difference between the rollercoaster emotions of a child, with its many highs and lows in even just one day, and equanimity and wisdom that adults (ideally) develop about changing life circumstances."[10]

As the student embraces complexity, they also build their capacity to handle uncertainty and their ability to be resilient. Resilience is a complex topic. No one wants to be celebrated because they withstood harm, and yet we must celebrate the body's incredible ability to survive and even thrive post trauma. According to Resmaa Menakem, the author of *My Grandmother's Hands*, resilience is a term that is often misunderstood. He writes,

First, resilience is both intrinsic and learned, a combination of nature (what you're born with) *and* nurture (the circumstances you encounter, especially as you grow up). Second, resilience manifests both individually and collectively. Sometimes it does take the form of a personal, individual act. Often, however, resilience is expressed communally by a group, a family, an organization or a culture. . . . Third, resilience isn't just about responding to—or getting through—a difficult experience. Resilience also manifests in a form that's more about being than doing. This aspect of resilience helps us stay grounded and settled, no matter what happens to us.[11]

Core Concepts

- Yoga is an effective modality for trauma healing because it incorporates the whole mind-body system.
- Grounding, presencing, sensation awakening, and relaxation techniques within yoga practice are what relieve the negative impacts of trauma such as dissociation and hypervigilance.
- Trauma-informed techniques and practices should be applied extremely slowly so as not to overwhelm the nervous system or leave the student feeling defenseless.
- A key technique in the presencing practice is the three-pointed focus, Tristana, which involves focusing the gaze, listening to the sound of one's breath, and feeling being in the body.
- Instead of holding all three points of Tristana, a trauma survivor may decide to choose the point of concentration that is most soothing or safe for them.
- Relaxation can lead to clearer mental capacity, strong decision-making, and a strong and articulate speaking voice.
- Yoga can help us distinguish between our thoughts and our unchanging nature and, in doing so, reduce our attachment to negative thinking.
- Trauma sensitive yoga can also assist in confidence and boundary building because it puts the student in charge. This in turn increases the student's capacity for discomfort and uncertainty and strengthens their resilience.

A yoga practice can build resilience through understanding, acceptance, and perhaps embracing complexity, change, and impermanence. Transformation can be deeply profound. It doesn't mean that we won't ever break down again. It means when we do, we are able to rise up again. We can recover because our deep inner support structure is not weakened by outer conflict. It is "*sthira sukham asanam*" (Yoga Sutras 2.46), steady and at ease.

3

Becoming a Skilled Trauma-Informed Yoga Teacher

Non-striving is trying less and being more.

—JON KABAT-ZINN

YOU DON'T BECOME A TRAUMA-INFORMED YOGA TEACHER BY learning a special yoga sequence or committing to memory lists of poses to teach to—or not to teach to—those who have been through trauma. It would be easier if you did, of course; I get these requests again and again from students in my trauma-informed yoga teacher trainings. They want me to bundle the trauma-informed yoga teacher experience into a neat little package so it can be unpacked piece by piece.

Unfortunately, learning to teach yoga doesn't work that way.

Becoming a skilled trauma-informed yoga teacher arises from our own internal work and self-awareness. This work includes nervous system regulation, both ongoing and when we enter the classroom. It means diving into our own personal development and considering how our childhood caregiver relationships, or absence thereof, have influenced us as teachers. It includes recognizing our identities, privileges, assumptions, and how we are perceived by others. It means extending this understanding of identity to gain a greater understanding of others. In this chapter, I offer some essential ways to approach this lifelong work. Self-development cannot be contained in one chapter; personal development practices would—and do—fill hundreds of other books. This chapter is an overview with inroads into a lot of the work that goes into being a skilled yoga teacher beyond a teacher training program. The benefits of doing the work laid out below go far beyond becoming good at teaching yoga. They will make you a more effective facilitator in any field or aspect of life. They are also the same skills you need to prevent burnout, resentment, and vicarious trauma that may come from commitment to this work.

Working toward Coregulation

So much of teaching yoga is about coregulation, balancing our nervous systems so that others in our presence may naturally do the same. When we are calm and not easily aroused in the yoga space, it helps others to do the same. If you are working in a trauma-survivor-specific space, you can assume many of your students are hypervigilant. This means their bodies use neuroception, the ability to sense the outer world and determine safety or risk of danger, more than average. We have to let them know by our very presence that they are safe, as nothing positive can come out of the yoga experience until that safety is established.[1] As the neuroscientist Stephen Porges explains in his book *The Polyvagal Theory*, "In the presence of a safe person, then, the active inhibition of the brain areas that control defense strategies provides an opportunity for social behavior to occur spontaneously."[2] When we arrive in class as a friend, ready to support our students by standing by them, sharing their vision for their future, students can become more at ease with closeness.

How do we become that safe person for our students, which will be the most necessary part of enabling our students to open up to the practice? According to a number of studies on startle reflex, a person is perceived as safe based on their ability to make eye contact, vocalize with appealing and appropriate vocal tone, and express understanding and care with their facial muscles. It's not enough to appear neutral. Evolutionary biology makes it so that others read flat facial expressions as potentially threatening. How do you develop a compassionate gaze, facial expression, and vocal tone? It comes from an embodied understanding of the depths of our human connection and the vast differences in our human experience. As you do *svadhyaya* (self-study, or studying yourself in connection to all beings), you begin to understand your own nervous system and how it is likely to react to stress triggers as subtle as the nonresponsive face of another person. Eventually you may be able to override those reactions due to your own practices whether they be yoga, meditation, mindfulness, pranayama, somatics, or some combination. Where you are unable to override, you can name, understand, and have compassion for how the human nervous system works and model that compassionate mindfulness for others. This is subtle change that happens slowly. What can you do now to begin? Below are some initial ideas.

1. **Self-evaluate your privileges.** What is your race? Is your skin light or dark? What is your gender? Is it the same as the one you were assigned at birth? What is your sexuality? Are you thin? Conventionally attractive? Young? Able-bodied? Do you have obvious or hidden health challenges or are you in good health? Where do you live? Did you grow up with two parents? What was your access to education and what degrees did you receive? Is English your first language? All of us have privileges that grant us unearned access to certain resources. How do your answers to the above prompts help you understand the resources society has granted or denied you? How do you use yours to pass those resources along to others?

2. **Get interested in folks who have had different experiences than yours.** Read books, watch shows and movies, and listen to music and podcasts from people with different backgrounds and perspectives than the ones you were socialized to. Listen when folks who are not the same as you have something to say—and get curious—instead of assuming a shared experience.

3. **Practice softening.** Ask someone you trust how you appear when you walk in a room. Record yourself teaching. Look for the places you might be overly assertive. Step back and let others take up more space.

These are just a few ideas for starting this process that takes a lifetime and that many others have written about more eloquently. Let this be a starting point.

Due to the American story line and its belief in stark individualism, as well as a number of other factors such as inadequate social safety nets and support, many people in this country tend to operate in survival mode. This causes people to think primarily about their own needs, experiences, and personal story first. Waking up to the experiences of others and appreciating how different they often are from our own is a sorely needed life skill. This awareness helps people see how they might be making miscalculated assumptions about others who share this world. When one awakens to the fact that the other is us and we are the other (another definition of *yoga*, or "yoke"), it is a kind of enlightenment that changes us forever. This cannot be taught, but one can be led to it. Many great teachers are guiding this kind of awakening, and many of them are quoted and listed in the resource section in the conclusion of this book.

I urge you to seek them out to pursue this most necessary aspect of your training in trauma sensitivity.

When you walk into the yoga room, your nervous system affects the others in that space. Is it exhausted, tuned out, and sleepy? Have you just run from a subway train, nearly late for class? Maybe you're annoyed that you have to be there or distracted by something you have to do when you get home. As yoga teachers, we have all arrived at a class distracted or conflicted, but where the effects of trauma are present in our students, we must aspire to shift our energy and enter our class with aliveness, awareness, patience, and curiosity.

MAINTAINING YOUR OWN PRACTICE

As a trauma-informed yoga teacher, your first responsibility is to your own vagal tone. You must have strong daily habits that train your body to regain balance after dysregulation and practices in place that boost self-regulation before you enter class. Make sure you carve out time for your own practice, whether it is five Sun Salutations, a round of Nadi Shodhana (alternate nostril breathing), or ten minutes of mindfulness meditation. Be as clear and diligent about your practice time as you are of your students'. Not only can your students feel the difference if you are not practicing, but you will soon become depleted if you are working with others and not taking care of yourself.

Before You Teach

Tune inward and notice how activated or aroused your body is. Is your heart beating fast or slow? What is the quality of your breathing? Is your body tight or loose? Checking in is the first step in being ready for class. Additionally, you can help to move your system to its best state for teaching with a few small exercises. Here are some helpful options:

CULTIVATING ENERGY

Is there something in you or outside of you that has a quality of calm alertness and friendliness? Maybe it's a feeling of warmth in your chest or the image of a breeze hitting the trees. What we put our attention on grows. See if you can identify something pleasant you are experiencing right now. Connect more deeply to that sensation and see if you can expand it to fill your whole being. This is a simple, reliable tool for preparing to teach a class.

SHAKING IT OUT
Good for both before and after class, this exercise dispels excess energy. When you need a quick way to get rid of a nervous or anxious feeling before class, you can shake your body rapidly, from your hands and wrists down to your legs and feet. Give your head a good shake, too. Thirty seconds of rapid shaking should help you feel calmer and offer a pathway into more focused energy.

WAKING UP
One of the greatest tricks for waking yourself up is squeezing your ears from top to bottom, gently pulling them away from the body as you do so. You can also use this method of squeezing and pulling on your hair, starting from the roots. You can even use the same gestures to pull on your fingers. All are great ways to wake up when feeling sleepy before class.

Embrace the Beginner's Mindset

Yoga teacher training or an ongoing experience teaching yoga may have you feeling like an expert, but a self-study journey will help you come to realize how little you really know, especially about what goes on inside the minds and hearts of others. This humbling crossroads is a sure sign that you are on the right track. If you are truly lucky and even more so prepared, you can retain this perspective throughout your teaching journey.

A skilled trauma-informed yoga teacher refuses to fall into the role of the all-knowing yoga master. They never claim unquestionable certainty. They acknowledge that the pose they believe will help a student feel better or heal may also not be the best choice. They are in constant conversation with their students, graciously asking for feedback and offering alternatives to each and every pose. They eliminate all assumptions and resist the urge to tell a student how a pose will feel, even if they have been taught that it creates a certain feeling or result, or even if they have read studies or performed research.[3]

Let Go of Teaching Clichés

Beginner's mind is a practice a teacher can develop, but it takes work. Part of the work is taking familiar teaching tropes out of circulation. "Forward folds will calm you" and "unresolved relationship issues will release when you open the hips" are just two of the results-oriented proclamations I've heard in dozens of yoga classes, repeated like talking-point loops that no one knows the origin of but everyone accepts as true because everyone is saying them. Few teachers dare to challenge these clichés. Instead, they continue to offer them, causing students to either assume the feeling via suggestion or believe something is wrong with them when they aren't experiencing what they "should" be feeling. You can see the danger in both these outcomes, especially in a trauma-sensitive environment.

Teachers who test these yoga "truths" may experiment with and note how the poses feel in their own bodies, assuming their students will feel the same. While well intentioned, they fail to realize the privilege assumed: what they experience in their own body may be wildly different from what another person experiences in theirs. This assumption is similar to the ignorance we see in the privileged trying to use their own life experience to downplay the legitimate complaints of others not like them. We cannot know the pain of another human since we can't get inside their body. We must listen, connect, and then try to sense what they are going through instead of assuming we know what they feel based on our own limited experience.

Recently I heard a teacher say, "Downward Dog is meant to be a resting pose." In a trauma-informed yoga class, telling a student what they will feel is not only unhelpful but can also be harmful, and it absolutely contradicts the spirit of the class. Our goal as trauma-informed teachers is to help our students reconnect to their bodies and what they are feeling, which only happens when they get to decide to be with and identify the sensations they experience on their terms. There are no rules for how a pose "should" make a person feel.

Observe with All Your Senses

Your goal is to be fully attentive to your students in each and every class so that you are able to give the right kind and amount of support when they need it. You must be able to see when the words they are saying do not match up to their downcast eyes, note when a shoulder that was once raised now drops with relaxation. This requires ongoing curiosity and commitment to a beginner's mindset. Even if a student was happy in a pose a week ago, they may find it triggering today. You must be ready to see, accept, and respond to that shift with kindness and concern.

LIVING AND TEACHING WITH COMPASSION

Curiosity and beginner's mindset go hand in hand with compassionate nonjudgment, which is often referred to as the other wing, alongside mindfulness, of the Buddha's two-winged bird. When I am curious, I meet life's sensations and experiences with a bit of distance, nonreactivity, and perspective. When a negative thought comes into my mind, instead of immediately believing it and by consequence acting on it, I ponder, *What's bringing this to mind?* or *Is what I'm thinking real?* and *Is there something more here I'm not seeing?* I might even think, *Interesting, how did that thought get there?*

Often, upon reflection, I can begin to see how many external factors influence my inner dialogue, including familial programming, country of origin, schooling, media, and even evolutionary biology. With this knowledge come understanding and compassion for myself, which extend to others who are so often fighting free-radical thoughts we never wanted put in our heads.

Compassion can be cultivated through practices such as loving-kindness meditation, self-study, and deepening one's knowledge of the experiences of others. As we come to understand ourselves and our desire to be loved and accepted, we begin to see how this desire is in everyone and at the root of what each of us says and does. As we increase our sensitivity to this deep need, we see more clearly how we have made mistakes in pursuit of it, perhaps causing harm to others. At the same time that we see our mistakes, we open to self-compassion around those mistakes, recognizing that we were oblivious to the harm we would cause and that we were following the natural tendency of the self to do what it thinks it needs to do to survive. As self-compassion grows, so does our compassion for others and our sensitivity to what they are going through as they pursue their same human desires. We feel more intensely for the ways others have been harmed.

Developing this understanding of human nature and compassion for ourselves and others is critical to becoming effective healers and teachers.

Exercise: Belief Investigation

Start with a negative assumption you have about yourself. Maybe you're convinced you're lazy or boring or can't learn fast enough. If you can't think of anything, watch your thoughts in meditation and notice what comes up. Are there voices in your head about being forgetful or needing to be more productive? When you notice one, instead of riding with it in belief or berating yourself for having the thought, get curious about it. Allow the curiosity to lead you to questioning the nature of all your thoughts and your responses to thought.

Once curiosity becomes a habit in your personal practice, watch how it bleeds into your whole life. When something doesn't go right when you are leading class, instead of getting down about it, your response will now be one of inquiry. Your students will see this behavior modeled in you and are more likely to take on this approach in their own practices and lives.

The next step is to start adding the all-powerful practice of "What if . . . ?" Ask yourself questions such as *What if I decided not to believe this thought?* or *What if I replaced this thought with an opposite one?* This experimental way of thinking will also inform your teaching style.

Finding Peace with Goallessness

I don't believe our growth as human beings is linear, nor in my more than two decades practicing and teaching have I witnessed the yoga experience to be a stair-step climb to some final peak. My perspective on growth is that it often takes a spiral shape, wrapping around and dipping down as it climbs. It can also be random, torturously slow, and change in an instant. If you are working with trauma survivors, it's even more important to know that your experience healing trauma with your students will not show linear progress. You will start anew again and again, day after day, in each moment. For this reason, learning to share yoga with a sense of goallessness is important. Your commitment to showing up without achievement goals in mind—except to be present, compassionate, curious, and nonjudgmental—is important for each class and for the long-term experience of working with the student or group. When expectations of how we want things to go are eliminated, joy and purpose arise. We have to let the unique moments of safe exploration and positive relationship building be enough and not strive for something different.

It is a misfire to create goals for the student they don't have for themselves or to assume a student's goals won't change over time. Encouraging an attitude of goallessness among the students is preferable to

It is common in our trauma-informed classes for students to have limited awareness of bodily sensation. One time, a teacher at our New York Harm Reduction Educators site asked a student what they were feeling in a posture. The student answered, "Nothing." They could not describe any sensations because they were disassociated from feeling *feelings* in their body. The teacher normalized the situation, letting the student know that it was okay and not unusual to be disassociated from feeling after a trauma and encouraged them to stay present and curious as to what, if anything, showed up in the form of sensation now or later. "What does nothing feel like?" he asked. Sensing the student's willingness, he encouraged them to stay in the posture, not rushing to change or fix the situation. Later, the teacher asked more exploratory questions, sensing when the student had become more comfortable. Responses to questions such as "What feelings does this posture seem to suggest?" and "What happens if you (alter one suggested element of the posture)?" can be informative and helpful. All the while, we remind the student that there is no rule they must feel anything. It's enough to be present with the experience they are having, just as they are.

emboldening goals they may harbor without full knowledge of yoga processes and timelines. Students may not understand that the process is not linear. They often overestimate how regularly they can show up for weekly class. They shouldn't have to face feelings of defeat or disappointment around yoga, a modality that we hope will support them in the full expression of their lives. Reassure students that anytime they show up for practice is wonderful, and they are welcome anytime—without pressure.

When you, as a teacher, release yourself of goals and expectations beyond presence, nonjudgment, and compassion, you will also be rewarded with a more expansive and less stressful feeling in your teaching. You can concentrate on the moment and the people in front of you, and you will feel more ease. Then you can do the work that is necessary to meet the needs of the moment with no agenda. No agenda doesn't mean no lesson plan; come prepared with many and a multitude of poses and exercises, stories and metaphors within you that can be accessed when you pivot to the needs of the moment.

A Note on Reading the Room

Practice checking in with your senses each time you enter the teaching space. What do you see, hear, feel? Do participants greet you or do they seem distracted? Are there clusters of conversations or is everyone unified? Check in with your own body's sensations as you ground into awareness in the space. Does the centering of your energy affect the others? If not, you may need to help the group expel more energy first. Learn to note the energy at the beginning of each class, ranking it with a number or a color, or writing a few notes down about what you sense, so you can detect differences from week to week. This allows you to be more immediately aware if pivoting is needed. Instead of launching into grounding or asana, you might need to introduce a shaking-off practice or start with a squeeze-and-release exercise to shift and expel energy. Or the group might need a long check-in and time to talk.

REMINDING STUDENTS OF THEIR AGENCY

The biggest challenge on the road to becoming an effective trauma-informed yoga teacher is unlearning the way you've likely been taught to teach. No longer will you give instructions to be followed dutifully and rally an attentive class into unified asana. Instead, you will suggest and invite, staying open and curious as you do so to all responses, especially and including resistance. You will not be used to this way of teaching if you've primarily led studio classes, performing in the role of yoga master and entertainer.

In the studio class, you were in charge. Now, with your trauma-sensitive understanding and mission, you are obliged to create an atmosphere where the student is in charge. The student is completely empowered to tell you when anything you suggest feels wrong, to let you know what they need and don't need, and for you to not just be okay with but love receiving this feedback. At first this may seem like a challenge to the ego, but you will soon find it is a relief not to have to pretend to know everything. It also is a more exciting and rewarding way of being in relationship with students in your class.

Once you recognize that the student leads, you can focus on developing your ability to show them that they can. Your role is to prove to each student that they are the one and only appropriate leader for themselves. You do that by telling them so and by reinforcing this in all the ways you respond to them in class.

You can transition easily to becoming this kind of teacher if you know your answer to this one question: What is yoga?

Exercise: What Is Yoga?

Get a pen and some paper or a journal. Find a position you can be still in for a little while. If it is comfortable for you to do so, close your eyes; if not, gaze softly down at a neutral spot in front of you. Turn your watchful gaze inward. Ask yourself, *What is yoga?* Let the question sink way down deep. Maybe no answers come at first. Perhaps a feeling or an image surfaces. If so, look at it more deeply. Notice what answers arise. Maybe a definition from your yoga teacher training or something you saw along the way in your yoga journey. Be honest with yourself about what thoughts about yoga are coming up because whatever they are, and however hard you try to hide or deny them, they will always be known by those you teach. Write down everything that comes to you. Note where that definition of yoga was first introduced to you and what makes you believe or disbelieve it today. It's better that you have an awareness of the programming that influences you than acting without knowledge of its influence.

You may find you need to let go of a definition that does not serve you or your students. Write this down: "Yoga is a practice by which a person can come to know themselves more fully and, in doing so, increase their agency and therefore ability to make informed and empowered decisions in all areas of their life." Try saying it aloud. Now say it again. Consider writing and vocalizing this understanding of yoga daily. Once you have internalized and believe this definition of yoga, you are ready to be a great trauma-informed yoga teacher. When you find yourself teaching or correcting a pose, you can ask yourself if what you are doing is contributing to your student's ability to know themselves. If not, you will stop or alter what you were going to do.

ENLIGHTENMENT AS COMMODITY

Most yoga teachers have been trained to believe that yoga is a physical practice that involves moving through a series of postures and that the better we match our imitation of these postures to the practice of some nonexistent thin, white, flexible woman, the better we are at yoga. If you believe this, it's not your fault. American yoga classes and yoga content (published or produced) in mainstream media tend to focus on the physical and superficial aspects of the yoga practice. To sell you yoga, the industry highlights the physical and aspirational qualities of the practice, convincing you that you too can look like an eighteen-year-old gymnast and never feel negative feelings again, if you practice hard enough. Those who aren't persuaded by the sell are often so turned off by a portrayal of yoga that cannot possibly include them that they dismiss yoga altogether. To me, this is the most devastating consequence of yoga as commodity.

You may think you believe differently, that yoga is yoking mind, body, and spirit, or a way to come into oneness or connect to something eternal. But if you perpetuate the teaching habit of constantly "fixing" postures—your students' or your own—you are demonstrating that that is not what you believe.

If you hold on to the harmful notion that a deeper backbend or more straight-legged Downward Dog makes you a better yogi, that notion will be felt in the yoga room. It will be revealed in the physical adjustments you give your students. Often we apply these adjustments out of genuine concern for alignment, which could lead to injury. But through the lens of unlearning, why not also question alignment cues. Many are passed down from senior teacher to junior teacher with a sweeping uniformness and no sense of origin. Is it really *dangerous* to plant your feet closer than hip-width apart on the mat? To allow the bent knee to drift past the ankle in a lunge? Most movements are not injurious if not overly repeated, and most students will adjust movements to comply with their personal bodily safety if they are in an environment in which they feel in control and free to do so. Let your primary goal be creating that environment.

HONING YOUR INTENTION

Finally, the most crucial component to becoming a skilled trauma-informed yoga teacher is how you see yourself in relationship to the students you teach. Who you are, or who you believe you are, influences how you enter a service situation to share yoga. If deep down, hidden far from where you think people can see it, you believe you are better, smarter, and superior to the people you have come to share with, they will feel that arrogance, distrust you, and could become even more negatively impacted from their trauma. If you see yourself as a savior of the downtrodden and you try to fix or "save" your students, you will likely end up burned out, bitter, and doing more harm than good.

The first thing I ask of my yoga teacher trainees on day one of their training is to think about what drew them to this work and what keeps them committed to it. Most want to help others, some because they've been lucky in life and others because they too have experienced trauma. I ask them to consider how their feelings might shift upon realizing that their students are as likely to teach them as they are to teach their students. What's the context for this shared, dynamic yoga experience? How might they reconsider their role once they realize how much exchange of knowledge there is likely to be?

Exercise: Finding Your Why

Take some time to investigate your intentions as a yoga teacher and look specifically at why you want to cultivate trauma-sensitive practice spaces. Write down what you come up with in your journal. The body's response to trauma is normal, necessary, even genius. If your intention is to provoke change, have you considered that this could instead cause additional harm? What are some ways you could reframe that intention? Perhaps it's assisting practitioners in their self-exploration with thoughtful questioning or supporting practitioners in their choices, even those that on the surface seem to you unwise.

Though you can learn some things about trauma sensitivity from reading books and studying, no one discipline or expertise can train you to be a skilled trauma-informed yoga teacher. It's an inside job, so to speak. You'll have to befriend and resolve the parts of yourself that carry a savior mentality or that harbor secret judgments or assumptions about others. You will need to examine your views on yoga and the ways you've been programmed to strive for perfectionism by the media and other influential figures in your life, and dive deep into your personal intentions. This work is the most important work of this style of teaching (and arguably for living an intentional life), and it must be done on your own. None of us enters the yoga room with much more than a bit of knowledge about yoga and even

Core Concepts

- There's no single, surefire step-by-step yoga sequence that makes a class trauma sensitive.
- An essential skill for teaching a trauma-informed class is learning how to regulate your own nervous system. This must be done in the moments before entering class and ongoing by making sure to keep up your own yoga practice.
- Embrace a beginner's mindset with your students and never assume you know how they feel in any particular pose or situation.
- Do the inner work to get to know your own privileges, beliefs, and assumptions—and challenge them.
- Reflection on how you define yoga and your intentions for teaching is essential to becoming a trauma-informed yoga teacher. Self-study and integrating new perspectives on your habits and assumptions are ways to avoid inflicting more harm on students.
- Once you rewire your understanding of yoga's core meaning, you will let go of goal-oriented teaching. Instead, you will offer your knowledge with compassion, curiosity, and a beginner's mindset and let your students lead the way. This is the key to avoiding burnout and to remaining in service for a lifetime.

less about the depth of experience of the humans we endeavor to teach. We must train ourselves through mindfulness and compassion to stay in awe, remain humble, and be in a space of learning. Using these tools, we can help create and maintain a safe, healthy, meaningful yoga environment.

4

Building a Safe Trauma-Informed Yoga Class

Our longing for safety and for what's comfortable
is very deep; it's hardwired into us.

—SEBENE SELASSIE

YOU ARE FINALLY ALMOST THERE, READY TO EXPLORE WHAT you can bring to the world as a trauma-informed yoga teacher. Now you need only add the necessary techniques and best practices to your foundational knowledge and self-work to compose the right structure and parameters for your class. There are several techniques you will need to apply when teaching every class, and each one of them is essential for one overarching reason: safety.

In trauma-informed yoga, the definition of safety encompasses the physical, emotional, and psychological aspects, including the perception of safety. As laid out in chapter 3, our role as teachers of trauma-informed yoga is to guide individuals to use the practice to know themselves more fully and, in doing so, make informed and empowered decisions. Once that mission is established in our mind and heart, the next logical inquiry is *How do I do this?* The answer: we do everything in our power to create a practice environment that allows for the highest level of agency from our students. **A person cannot embody a sense of agency without a sense of safety.** In fact, the deeper our sense of safety, the more widely we can explore choice through creativity and risk-taking—mentally, emotionally, and physically.

The fastest and most secure way to get to agency is via a reliable and embodied experience of safety. It is only in this state that students have full access to all of the choices available to them. When we are fearful, this is not the case. We quickly act or react without thinking at all. In fear mode, we stay in uncomfortable postures, afraid to speak up, and cause self-harm. Or we refuse to do a posture or get angry about being asked to do it, and disrupt the class or leave. Contrast this with a person who feels safe. This person will recognize they have options. They can adjust a posture, take breaks, ask for advice, or move into the posture creatively with no fear. As the therapist and yoga teacher Hala Khouri states so clearly in her book *Peace from Anxiety*, "When we are centered, our sense of self and our center of power is inside of us, regardless of what is happening around us. We have a sense of personal agency and self-efficacy in our life. Although we may not be able to control everything that is happening around us, we are able to manage our own emotions and behavior."[1] She goes on to remind us that our safety may not always be in our hands alone. When working with your students, it's important to have this front of mind. If your students are experiencing immediate danger, it may be necessary for them to focus on the danger and how to protect themselves. At the same time, if stressful and dangerous situations are ongoing outside of class, your students may be empowered to find moments of calm and inner safety in class.

Safety is experienced when two factors come together: the reduction of external threat and the establishment of an inner feeling of security. Together, these factors are nurtured by resources both within a person and in their environment, which calm the body when a threat or perceived threat is present. We learned in chapter 3 how teachers can use facial expressions and vocal tones to create a safe environment. In this chapter, we examine other ways we as teachers can build external safety and help our students explore feelings of safety within.

Establishing External Safety

In a yoga teaching environment, three main external categories can build feelings of safety: class location, room setup, and teaching technique.

Class Location

External safety is heightened for your practitioners when you come to them in a location they are familiar with and comfortable in. With this fact in mind, it is the model of Three and a Half Acres to partner with organizations that are already providing services for trauma survivors and to use their facilities for yoga classes (instead of a traditional yoga studio).

Ten Key Factors That Ensure Security in a Yoga Class

Below are ten factors that aid in creating a feeling of safety for others. Consider carefully how you will build these into each of the three core categories: class location, room setup, and teaching technique. As an exercise, write down your insights and reflect on any new insights that arise as you begin to teach. We will revisit these factors throughout this chapter.

1. **Predictability.** Students are able to guess accurately what is going to happen in class.
2. **Clarity of expectations.** Students understand what is expected from them in class.
3. **Boundaries.** Having students' boundaries recognized and honored through conversation and action.
4. **Consistency.** Knowing the teacher's behavior aligns with their words, experiencing their reactions and energy as unchanged during class and from week to week.
5. **Articulated options.** Clear choices about what students can do to express each posture.
6. **Freedom.** Ability to experiment with postures at will and to voice opinions within the terms of the group agreements (see page 71).
7. **Contribution.** Suggestions are encouraged and integrated into class.
8. **Opportunity to opt out or leave.** Feeling completely able to leave class or choose to sit out any posture with no response except to be celebrated for making appropriate choices.
9. **Experience of acceptance.** Knowing that all students and all they feel and experience is welcome in this space.
10. **Receiving understanding.** Having students' needs anticipated in advance, being considered ahead of time, and having their differences cared for.

Arriving in someone else's space immediately establishes you as a guest. This is a healthy, humbling, and appropriate role for a yoga teacher. Being a guest pushes you into your vulnerability and disrupts any authoritarian habits absorbed from the culture of some yoga studios.

When you partner with nonprofits and community organizations, it is unlikely that you will have a dedicated yoga room. Classes may take place in a conference room, meeting room, dining room, or even a kitchen. You must do your homework before arriving. Find out as much about the space as you can, touring the location before your first class if possible. Where is the best entrance? Do you need ID to enter? What are the mask, vaccination, and other public health policies? Is there storage space for mats and other basic yoga props? Do floors need to be swept before class? If so, will that be your job? Where are brooms located? Will there be wipes and/or disinfectant available to clean mats?

Before the first class, consider discussing with your partner organization what types of clothing you can expect the practitioners to arrive in. Students are not likely to wear yoga- or fitness-specific clothing to these types of classes. Having a sense of their street clothing could help you design sequencing as some postures are difficult or uncomfortable in jeans or dresses and skirts. For transgender-specific groups, you may also want to account for any binding or surgeries that students could be managing. Finally, it is perfectly common that folks won't want to take their shoes off for class. Never insist they do. Prepare your classes with this in mind.

Setting Up the Teaching Space

No matter where your classes are held, you must consider the way you will set up the space as your yoga room. Be sensitive to the fact that a small change in the practice environment can make a big difference in the student's ability to relax and settle in. Creating feelings of safety in your practice space can evolve based on how students' needs develop and shift. Below are several suggestions to launch your planning.

EXITS

The most important factor in orienting your students within a yoga space is considering where the exit is. When possible, all students should be able to see the exit and have easy access to it when they are on their yoga mats or practicing. If this is not possible, make sure at least some of your students will have this option. The exit should not only be in view but should remain unlocked and unblocked. This accounts for factors 6 and 8 on page 67, promoting freedom and making it easy for students to leave at any time they feel the need.

MAT PLACEMENT

Once you've established the direction your students will face, consider how you will position them within the class. Though orienting mats in a circle has its benefits and has become a popular setup in many modalities, it does not work well for instructing yoga asana. A circle poses difficulties for following left and right instructions and inhibits space for arm and leg extensions. Rows or staggered rows are ideal, with the instructor remaining at the front of the space. This orientation establishes personal space and allows the students to see the instructor clearly. Taking care that mats are positioned in this way promotes healthy boundaries (factor 3) and aids clarity of expectations (factor 2), since a practitioner can more easily do the posture suggested when they can see you clearly.

PROPS

Provide each student with a chair and a yoga mat so they can use either or both from pose to pose. Even if a student expresses that they plan to remain seated, place the chair on top of a mat. This has many benefits. It keeps the chair from slipping during asana, which could lead to feelings of instability or injury. It also ensures that the practitioner doing chair yoga will have personal space equal to others using mats. It also makes it easy for the practitioner to change their mind and use the mat without needing to ask for one later. Providing the mat in advance results in wider choice and agency, as a student might choose not to ask for a mat if they perceive they would be disruptive to the class by doing so. This is a way of showing understanding, the tenth factor for creating safety.

LIGHT, SOUND, AND SMELL

Sensory input heavily influences your students' perception of safety. Lights should be kept on at all times. With permission, you may dim sharp lights slightly, but never more, because altering the lighting without warning could be triggering. Playing music also comes with many challenges. In addition to its risk of becoming a trigger, it also pulls attention outward when we are aiming for internal focus in the yoga practice. I suggest working without music. Let the sound of the breath be the music the individual focuses on. Finally, make sure to consider the scents that could be present in the yoga space. Smell is one of our most powerful senses and the one most deeply connected to memory. Avoid wearing perfume and other scented products such as oils and strong-smelling hair products. Smells and unwanted sounds may be present. Instead of ignoring them, do your best to work these into the class by acknowledging their presence. After that, you have the option of shifting the class's attention so those stimuli become background elements or getting curious about how our minds react to unwanted sounds and smells. Either approach can be helpful for self-discovery and agency. Where there is seemingly no choice, as in the case where cooking is present in the yoga classroom, we may come to realize that there are some choices as far as where we focus our attention and how we respond to the irritant. This discovery is then applicable outside the yoga classroom. This doesn't mean we should try to increase scents and sounds. Removing as many potential triggers as possible creates predictability, the first of the ten factors for creating safety, and it shows understanding, the tenth. You don't want to activate a student's memory unnecessarily in class.

Teaching Techniques

Below are a number of teaching techniques that make up the bulk of trauma sensitive teacher training. These can be practiced by simulating a class at home, with friends and family who will be your students, in your current classes, and by taking a trauma sensitive yoga teacher training. I recommend practicing all these ways so you have many different experiences using these tools. You may also want to observe teachers who have mastered them, especially when it comes to group agreements, as facilitating group discussions requires some additional skill sets.

POSITIONING YOURSELF

When teaching, always position yourself in front of the students, where you can be seen clearly. If you instruct a pose in which the students shift their orientation to you and the room, such as when they step out to the side or to the back of the mat, you should also shift so that you remain in front of them. Use the mirroring technique when you demonstrate: use the opposite side you are verbally cuing. For instance, when you say to your students "Lift your right arm up," you lift up your left. Avoid walking around the class while teaching, except to reorient to be visible. Many practitioners feel dysregulated and distracted when someone is walking around a room.

In addition to staying visible to your class, it is also important to align yourself at eye level with your students. In general, it is best to sit when they are seated and stand when they are standing. Never stand over your students, especially when they are in Savasana or any resting position.

This feeling of being loomed over is highly triggering and has the potential for setting off flashbacks. Staying in view of your students takes care of many factors of safety, predictability, boundaries, and understanding, among others.

SETTING GROUP AGREEMENTS

Group agreements are terms that the class and instructor create together and agree to for how they want to show up in the space. They are an attempt to prevent harm, especially types of harm that may not be easily predicted by the teacher, and to create space for folks' needs to be affirmed before they agree to participate in class. The practice of establishing group agreements represents a big shift from typical studio yoga classes in which students are rarely asked their needs and desires and classes often vary from week to week and from class description, most commonly with beginner classes being far from introductory level.

Though you have carefully considered as many variables as you could anticipate before class begins, incorporating group agreements into your class acknowledges that trauma triggers and safety needs are unique to each individual.

Launch your first day of any new class by asking the group to suggest and agree to collective guidelines that would support everyone in feeling safe for the duration of the session. Guidelines can be as simple as each student staying on their mat or in their practice space, waiting for dedicated times to comment on the yoga experience, and keeping comments in the "I" perspective and about one's own practice. This is also a good time to share your pronouns and offer others a chance to do the same. Group agreements should be written out and can be displayed during class, so make sure to have a large piece of paper, marker, and tape available. Having group agreements takes care of many of the ten factors of safety including predictability, clarity of expectations, boundaries, and contribution.

When partnering with organizations that are already running groups, you may ask them for their group agreements so you can work in tandem with community standards. However, also collaborate with your group in real time to come up with new agreements and revisit ones they've created in other contexts. This is a good opportunity to inquire if they feel supported. In this way, everyone is not just involved in the process but also invested in it.

You can also use this time to articulate your role in the yoga space in more detail—for example, you will explain and demonstrate all postures,

Creating group agreements will be a profound learning process. You will discover something you do (likely something you had never noticed yourself doing) that makes someone in the group feel unsafe. That insight is a gift; you will become a more aware and stronger teacher if you allow yourself to be changed by it.

you will offer many options, and you will never make anyone do anything they don't want to do. You can be clear about how you interact with students after class, such as whether you can stay for questions and for how long, and other related boundaries you draw around contact outside of class.

Remember that for a variety of reasons, trauma survivors often have difficulty intuiting and holding boundaries. Having clear agreements helps establish boundaries but does not ensure absolute safety. There could be (and often are) conflicting needs within a group. Talking through conflicts that are likely to come up means resolutions may be anticipated and can be referenced when disputes arise. One student may need to yell, joke, distract, and deflect to feel safe. Another student may feel unsafe around outbursts of emotion. Learning to work with your students to find creative solutions for these moments is part of being a skilled group yoga teacher. It creates an experience of acceptance and understanding.

BEING CONSISTENT

You've set up your room and welcomed your students in. Now it's time to think about the ways you will teach. It is in this realm you most bring consistency.

Many survivors of trauma have suffered some form of abandonment, and often multiple forms. Being abandoned may have been the inciting trauma. Or the abandonment may have come from friends and family members after coming forward about a traumatic incident. Or a supportive person may have left their life, creating an emotional void. Often in our society, caretakers burn out from being overextended or underpaid, leaving organizations abruptly and causing further trauma to the members they serve. Lack of funding and other resources can lead to service establishments closing suddenly and without any transition time for those who have grown to rely on them for essential services. It is therefore critical that you vow to stop this cycle by honoring your teaching commitment. Be meticulous in your efforts, showing up not

Co-teaching for Continuity

Assigning two teachers to each class helps address abandonment. If one teacher needs to step down, a familiar second teacher is still there for continuity. Your co-teacher or teaching partner teaches class with you. One teacher can cue students who are practicing in chairs and the other can focus on those who are standing or using mats. Alternatively, one teacher can talk and the other one can demonstrate. Sometimes one teacher leads the opening half and the other the second half of class. Co-teaching partnerships benefit from meeting or talking on the phone before class to discuss the flow and determine each other's strengths. It may be helpful to have additional substitute teachers attend class with you, too, so the community gets to know them. Spend more time with your substitute than you normally would when preparing them to take over your class.

just on time but early. Allow extra time before class so that folks who want to can talk to you privately about needs and concerns. Even if it's not your best day, make sure you are there. Sometimes our showing up is what is most needed. However, be prepared for a time when you may be ill or need to take leave by having a teaching partner and a list of substitute teachers who can be ready to relieve you.

Be consistent in your mood and attitude. We all have good days and bad days, and while you don't have to hide all emotion and become a positivity robot,[2] your trauma-informed yoga class isn't the place for dumping your personal struggles. You can establish a balance in which you can be real without oversharing.

PREDICTABLE SEQUENCING

Teach similarly, if not identically, from class to class. Unlike your typical class at a yoga studio, the best trauma-informed yoga classes do not call for fancy sequencing. Offering the same poses, in the same order, each class gives your students *predictability*, one of the ten factors for creating safety. It also ensures your students won't miss out on something new when they cannot come to class, which can be common for students who have unstable living environments and other hurdles. A set sequence also makes it easier to share lesson plans if you must have a substitute or bring in a replacement teacher.

Rhythm of a Trauma-Informed Class

Classes should start with grounding, breath awareness, and
   awakening sensation in the body.
Next, add small movements, matching them to the breath.
Once this connection is established, begin Seated Sun Salutation.
Add classical standing poses such as Triangle and Extended Side
   Angle taught from the chair.
Bring in Warrior poses and balancing.
Invite folks to stand or remain seated, with the option to stand,
   while you repeat this sequence.
Add forward folds, twists, and gentle hip openers.
Add Boat Pose to engage the core, the center of our willpower.
Offer gentle heart opening, always followed by a forward fold or
   rounding posture that counters that opening with protection.
Start your closing series with Legs Up the Wall or Shoulderstand
   and end with a trauma-sensitive body scan or squeeze-and-
   release exercise.

BREATH INSTRUCTION

Breathing in, I calm my body and mind. Breathing out, I
smile. Dwelling in the present moment, I know this is the
only moment.

—THICH NHAT HANH

Our breath is the link from our inner world to our outer world, and it is
our lifeline. It is critical that the breath be free, not restricted, for trauma
survivors. Never suggest breath retention practices. Also avoid breathing
techniques that increase breath rate as they can trigger a panic attack.

   The best suggestions you can give your students when teaching class
is to observe their breath, or even better, to feel their body breathing.
If they are comfortable and able to do so, you can invite them to gently
close their mouth and allow the breath to come in and out through their
nose only. Just this small change can cause anything from relaxation to
discomfort to panic. Observe your students with all your senses to make
sure they are breathing freely. Remind them that they can open their
mouth at any time if nostril breathing becomes too difficult. Or bring

their attention to something more pleasant to see if that alters the experience. For those for whom nostril breathing is not problematic, you can offer the option of Ujjayi Pranayama.

The way I teach Ujjayi Pranayama has been described by students as uniquely open and freeing. Once they have established nostril breathing, I invite students to bring a little more energy and attention to their breath. I then have them lift the roof of their mouth slightly and imagine they are breathing in through their cheekbones, or even their eyes, on the inhale, making a little sound with the breath. I offer that it should feel as if their face is breathing. The exhale I describe as breathing as if they were fogging up a mirror but with their mouth closed. I explain that they are working toward eventually an inhale and exhale that have the same sound and duration, though this could be a lifetime project.

Many people ask about instructing Nadi Shodhana, alternate nostril breathing, in their trauma-informed yoga offerings, because it is popular in conventional yoga classes. Alternate nostril breathing *without breath retention* may be taught by experienced teachers. They should recognize that this breathing technique may feel restrictive to practitioners, even without retention. Therefore I recommend teaching the method in which you use just your intention to bring the air up one nostril and out the other. This works surprisingly well and is perhaps more sophisticated a practice since it works with the subtle body. If you do teach with fingers closing alternate nostrils, strongly encourage students to stop and breathe freely and naturally at any time they feel uncomfortable.

Asana Instruction

It's not just what we teach but how we teach it that creates an experience of safety for our students. To optimize safety in asana instruction, use this three-step process: explain, demonstrate, invite. This method of yoga explanation is sometimes used in mainstream yoga classes but is not practiced reliably. Teachers often jump into their own practice and students try to follow along. Other times teachers offer partial instruction and/or don't demonstrate at all.

For each pose or movement, begin by letting your class know what you are about to ask them to do. Explain the pose or movement that is coming up next while looking around the class and searching for signs of recognition. Next, demonstrate the pose or movement you've just called, describing it step by step as you do it, this time with some added details and variations. Then give options: invite folks to join you, watch again before joining, take an alternative posture altogether, or sit this one out.

Practice: Talking through Linking Breath with Movement

It is often helpful for students for you to talk through linking breath with movement. For example, after teaching Ujjayi Pranayama, you might explain, "Now we are going to work on matching our movement with our breath pace." Let the students know that you are going to soon suggest they lift up their arms over their head. They will have the option to press their palms together or conclude the upward movement when their arms are shoulder-width apart. Their gaze can be up at the hands or ceiling or straight ahead. Encourage them to deepen awareness of their breath by lifting their arms just as the inhale is initiated and arriving at the uppermost arm position as the inhale ends. Similarly, they should begin the descent of the arms with the start of their exhale, completing this movement as the exhales concludes. Offer those who prefer smaller movements the option of turning their palms up on the inhale and down on the exhale.

Next, suggest to your students that they watch you as you reach your arms up with your inhale. This time you can offer additional options, such as pressing their fingers tightly together or stretching them wide apart. Open up the possibility that when it's time for them to move, they explore all the arm and hand positions offered and discover how the differences in posture influence their state. Teaching asana practice in this way brings *freedom*, *contribution*, and *opportunity to opt out* into the space.

Finally, invite in those who want to try this practice. Those who don't want to can sit out, choose an alternative, or visualize the posture in their minds, a practice that also has calming results. Continue to demonstrate as long as needed for all students to get the hang of the posture or motion. Stop demonstrating if you have a co-teacher who can continue or when the class is able to do the moves on their own, so that you may more deeply observe each student.

Demonstrating is a necessary part of teaching trauma-informed yoga, but it can come with adverse side effects in students, such as thinking they should look like you do in the pose. Resist demonstrating the version of a posture that requires the most flexibility or strength, and remind your students often that everyone's bodies are different and will look different in the pose. Let them know that what they are observing is a general shape showing where the arms and legs and other parts of the body might be in the pose. No one should try to replicate your exact posture. Encourage them to move their eyes to their drishti after they've observed the posture so they can return their concentration inward.

Word Choice and Semantics

Word your instructions so that they are truly invitational, offering options and honoring choice. You can do this by using phrasing such as "If it feels right in your body today . . ." or "If you'd like to try . . ." before suggesting an exercise or position. Offer the most accessible version of any posture first using language that reflects how powerful the most simple and accessible postures often are. When incorporating more challenging postures into a sequence, use language such as "If you're feeling like a little more of a challenge today . . . ," which is gentle and inviting. Never use stock phrases such as "the full expression of the pose" to describe a challenging variation, as it suggests other expressions are less than. Always vocalize the option to do something else or nothing at all.

When students are in the posture, do not focus on alignment but use cues that invite your students to explore their minds and bodies and build self-awareness. Examples of this are:

> "Bring your awareness to your . . ."
> "Notice what happens when you . . ."
> "Explore if you are holding any unnecessary tension in this posture."
> "Pay attention to any thoughts arising as you take this shape."

Address verbal cues and observations to the whole class instead of isolating individual students. Keep your language and cues gender-neutral, referring to the class as folks, humans, or practitioners instead of guys and ladies, as students may identify as nonbinary. If you refer to someone personally, make sure you know their pronouns or use their name. As the digital strategist and equity-inclusion facilitator Tristan Katz states in their article "Creating Trans Affirming Yoga Spaces," "Using thoughtful language and not relying on gender assumptions is as an invitation to be more fully aligned with our identities. Gender stereotypes have kept us all in contracted states, whether we identify with the sex we were assigned at birth or not."[3]

Finally, think about the words you tend to use when you teach and consider how alternatives may change the feeling of what want to say. For instance, how does the word *posture* feel instead of *pose*? What about *shape*? It's okay if you don't know. You may want to ask around. Words resonate differently with different people.

STEADY BREATH COUNTS

Always let your students know how long you will be asking them to stay in a pose. You can suggest three, four, or five breaths, depending on the class and their ability to be in stillness. However, it is not enough to let them know the number of breaths. They must get to know and trust your breath count. This starts with the way you lead poses and count breaths on day one and develops as your students experience your consistency.

Many people who attend mainstream yoga classes have had the experience of being left in a pose for an unusual or imbalanced amount of time. Many mainstream yoga teachers pause the breath count to launch into long explanations about what various parts of the body should be doing in the posture. To make up for the deviation, the teacher rushes through the last three breaths to catch up. Another common occurrence is the teacher giving all the pose explanations during the first side, leaving nothing to say while students are in the second side, making that side's breath count much shorter. Some teachers don't count breaths at all. Many inconsistencies exist, all very dysregulating for someone who has been through trauma and relies on predictability and consistency to feel safe.

Folks who have survived trauma step into great vulnerability by endeavoring to practice yoga. Opening and reconnecting to their body can feel extremely triggering. Uncomfortable sensations can arise as the nervous system is tested. In those moments, the student needs to make the right decision for themself about whether they should stay in the posture. This is the exact awareness and agency that we are pointing them toward through the whole yoga process. In many ways, it is the point of the practice. The poses help the student recognize, respect, and perhaps one day widen their window of tolerance. How can they choose what is best for their body (and nervous system) if we don't give them the predictability of evenly spaced breath counts? This is the most crucial technical role of a trauma-informed yoga teacher and something that can be developed easily with just a little practice.

Exercise: Record Yourself Teaching

Teach a pose out loud to yourself or an imaginary student, instructing both the left and right sides. You can also do this exercise with a friend or family member as your student. Record it, if possible, using your regular cues for focus and alignment. Now play it back and, using a timer, see how long you spent on each side and between counts. Was the space between counting the first and second breath the same as between breaths four and five? Was the time you spent on the left side the same as on the right? You must be a metronome. Only then can the student know for sure if they are capable or up for stretching that window of tolerance for one more breath.

One trick I use to stay consistent with my counting is to have a little beat going in my head, like, "TA, ta-TA, TA, ta-TA, TA'tata tata taa taa taa." Use the same beat between each count to keep yourself accountable (pun intended). Another trick I use is to break up instructions into little bites that fit nicely and evenly between counts. For instance, I'll say, "One. Notice your breathing. Two. Check in with your gaze. Three. You can come out at any time," and so on, keeping all instructions to a similar length.

Try this exercise again using these tips and see if you notice any difference.

AVOID ALL PHYSICAL ADJUSTMENTS

Though touch can be extraordinarily healing, I do not recommend it in a trauma-informed yoga class. Touch has the potential to do more harm than good in this setting. It can be triggering to your students, and there are debates in the yoga world about whether touch from a teacher can ever be wholly consensual. Physical adjustments also risk pushing the body too far and injuring students. Finally, physical adjustments could suggest to the student that something is wrong with them, having not been able to do the pose completely or "correctly" on their own. For all these reasons, they are best avoided in this context.

Adjustments are just as effective via verbal cues. As mentioned earlier, when describing poses, always use inviting language and offer the option to come out of the pose at any time. Do not correct a student's form, except in an instance in which you suspect a student could injure themselves. The greatest protection from injury comes from the student themself. If the student feels welcome to come out of a posture at any time they feel the possibility of harm, then they will protect themself from getting hurt.

When observing a questionable expression of a posture, you may gently suggest, "It may feel more comfortable to . . ." or "You might want to try . . ." but resist the urge to fix your students or give too many alignment cues. Remember, the goal of yoga is not to attain ideal alignment but to show the student how to trust themselves and their body's signals.

If you encourage agency, they will self-correct. If you encourage "correctness," they will look to copy you and, ironically, may do so incorrectly, potentially causing harm. (For this reason, it is equally important to avoid individual praise. This may encourage the student to try to do postures in a way they think will please or impress you instead of in a way that feels right for their body. This can lead to injury.) Bring the essence of acceptance to every student and every class.

Address the Needs of Each Individual

Perhaps the biggest challenge to teaching group trauma sensitive classes is teaching folks with differing needs and abilities at the same time. This is one of the reasons we always try to place two teachers at each of our locations.

The best way to work with people with varying physical abilities and practice desires is to talk through all asana or movement options first. Explain what you are going to do and then demonstrate the simplest expression of the posture. Invite everyone to try this first option. Then you can explain and demonstrate a slightly more challenging expression and offer the group the option of continuing with the first version or trying the new one.

If some in the group seem ready or eager, you can offer a third variation and then everyone can choose one of the three, visualizing the posture, or nothing at all. More than three choices can cause confusion and feel overwhelming, which is proven to detract from decision-making. If you have further variations you'd like to share, you can do so while the students are in the pose. This works well for small changes such as lowering the gaze or stretching the fingers wide. I highly encourage offering subtle pose variations: the options are infinite and they can have big impacts on students.

Another approach to differing needs and desires in the classroom is to begin with the whole class in chairs. Offer a short seated sequence that can easily translate to standing. When the first round of the sequence is complete, give the option to remain in the chair and repeat the sequence. Others may try the same poses standing. Then, when the second sequence is complete, give all students the option to do a seated sequence in the chair or on a mat on the ground.

Avoid Triggering Postures

"What poses do I avoid?" is the most pressing question I get from all my yoga teacher trainees. Because the response to trauma varies so much, it is misleading to declare that any one pose is or isn't triggering. But there are general rules to consider. As the body generally wants to protect itself after trauma, I suggest using caution around heart-opening postures such as Cow, Ostrich, and Wheel. These postures may release trauma stored in the chest area, perhaps too quickly. Introduce these slowly and with care. Extremely constrictive poses in which the chest presses on the ground, such as Reclined Turtle (Supta Kurmasana), can also be contraindicated. When sexual trauma is present, avoid poses that draw attention to or expose sexual parts of the body, such as Happy Baby (Ananda Balasana). Child's Pose (Balasana) and Downward Dog (Adho Mukha Svanasana), poses I typically get asked about, can be incorporated depending on the group. They expose the back body, which could be problematic but isn't usually as triggering as exposing our front. Consider avoiding poses in which someone might fold toward the backside of another person practicing in front of them, such as Wide-Legged Standing Forward Fold or Child's Pose, if staggering personal practice spaces within the classroom is not possible.

If you are unsure about including a posture, leave it out.

Managing Silence and Meditation

Do not go silent for long periods, especially during final rest. Going suddenly silent is similar to turning out the lights. Silence is a kind of darkness. Though it may seem comforting or relaxing to you, it can be the opposite for a trauma survivor. Always let students know in advance if you plan to remain silent for a period and for how long. I suggest keeping it to under sixty seconds. Too much quiet will trigger vigilance, the opposite of relaxation. In contrast, hearing a calm voice can be an anchor, grounding the student in safety and giving them the freedom to rest. For this reason and others, never leave the room during Savasana. Instead, stay and talk through a body scan, stress-and-release, or presencing practice (see page 33). Avoid the temptation to lead visualization or gratitude meditations. Though they seem positive and helpful, these types of exercises can have harmful effects. You may find the beach a calming visual, but it could be the setting of a bad memory for a student. And while gratitude journals and meditations work for some, for others they bring to the surface how little they have or what is missing. Both of these practices move your students away from the present moment, which is where we most want to anchor in our practice.

All the instructions above are ways of reducing exterior threats and thus creating an experience of safety for your students. These practices are critical, but they cannot accommodate and provide safety outside the class, where your students live. While no one can ever promise that an external space or environment will be safe to everyone at all times, you can encourage your students to develop an internal sense of well-being through the yoga practice, which will support them in feeling safe from the inside out.

SPECIAL CONSIDERATIONS FOR TEACHING ONLINE

If you are teaching classes online, you must consider some additional elements when shaping and staging your teaching space.

As a teacher, you'll want to be clearly seen in the frame of the camera. Be very mindful about what is seen behind you: avoid having pictures, personal items, alcohol or other mind-altering substances, and anything else that could be distracting in your camera's view. Natural elements such as plants, candles, or a view to the outdoors are enjoyable and recommended for enlivening a virtual environment. If you can, have a plant near your teaching space, within the camera's view. Photos of plants and the color green have been proven to bring down our sympathetic responses and increase relaxation.

Think of ways you can contribute to calming your students, who have the extra barrier of the screen to get through. Make sure the room you are in is as devoid of as much outside noise as possible. Let other members of your household know you are teaching and encourage them to have quiet time in a room away from your streaming room.

When teaching online, I recommend setting up two mats in an X or T position to make it easy to demonstrate poses from different directions and angles. Teach all chair, standing, and mat poses grouped together so students do not need to adjust their cameras more than once when moving up and down. Have your chair and any other props you are using immediately accessible so you don't have to disrupt class or leave the frame to retrieve them.

Be considerate in what you choose to wear when teaching online classes. Wear functional, clean, neutral clothing and pull your hair back so people can see your face and read your expressions. This is also true of in-person classes, but I sometimes think it needs extra noting at home where we can sometimes get overly casual.

Extra Equipment for Virtual Teaching

I suggest all teachers invest in three home studio items, all of which can be purchased inexpensively.

- A wide-angle lens slipped over your computer's camera immediately widens the view of the room, allowing you to show your whole body in a yoga posture even in a small space.
- A ring light will make sure you are flooded in light. This or other lighting facing toward you will improve your visibility. Avoid backlight, any light that may be coming from behind, including from windows and doors.
- A wireless Bluetooth earbud/microphone combination will make your voice steady and clear for your students.

Remember that your students may not have special equipment themselves, so the more professional you can make the experience for them, the better. Also keep in mind that not all folks eager to participate in yoga have yoga-specific clothing. Consider what your students are wearing when you choose poses that will be viewed on-screen.

You may find when teaching online classes that some students choose to turn off their video. Though, no doubt, video makes it easier for the teacher, many practitioners find practicing from (or being seen at) home a sensitive experience. The option to remain anonymous may be what gets your student into the online class. Say hello and let them know they are welcome to participate however they are most comfortable. Encourage them to ask questions if they need help as you will not be able to assess that visually.

Online classes can both increase and limit accessibility. A smartphone, computer, or laptop is needed by both teacher and student, as well as a strong Wi-Fi connection and sometimes an online class registration and Zoom or other streaming subscription. Some of our partnerships at Three and a Half Acres Yoga have had to pause classes because of the limitations, while others have found ways to make it work (sharing subscriptions, offering recorded content, or streaming via Facebook instead of Zoom, for example). As with so many aspects of trauma sensitive yoga, there is no one right way to offer online classes. It is a work in progress and a partnership. Listen to the needs of your students and allow for solutions to emerge.

REGULATING INTERNAL SAFETY

The last piece of the puzzle, once you've accounted for as much external safety as possible, is making sure that the entirety of your trauma-informed yoga class is designed to promote and help strengthen an internal feeling of safety in the student's body. It is your job to guide your students with slowness and care toward movements or positions that may challenge that feeling of safety and help them discover methods for finding it again.

The interplay of moving into and recovering from stress builds the body's resilience and stress capacity, which is why yoga is so supportive of trauma recovery. It provides the practitioner with an understanding of what they can handle, how much sensation, and in what context. This allows subtler understanding around sensations of stress, allowing the individual to figure out for themselves what kinds of stress they can and want to work with and what kinds to avoid. All of this leaves the practitioner with more choice and debunks the unhelpful notion of the stressed/not stressed binary.

Here's how it works. Throughout each practice, you invite students to put their body in a shape (a yoga pose) and give a variety of options for that particular shape in no particular order and with no hierarchy. Then you encourage them to choose which form (or no form) to take. While in the pose, you invite them to notice any sensations they are experiencing in their body and perhaps how those sensations are affecting their thoughts. Then they have the choice of staying in the position for the remainder of your very clear and predictable breath count or coming out of the posture if the sensations take them too far from a feeling of safety.

Should they choose to stay in the posture, they are encouraged to bring their attention to the present moment using the three-pointed focus of breath, gaze, and feeling of their body. Using this focused attention, they may watch and see if the sensations they are experiencing increase, decrease, leave, remain the same, or morph in any way. It is not uncommon for uncomfortable sensations to disperse when they are met with intentional breathing, though this is not always the case. Whatever happens, learning to stay with uncomfortable feelings even for a short while can be empowering for trauma survivors. They learn they have the strength to stay present through tough emotions and sensations. They grow to differentiate between false alarms in the body and real danger. And they learn to use the breath and all parts of the three-pointed

Core Concepts

- The experience of safety is physical, emotional, and psychological, and all facets must be addressed in teaching.
- It is impossible to experience agency without safety.
- Predictability, expectations, boundaries, consistency, options, freedom, contribution, opt-out, acceptance, and understanding are ten factors that can lead to an experience of safety.
- These factors can be built into all elements of the teaching practice, from room setup to instruction style, to create a safe-as-possible environment.
- Certain exercises and postures should be avoided in trauma sensitive yoga classes, such as breath retention, Happy Baby and other genital exposing postures, and guided meditations. Aside from these restrictions, the teacher must make subtler omissions based on the specific needs of their students.
- Once the outer components of safety are established, students can invite in moments of challenge and reregulation, which are necessary for long-term healing.

awareness to calm the body and increase a sense of inner safety when no real danger is present.

What *doesn't* help create safety and can derail progress is pushing students to stay present with sensations that are too intense for too long. To avoid backsliding in healing, your students must feel empowered to disengage at any time.

All responses to trauma are normal and are a necessary way to get needs met and protect the self. It's important not to judge or feel critical of what's going on while you aim to meet the needs of your students. As a new teacher, you will make mistakes, and that's okay. When you do, acknowledge them and work sincerely to repair damage. Admitting to mistakes and gaps in knowledge models to students that you are not seeking perfection in yourself or in others.

5

Trauma-Informed Yoga Sequences

THIS CHAPTER CONTAINS FOUR COMPLETE YOGA SEQUENCES for trauma sensitive yoga classes. In many ways, these sequences are similar. They are derived mainly from the Ashtanga yoga primary series with influences from Kundalini and other traditions and follow the structure and arc laid out in the previous chapter. The sequences represented are not typically done in their entirety on the first day, month, or even year of practice. They represent an expression of where a class might go after many sessions together.

Doing less is often more powerful, especially when digging into the subtleties of each position. When teaching, I often choose a few poses from the sequence and repeat them with alternative focuses. I do not offer everything at once.

In each section, I note where poses may be dropped to shorten the sequence, whether for time constraints or greater accessibility. The sequences are flexible and open to modifications, so you may take liberties with them. Ultimately you will bring your own voice and adaptations to your particular community and to your teachings.

The main thing to consider as you adapt the sequences to make them your own is retaining the arc of the sequence, including all the elements introduced in chapter 2 that make yoga so healing for trauma. As a reminder, these are:

- Grounding
- Presencing via the Tristana (three-pointed focus of breath, body, and gaze)

A Note on Props

You will find limited instructions around the use of props in this book. This is because for many of the Three and a Half Acres partnerships, there is rarely space for storing props. We rely on our bodies, chairs, and sometimes the wall for support. This does not mean you cannot use props freely, adding them to make any posture more accessible or comfortable. If you don't have yoga props, household items such as books and towels can often substitute. For more detailed instructions on incorporating props into your yoga teaching, I suggest Jivana Heyman's book *Accessible Yoga*.

Chairs, however, are invaluable in many settings and can be a dramatic way to make yoga more accessible to students. Folding chairs can be stored on hooks or stowed away in a closet to save space.

- Awakening awareness by matching movement to breath
- Bringing in balance to work with the body to find calm in times of imbalance
- Adding challenging poses that are fun and build confidence
- Slowing the body as you near the end of class, giving a chance for reflection and body scan before rest

Remember that *how* you teach, not *what* you teach, is most important. Throughout, make sure you remain steady with metronome counting, using invitational language, giving options (including chances to opt out), demonstrating by mirroring each pose, and using all the other tools and recommendations for creating safety for practitioners in your classes.

AN INVITATION TO BEGIN

In all sequences and classes, start by checking in with your students and giving them a chance to express any present needs. When they are ready, encourage your students to find a comfortable and still seated position. Remember that they may not be aware of all the options available to them, such as sitting back in the chair or placing blocks under their feet. You empower them by giving them choices. Dive into that by exploring, for example, the many ways one could sit in a chair. Have your students sit at the front edge of the seat and then farther back. Give them a chance to feel their back against the chair and then sitting upright without that support. Encourage them to note any changes in sensation and then ask your students to choose the position that feels best for them.

Standing Strong

If you are working with a class that is standing, explore instead the differences in sensations when position and weight-bearing changes. How do folks feel when their feet are together instead of hip-width apart? Play with where the weight is in the feet by inviting folks to lean forward and back, then side to side. Ask your students to lift their toes up and spread them down into the floor. Invite them to stand on their heels. Shift weight between the inner and outer parts of the feet. Then ask students to choose their position and move into stillness.

Settling In

Introduce grounding by suggesting students allow their weight to drop into the support below them. Using invitational language, move awareness to the parts of the body engaging with the chair or floor and ask students to explore what it would feel like to give in to the support of those surfaces with more intention. Invite them to feel for unnecessary muscle engagement holding them up and to release that extra tension, allowing the floor and chair to support them fully.

Staying Present

Next, move into presencing. Walk through the importance of keeping a drishti, or soft gaze. Practitioners can look softly down at the tip of their nose or at an unmoving spot on the ground a few feet ahead of them. Remind them that they may be tempted to shift their eyes while in a posture. Explain that this is a form of disengaging and that it is available to them if they choose. However, they may want to see what changes when they go against instinct and keep their eyes still.

Scanning the Body

Next, guide your students to turn their attention to different parts of their body, from their feet touching the ground all the way up to the top of their head. Make sure to include the back and sides of the body, and always skip over sensitive areas of the body that might be triggering. The scan helps quiet the body and bring students into the present moment. It also helps awaken bodily sensation. In addition to inviting the mind into different parts of the body, saying the name of the body part also encourages students to feel into the three-dimensionality of the body and how much weight and space they take up in the room. Becoming comfortable with taking up space can be very empowering. While in a neutral seated or standing position, we encourage them to notice any thoughts, feelings, or sensations that arise as they keep the eyes steady.

Finally, you can introduce awareness of breathing. Start by bringing attention to the breath. Then, as an option, invite students to explore breathing in and out through their nose only, if it is available to them. Mouth breathers may find the shift to nostril breathing dramatic and may decide to keep working as is before trying a new step. When nostril breathing feels comfortable and steady, invite in more attention and energy to the breathing to create a soft, audible sound. Sometimes new students find this difficult at first. In those cases, encourage them to let go of the prompt and focus on the natural breath. Remember the *awareness* of each breath is most important. When the mind wanders, as minds do, we discover our ability to redirect it by guiding it to listen to the breath.

From Stillness into Movement

From here, you can add small movements that encourage your students to match the initiation of the movement with the start of the inhale and complete the movement before the pause to exhale. Then the start of the exhale begins the next movement, usually a downward position or a return to the starting position.

For example, you may prompt your students to lift their arms up overhead with an inhale and return their arms down to their sides with an exhale. After a few rounds of this movement cycle, you may modify it by suggesting that on the next exhale, the arms come down and the body twists, alternating between right and left sides.

The Rhythm of a Sequence

Most often the sequences in this chapter follow a pattern. After pairing breath with movement, we transition into Seated Sun Salutation and fundamental poses. Then come balances and perhaps chair and Warrior poses. The initial sequence is then repeated, this time with the option to do the sequence standing. Otherwise, students can repeat the poses from a seated position, noticing how each posture feels a second time.

After each posture, bring your students to a neutral position, such as seated with hands on the thighs and feet flat on the floor or standing with feet hip-distance apart and arms at the sides. Invite them to check in with how they are feeling. Encourage them to take this moment to note and imprint any pleasant feelings or changes. Sometimes folks need practice remembering and getting comfortable with feeling good. Remembering how to access and become comfortable with positive sensations is as important to growth and well-being as being able to stay with challenging ones.

If there is time after the sequence is repeated, move into seated poses, which your students can do in a chair or on the ground. These can include forward folds, hip openers, twists, and a peak or challenge pose, such as Boat Pose (Navasana). Next, if the class is ready for it, offer backbends before moving into inversions and closing postures.

You can end your class by inviting your students to find a comfortable seated or reclined position, then offer a second body scan. During this scan you again invite your students to bring attention into their feet, ankles, calves, knees, and up their body to the crown of their head. Again, omit cues to potentially sensitive parts. Invite your students to notice if any tension lingers in any part of their body and see if they can use their mind to let it go. An alternative to a body scan is to use a squeeze-and-release exercise: invite students to tense and release muscles in individual parts of their body, one by one, beginning at the toes and traveling up to the crown of their head. Finally, they tense and release the muscles of the entire body. Cue your students into stillness after the body scan or squeeze-and-release exercise. Then ask your students to sense the feeling of their whole body in the present moment and notice any changes that may have occurred since the beginning of class.

Closing Rest

To conclude class, invite your students to rest in stillness. Remember to always give the option to keep the eyes open in rest and not to leave more than a minute of silence after the body scan is complete. Long periods of

Common Variations for Any Posture

In a trauma sensitive yoga class, you may want to be prepared with gentle variations to incorporate into every pose you offer. These are always available to students, and they should be cued aloud regularly throughout class. Both you and your students will enjoy discovering ways to adapt familiar poses to a more sensitive sequence:

· Turning the head to gaze downward instead of looking up
· Taking the hand to the waist instead of extending the arm straight
· Keeping the hands shoulder-width apart instead of pressing palms together
· Sitting or lying down instead of standing
· Sitting on a chair instead of a mat
· Crossing the legs at the ankles or sitting on the heels instead of taking an ankle to a knee or into Lotus
· Holding on to a wall or chair instead of balancing hands-free
· Practicing Child's Pose instead of Downward Dog
· Taking opposite elbows or holding clothing behind the back instead of Reverse Prayer Hands or binding
· Keeping legs bent instead of straight
· Laying on, sitting on, leaning on a block or blanket

silence can be dysregulating for trauma survivors who may become hypervigilant when nothing is going on. When thirty to sixty seconds have passed, guide your students' awareness back into the room, thank them for being there, and open up the room for students to share observations and feedback or ask questions.

SHOULDERS AND HIPS SEQUENCE: A DYNAMIC FLOW WITH TIM

Often when teachers offer sequencing in a chair, they assume the prop alone makes it accessible. The Shoulders and Hips Sequence brings in additional support through use of blocks and modifications. There is great care in this sequence to establish a feeling of grounding, which is so fundamental to a healthy, sensitive practice. Additionally, this dynamic sequence illustrates how creative yoga can be with a simple block-and-chair setup and the way small movements can have big impacts.

In the following sequence, students spend time "waking up" each part of the body before launching into a flow. Pay attention to how Tim starts with simple exercises that tune in to individual parts of the body and gradually grow into bigger movements and more flow. The subtle and slow beginning sets the foundation for all that comes afterward and is not a reflection of physical limitation.

Tim's hips and shoulders are sensitive and tight. Working on these areas from different positions and angles and at various moments throughout the sequence can reduce frustration and opens the possibility for a breakthrough realization about how these joints can be accessed without force. This opening work is interlaced with powerful strength work, which has many benefits, such as joint stability and confidence building.

NOTE: The seated portion of Tim's sequence is highly accessible and would work well with most populations, especially elderly communities who could stop at or after Boat Pose or Warrior and either repeat or move into seated closing postures on the floor or chair.

Seated Equal Standing Pose (Samasthiti)

Ask students to start in a stable, supported seated position in their chair, with their feet on the ground or on blocks. Introduce the three-pointed focus (see page 33). Ask students to turn their palms faceup and notice how that feels. Then invite them to turn their palms down and take in that feeling as well. Allow them to flip their hands back and forth a few times, noting as much as they can about the sensations they are receiving, however unexpected. You may introduce questions to help build awareness: "Do you feel any changes in your chest when your palms are turned upward? How about in your feet?" Invite students to make a mental note of all they can sense, without judgment or at least with lightheartedness. Encourage them to choose the hand position that works best for them at

Sthira Sukham—Strong and at Ease

Muscle contraction and relaxation work well together. Contracting a muscle often teaches it how to relax even more deeply after the muscle is released. Similarly, building personal power can be as therapeutic as being with vulnerability. We don't have to avoid strength and physical challenge just because a sequence is trauma informed. Ultimately we are working to establish a balance between opening up and holding to our core values and boundaries. When building a sequence, it is just as important to give students a chance to lean into their strengths as it is to work on areas of growth. You will undoubtedly have some students in your class who excel at postures that require strength and others who are more flexible. Mixing both types of postures into your class gives everyone a chance to use their skills and focus on growth.

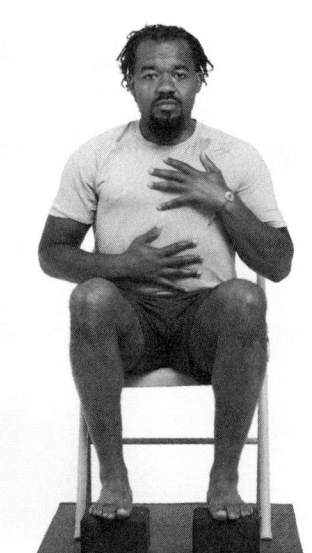

that moment and to stay there, focusing on their breath. Remind them that if it feels hard to remain still, they can notice that and reflect on the options available to them, such as staying with the uncomfortable feeling arising, remaining still but shifting their focus to something that feels neutral or pleasant in their body or surroundings, pendulating between awareness of uncomfortable sensations and more pleasant ones, or shifting their position altogether.

Students can remain with their hands on their knees or bring in more self-touch by moving one hand to their heart and the other to their belly. If they move their hands, ask them to breathe consciously into both hands and tune in to the temperature of the skin where their hands and body meet. Invite them to pay special attention to changes in their breath and heartbeat, which can be felt more fully with the hands in this

Seated Equal Standing Pose (Samasthiti)

position. Stay with this position for five to ten breaths. Ask students to switch hand positions, so the hand on their heart is now on their belly, and vice versa.

Neck Stretches

After the initial grounding and presencing work, it's time to add in simple movements, which address tensions held in the body. The head and neck can carry a lot of stress and tension, negatively affecting the rest of the body. Try these stretches with your students or substitute neck rolls or head and neck self-massage, or invite students to stretch the muscles of their face instead. The important thing is to start digging into isolated areas of strain.

Let students know that when using their hand to stretch the opposite side of their neck, they should not pull the head down. Instead, let gravity do the work and the hand be a gentle guide. Ask them to tune in to what is happening to any tension releasing from the neck. As tension releases, it often travels elsewhere, such as into the jaw, brow, or even the glutes. Invite students to tune in to the new location and redirect the energy again, this time down their body, out through their feet, and into the floor.

> Positions that involve compassionate self-touch often result in emotional release. As a teacher, it is important to consider the needs and bandwidth of your group before introducing self-touch in your sequence.

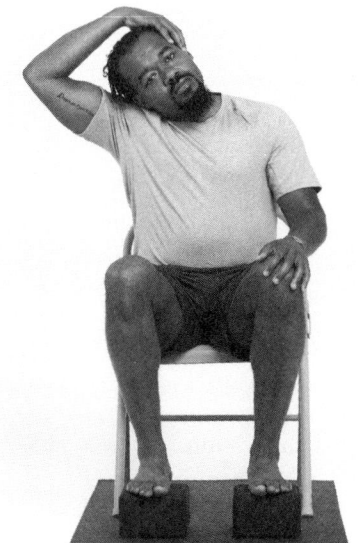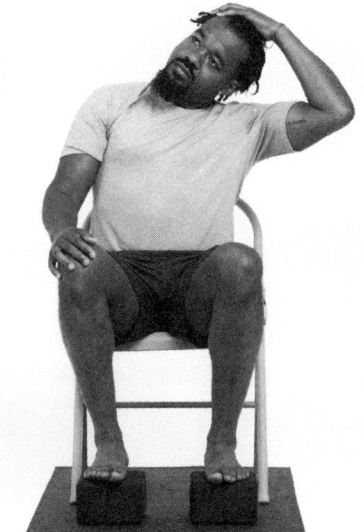

Neck stretches

Arms and Shoulders

Invite students to extend their arms in front of them, staying there for five breaths, gazing at their nose tip. They can hold a block between the hands or simply extend their fingers outward, stretching away from their body. Bring attention to the dichotomy between the strong, active positioning of the arms and any relaxation in the body. Ask students to play with the amount of energy they need to keep the shape active but not tense. Suggest they consider which is easier for them, muscle activation or muscle release.

Invite students to now reach their arms overhead. Again, they can hold a block between their hands or extend their fingers. Ask them to keep their gaze down toward the tip of their nose and their face soft and inactive. Suggest that they take slower and deeper breaths as they feel the intensity rise. Have them experiment with extending their shoulders up

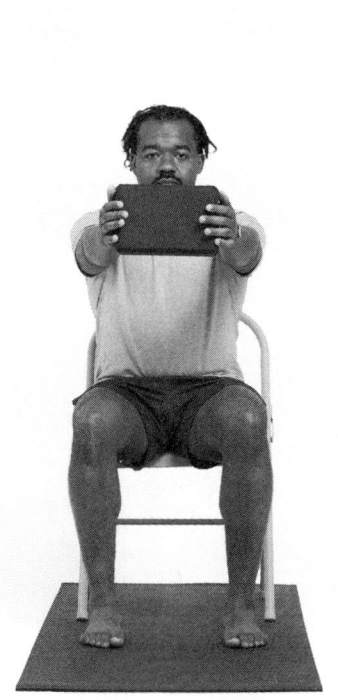
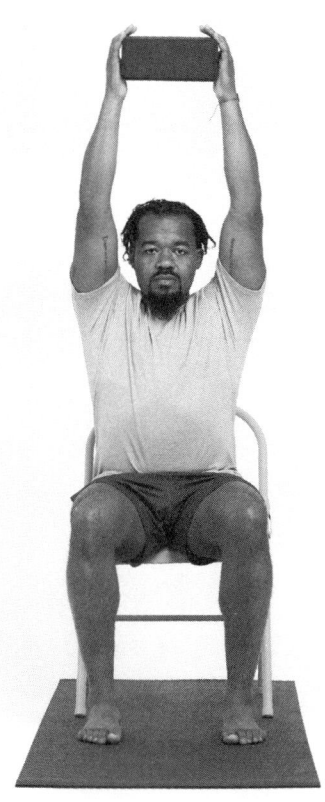
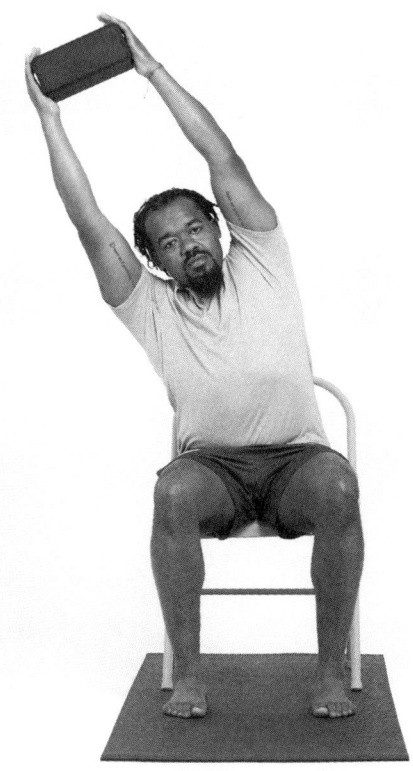

Engaging arms and shoulders

Grounding side stretch with block

toward their ears and releasing them down. Invite students to settle their shoulders in the down position and feel into the opposition created by their shoulders integrating down their back as their arms, elbows, and fingers stretch upward.

Suggest students ground down even more into their seat as they work with those opposing forces to stretch the side of their body. The more they can anchor down, the more they will feel the stretch as they reach their arms up and lean to the side, remaining grounded. Stay here for five breaths. Be sure they don't crunch the side of the body as they lean. When ready, reach upward again and lean to the other side, holding for another five breaths.

Seated Twist

Students who have a block can bring it to their right thigh and place their left elbow on top of it, turning into a twist. Students can bring their right hand to meet their left, pressing their palms firmly together to deepen the twist. Encourage students to point their top elbow toward the ceiling as they pull their prayer palms close to their chest. Bring their attention to their seat and invite them to ground again into the chair, keeping awareness around their lower body even as they twist. Count five full breaths in this position before switching sides.

If blocks are not available, you can create a gentle twisting position by asking students to hold the right side of the seat of their chair with their left hand and bring their right hand behind the back to the top of their chair. Offer the same instructions regarding body awareness and cue the twist on both sides.

Seated Cat and Cow (Bitilasana Marjaryasana)

With their neck and shoulders now open, students are prepared for Cat and Cow, the first series of postures that involve a flow. The undulation of Cat and Cow offers students a chance to feel into parts of their spine they might otherwise overlook.

Ask students to return to a neutral seated posture, this time with their hands gently holding the sides of the chair.

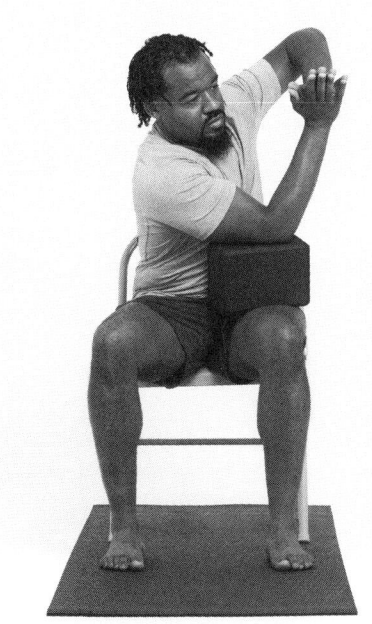

Seated twist with block

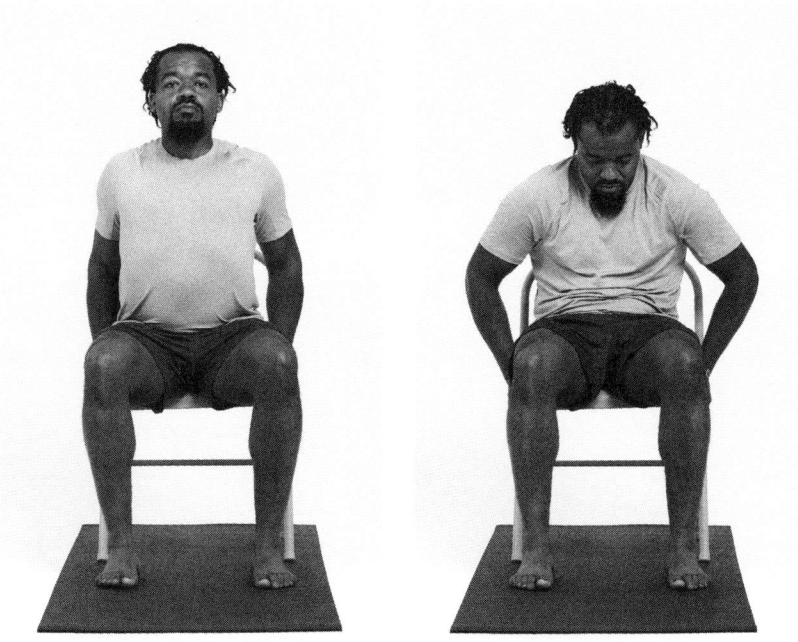

Seated Cat and Cow (Bitilasana Marjaryasana)

Moving with the inhale, invite them to arch their lower back and press their whole spine to the front of their body, lifting their sternum and puffing their chest. As they exhale, cue them to tuck their lower spine and curl until the top of their spine presses back, hunching the shoulders. Draw attention to all the regions of the back and spine, cultivating small, articulate movements. Suggest that it might help to visualize each vertebra, especially in the middle back. Cue them through two or three rounds and then invite them to continue, without cues, moving with their own breath cycles for five to ten more rounds.

Seated Balance

This portion of the sequence works the legs, bringing strength and awareness into the lower body. Low and controlled bent-leg lifts not only activate the thighs but engage the whole body as it calibrates balance. Encourage students to focus not only on their legs but also the parts of their body grounding into the chair, their core stabilizers, and their chest as it lifts and expands. Their gaze can be down to the tip of their nose if that is comfortable. Make sure to instruct both sides for five breaths each.

Many people don't realize how much you can play with balance from a seated position. Though students may not feel the dramatic impact of falling to one side, their bodies will adjust internally to keep them centered, activating the stabilizer muscles, as they take one foot off the ground. The more forward they are in their seat, the more their body will need to do to find that centering.

Invite students to repeat this lift on each side, this time extending their leg. In addition to trying to balance, their body now has the task of keeping their whole leg raised. How does that intensify the posture? Encourage them to lift their leg one inch higher and see what happens. Ask them to notice what the internal voices are saying, if anything. Bring them to awareness of their gaze by inquiring if their eyes have shifted. Remind students to keep softly resting their eyes on their nose or on their big toe if they prefer. Remind them to breathe.

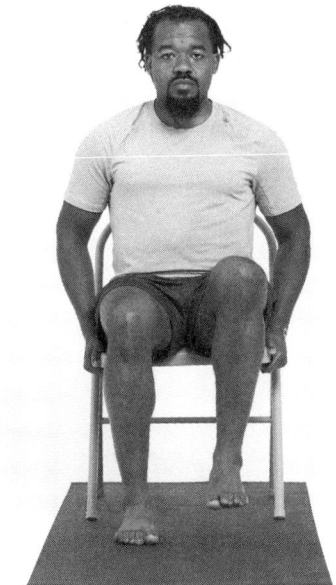

Seated balance

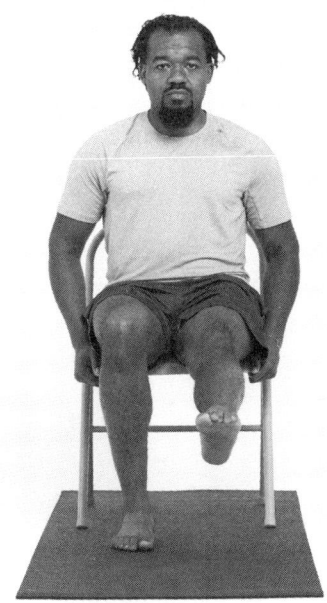

Seated balance with extended
leg variation

Seated Sun Salutation (Surya Namaskar)

Now the postures become more dynamic, pairing movement more closely to breath. The intention is for the student to become more articulate with the body and more knowledgeable about how the body and the mind are working together. Seated Sun Salutation is a wonderful, effective way to invite this intention.

Ask students to inhale and reach their arms up overhead. Their palms can be pressed together or shoulder-width apart. Their gaze can be upward or at their nose tip. As they exhale, invite them to fold forward and feel into the full body release. Remind students that their hands can reach toward the ground but they don't have to touch.

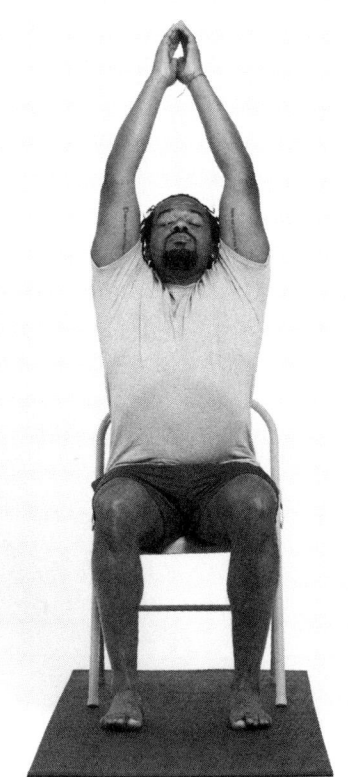
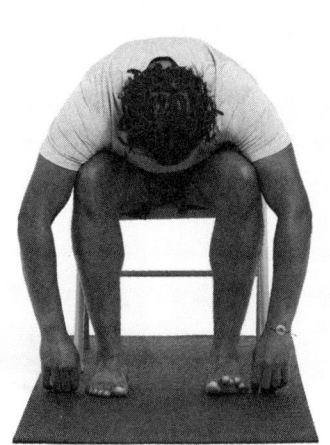
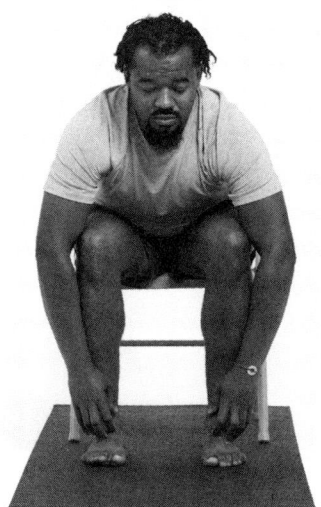

Seated Sun Salutation (Surya Namaskar)

On their next inhale, ask students to lengthen their spine and lift up their head. They can press their fingertips into the floor or against their shins as their chest rises. With the next exhale, instruct students to let their body fold forward more deeply, resting the weight of their torso on their legs.

Ask students, with the inhale, to lift up their torso and arms, extending their arms overhead, hands shoulder-width apart or palms pressed together. Invite students, with the exhale, to return to a neutral seated position. Suggest that they repeat the Seated Sun Salutation three to five times on their own, matching the pace of their movements with their breath.

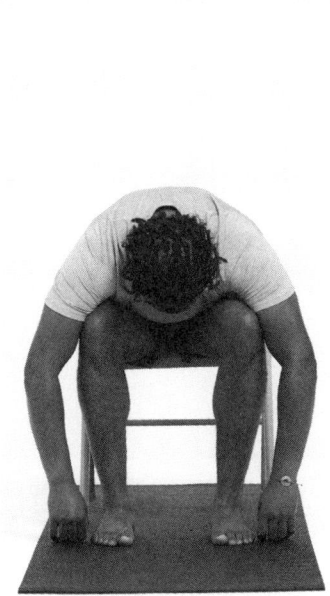
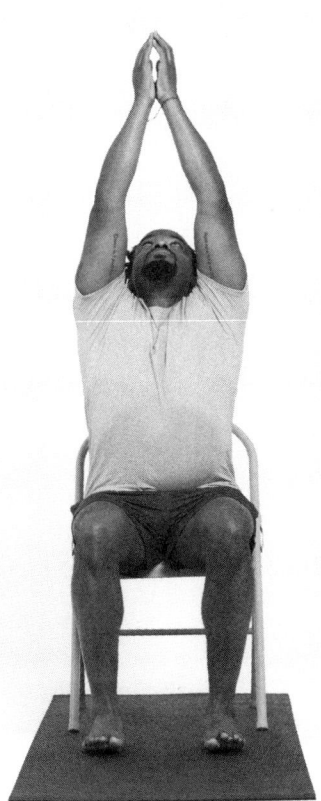
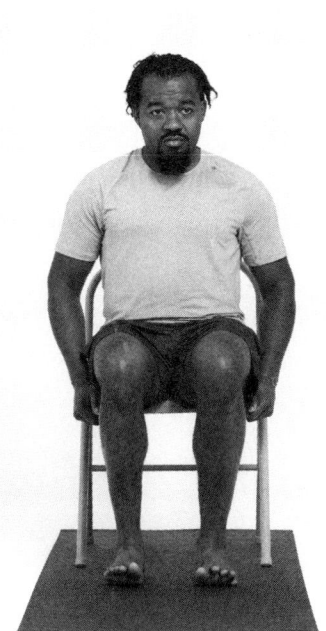

Seated Warrior 1 (Virabhadrasana 1)

Now that the body is warm, it's a great time to bring in a strong seated posture. Invite students to shift to the side of their chair for Seated Warrior 1. If working with a chair with arms, the student must sit at the front and center of the chair and reach one foot back under the chair as far as they can, or use the standing version of the pose, found later in this sequence. (Some chairs with shorter arms allow the possibility for sitting sideways and using the front of the chair such as in the Spacious and Opening Sequence: Expansive Flow with Nikki on page 130.)

Bring students to a seated position on the side of their chair, facing forward with their outer leg extended behind them. Their knee should be bent, and their toes should curl down into the ground while their heel points up. They can hold the sides of the chair for support or bring their palms together at their chest. Cue them to use internal core strength to actively lift their body so they almost feel like they are hovering. Invite students to take five breaths here, or if they would like to, with their arms up in the air. Their gaze can stay at the tip of their nose or turn up toward the ceiling. Repeat the posture on the other side.

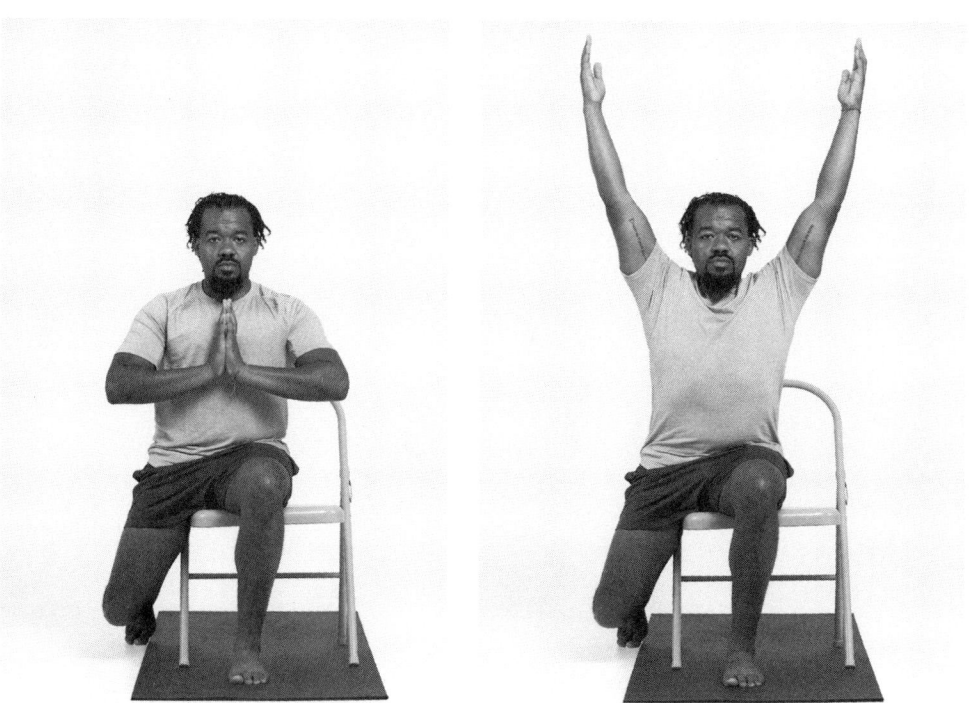

Seated Warrior 1 (Virabhadrasana 1)

NOTE: The intensity of Seated Warrior 1 is based on the student's positioning in the seat. If they move toward the edge of the chair, the pose becomes more challenging. Guide them toward experimentation and choosing what is right for their body. A block can be placed under the back knee to reduce intensity and add more support.

Seated Half-Bound Lotus Forward Fold (Ardha Baddha Padma Paschimottanasana)

After the leg strengthening work, we move into hip opening, taking special care if your students have any knee issues or injury. Make sure to ask students if they have any knee pain or have had knee surgery before initiating this posture. Invite students with knee issues to cross their legs at their ankles, put a rolled-up sock or towel under their knee, or try flexing their foot in this posture. Invite students to extend one leg in front of them and lift the other, rotating at the hip so their foot rests on their extended leg's shin. Encourage students to flex their lifted foot deeply to protect their knee. Invite students to hold the sides of their chair or rest their hands at their waist. Students may stay here or hinge forward slightly at the waist to intensify the stretch, keeping their back straight. Cue students to fold only until they feel strong sensation. Then they can stop and breathe and bring awareness to the sensation. If the sensation passes or changes, they can bend more deeply, but only so far as they can remain pain-free and with a straight back. Invite them to breathe five times, then return to a neutral seated position. Repeat the posture on the other side.

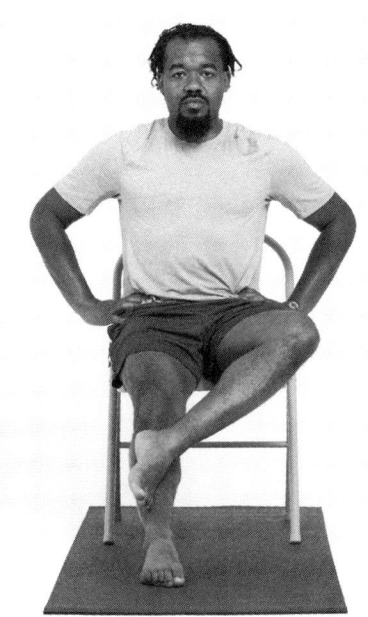

Seated Half-Bound Lotus Forward Fold (Ardha Baddha Padma Paschimottanasana)

It's common for many poses to feel different from one side to the other. Let your students know that this can be expected and to resist the idea that there is a "good" side or "bad" side. Our left and right sides have anatomical differences as well as adaptations to how they've been put to use. Those differences are likely there for a reason. Help them resist the urge to try to fix anything or feel they need to even out anything. Instead, ask them to stay with what is and observe the sensations as they arise.

Seated Ray of Light Pose/Sage Pose (Marichyasana A)

Marichyasana A has been associated with benefits such as improved digestion, reproductive health, hip and shoulder opening, and stress relief. Still, many feel they cannot access this pose because of an inability to sit on the floor or for other reasons. This chair version makes the pose more accessible for many. Feel free to introduce just the leg setup to start.

Cue students to place blocks or books under their right foot so their leg is high and their knee bends deeply. They can stay in this position and breathe. For those who want to continue, ask them to inhale and stretch their right arm forward. With the exhale, they can bend at the elbow and rotate their right shoulder, aiming to wrap the right arm around their bent knee. They can reach their other arm behind their back and try to take the wrapping hand. Remind them not to strain and that binding is not important; they can hold on to their clothing to help them stabilize. Students often hinge forward at the waist naturally in this position, but consider cuing a forward fold if they aren't there already, to get an extra stretch in the lower back. Invite them to sit for five deep breaths, visualizing they are sending breath into their hip socket.

VARIATION: SEATED MARICHYASANA A

If blocks aren't available or your students want another challenge, they can try Seated Ray of Light Pose/Sage Pose (Marichyasana A) with their

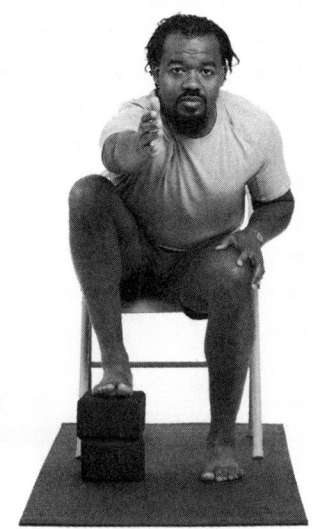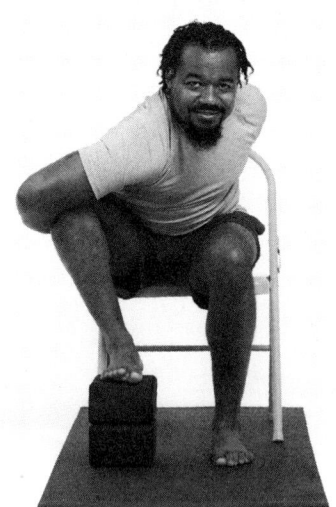

Seated Ray of Light Pose/Sage Pose (Marichyasana A)

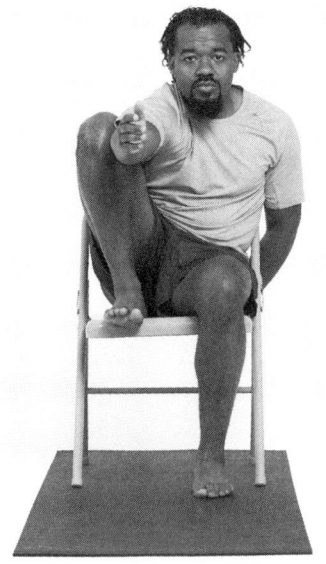 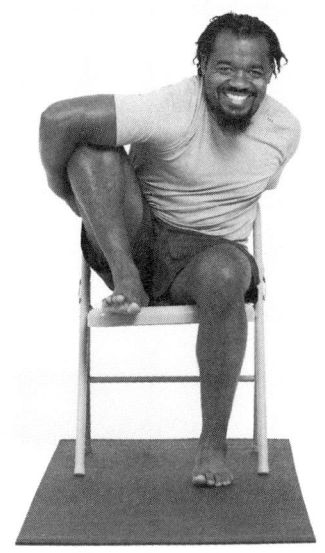

Seated Ray of Light Pose/Sage Pose (Marichyasana A) variation

Many practitioners appreciate the opportunity to look behind them, which may provide a sense of safety and security. Though they may wish to look back at other times during class, the opportunity is not always built into the sequence.

foot on the seat of the chair. Talk through the same steps to help students wrap their arm around their knee. You may want to encourage attention to the shoulder opening in this pose for these next five breath cycles.

Seated Marichyasana C

From Seated Marichyasana A, it's an easy transition to Seated Marichyasana C, which can also be done with the foot on a block or a chair. This posture uses the same leg position but adds a spinal twist. Ask students to bring their left elbow or upper arm to the outside of their right knee, trying to bring their knee in as close to their left armpit as possible without taking the opposite leg out of a right angle. The movement comes from the stretch of the left arm and the spinal twist. Invite folks to soften into the twist, without force, relaxing in the belly area. Students can use the opposite arm for support against the chair. The benefits here are spinal health, improved breath capacity, and eyesight improvement due to the stretch of the eyes as the gaze reaches behind them, plus the benefits from Marichyasana A.

Ask students to stay in this posture for five breaths. After Marichyasana A and C on one side, repeat these postures on the other side.

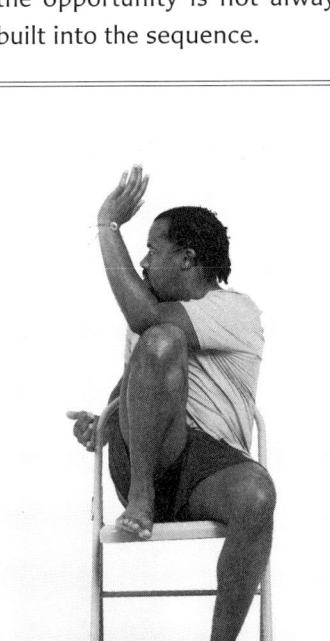

Seated Ray of Light Pose/Sage
Pose (Marichyasana C)

Boat Pose (Navasana) in a Chair

Boat Pose has many variations and just as many benefits, which is why you'll find it in most of Three and a Half Acres' trauma-informed yoga classes. This pose forces the mind to stay present. It draws attention to the abdomen, calling on our power center for strength while engaging and lengthening the spine. This combination leads many to feel more alert, focused, and centered long after taking this posture. For people who feel emotionally remote or tend to disassociate, Boat Pose can be powerful. You can choose all or some of the following four Boat Pose variations to share with your students, settling on three to five rounds. Invite students to choose which options they want to take. Consider repeating this pose multiple times in the sequence. Each variation begins with the student seated forward in a chair.

VARIATION 1: BOAT POSE (NAVASANA) IN THE CHAIR

The first option for tapping into Boat Pose is to lift both feet off the ground together. Invite students to pay close attention to what's going on in their mind, especially as they tap into the core strength needed to lift their feet. Remind them to watch their breath closely and resist the urge to hold it. Instead, challenge them to relax their breathing and thinking as

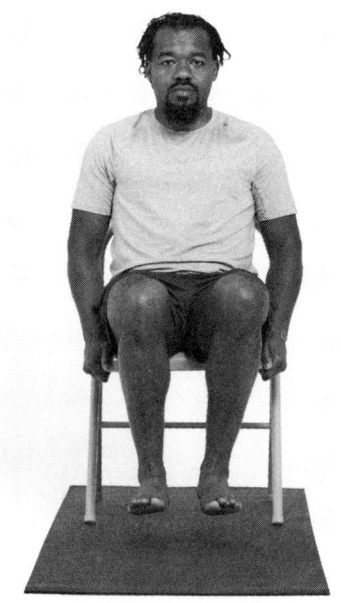 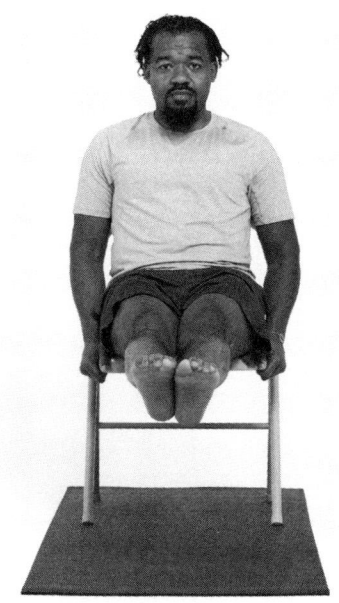

Boat Pose (Navasana) variation 1   Boat Pose (Navasana) variation 2

the pose gets more difficult. Where else can they pull strength from? Cue them to hold the pose for five full breaths.

VARIATION 2: BOAT POSE (NAVASANA)

Ask students to straighten both legs in front of them, continuing to observe how this position is impacting the rest of their body. Ask students to note if they are tightening their jaw or any other parts of their body unnecessary for making this shape. If the answer is yes, invite them to release the clenching and breathe. Count five breaths here, inviting students to lift up their legs again if they begin to drop.

VARIATION 3: BOAT POSE (NAVASANA)

Invite students to lift up their legs higher, with their knees bent. They can hold on to the chair or the back of their thighs for support or extend their arms out in front of them parallel to the floor. They can lean into the back of the chair, which will reduce effort, or lean away from it for a more intense sensation.

VARIATION 4: BOAT POSE (NAVASANA)

The final variation of Boat Pose is to extend the legs straight and at an angle. Students can hold on to the base of their chair or reach arms forward, parallel to the ground.

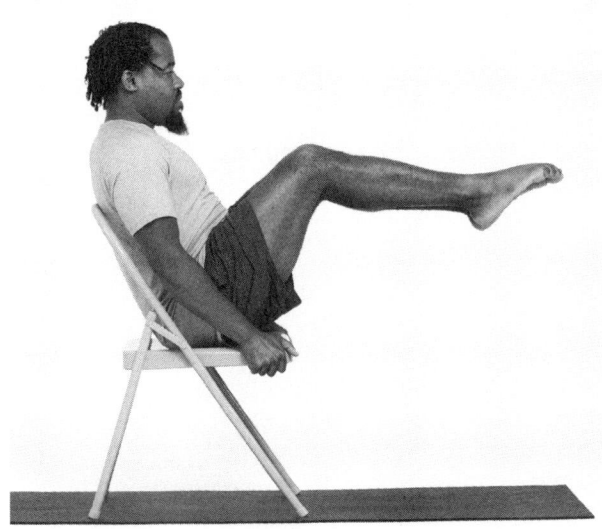

Boat Pose (Navasana) variation 3

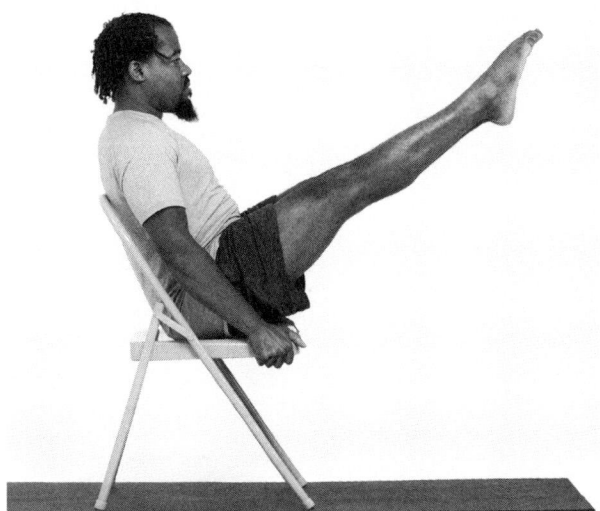

Boat Pose (Navasana) variation 4

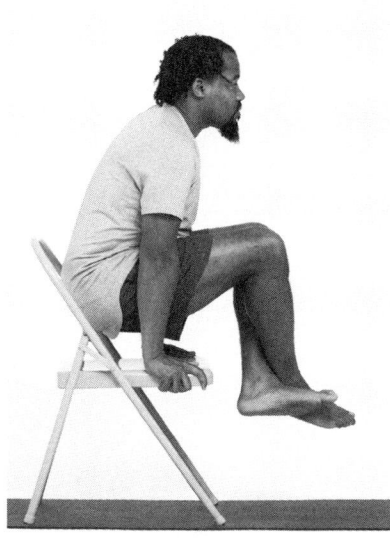

Uprooting (Utpluthih)

Uprooting (Utpluthih)

For even more fun and challenge, consider adding an Utpluthih lift between each Boat Pose. Sometimes this posture is so difficult the class actually erupts in laughter, an emotional release and side benefit of the asana. Stimulation of the solar plexus can make us belly laugh. Teachers can use this with art and purpose to release tension in class.

To instruct Utpluthih in a chair, ask students to cross their legs at the shins and lift their feet off the floor, bringing their knees in toward their chest. They can grip the sides of their chair with their hands. Students then take a deep inhale and, as they do so, press down and lift up from their chair. For an extra feeling of weightlessness, challenge students to bring their bottom to the seat on the exhale without letting their feet touch the ground, then lift legs directly into Boat Pose.

Many practitioners will not be able to lift their bottom up off the chair, which is expected, normal, and part of the process. They can still work their arms and build strength in their abdomen by pressing down and trying to lift. Also, students can keep their feet on the floor and press down into their hands, lifting their bottom out of the chair.

Utpluthih Variation: Knee Squeeze

A lovely alternative to Utpluthih is to invite students to stay seated in their chair, pull their knees in toward their chest, and wrap their arms around their knees, giving themselves a squeeze. This is an effective and creative way to incorporate self-touch, which is healing but can feel imposed if cued as a "self-hug."

Standing Mini Sun Salutation (Surya Namaskar)

Now offer students the opportunity to stand. Those who prefer not to can be reminded of the Seated Sun Salutation (page 100) and encouraged to repeat the sequence here. Before launching into movement, invite students to take the time to be with their stillness in Equal Standing Pose. Suggest they tune in to any shifts in energy that may have occurred since the beginning of practice. Propose they find their grounding again through bringing attention to the surfaces below them.

When grounding and the three-pointed focus have been reestablished, invite students to inhale while lifting their arms. As students exhale, ask them to fold forward, bringing their hands to the ground even if it means bending their knees to get there. On the next inhale, they can

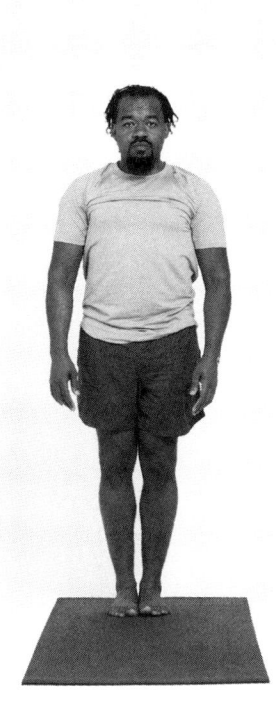
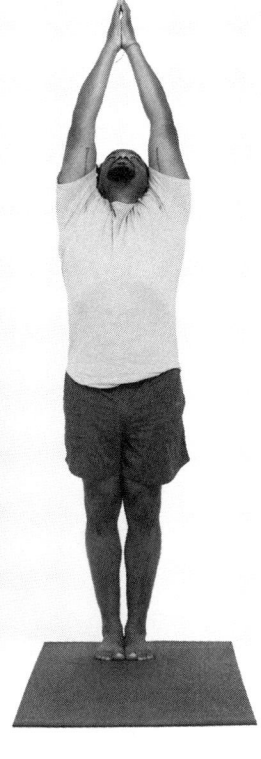
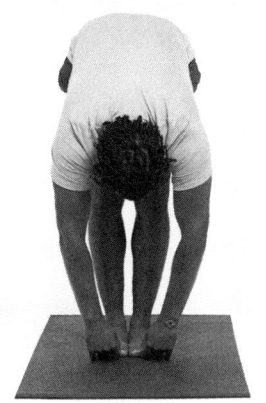
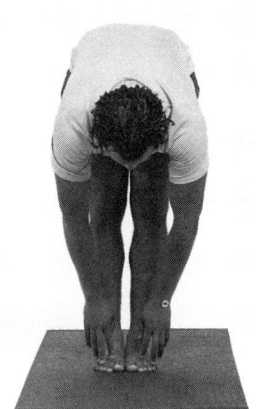

lift up their head and continue to reach their fingers downward. On the exhale, students fold more deeply forward and continue to keep their hands engaged with the ground.

Next, practitioners can inhale, coming all the way up to standing, reaching their arms overhead. Exhaling, they can bring their arms back to their sides.

Standing Mini Sun
Salutation
(Surya Namaskar)

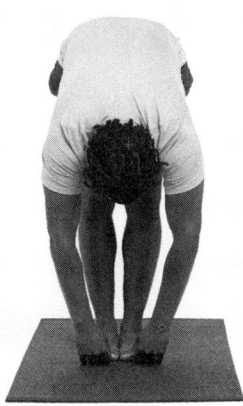
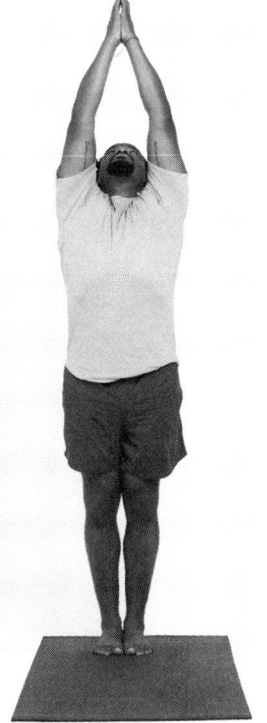
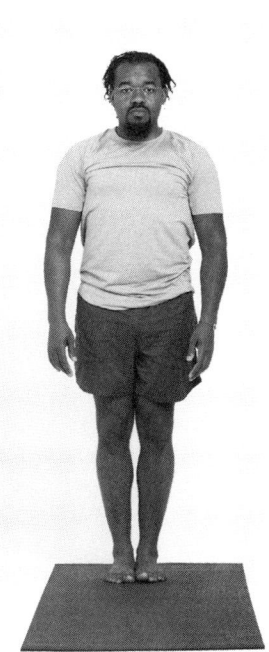

Downward Dog (Adho Mukha Svanasana) with Chair

Downward Dog is not included in the Standing Mini Sun Salutation, so you can introduce it afterward with support of the chair. Invite students to bring their chair to the front of their mat with the seat facing them. They can grip the top of the chair, extend their arms, and walk back slowly, hinged at the waist, to stretch their back and legs.

Those who have remained seated can reach out their legs and arms in a V shape for a Seated Downward Dog.

VARIATIONS: DOWNWARD DOG

In this expression of this pose, students rest their hands on the seat instead of on the back of their chair. Let students experiment with bent and

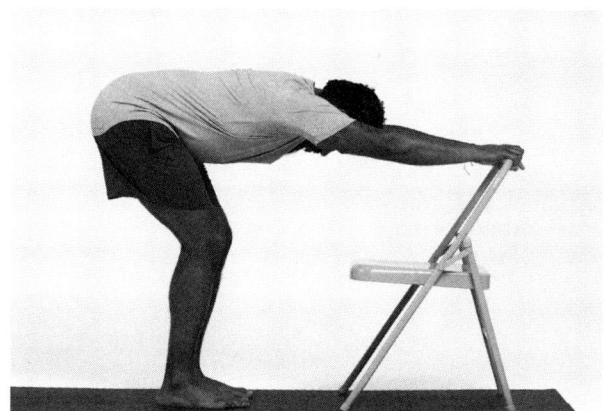
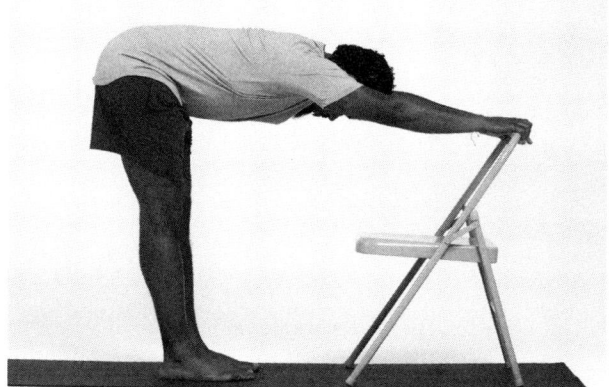

Downward Dog (Adho Mukha Svanasana) with chair

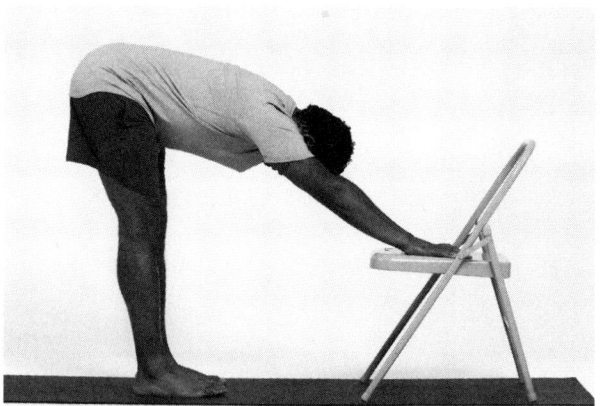
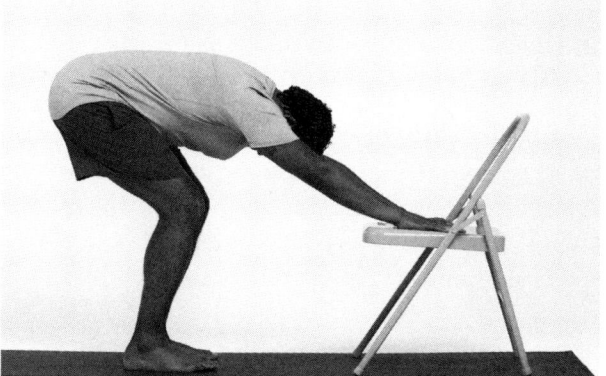

Downward Dog variations

Small adjustments can significantly alter where a student most feels the pose. Give options such as bending the knees to access more feeling between the shoulder blades. Let students tell you what they feel instead of anticipating it.

straight legs in this position, and then with the different arm positions available, before landing on one combination to stay with for five breath cycles.

Tree Pose (Vrksasana)

With the chair at the front of the mat, Tree Pose can be done with toes on the ground or the foot on inner shin or thigh. The height of the leg matters much less than the awareness the student brings into the posture. Encourage them to feel the subtle shifts the body makes to retain balance, to straighten the standing leg, to lift the sternum, and steady the eyes. Students can grip the chair with their hands, come to Prayer Pose at their chest, or stretch overhead. Challenge students to press their standing leg into the foot as the foot presses into the leg, aiding balance. Breath five times in each variation. Repeat the posture on the other side.

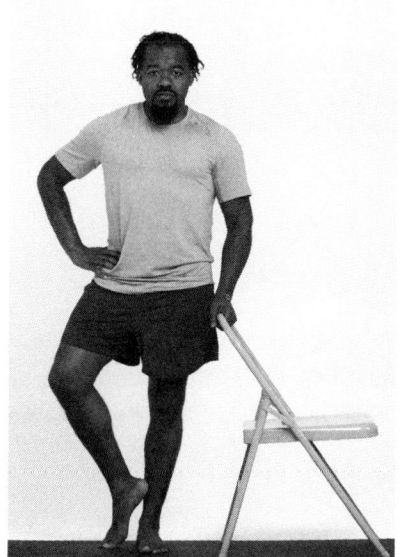 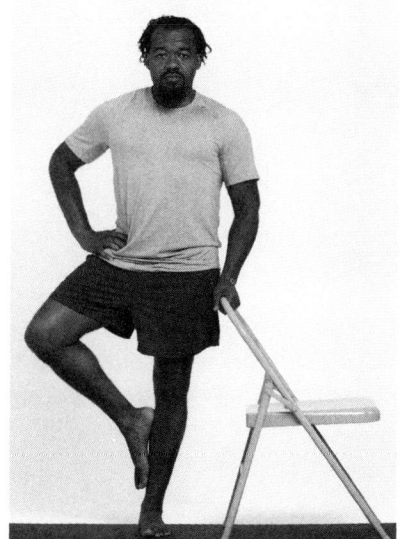 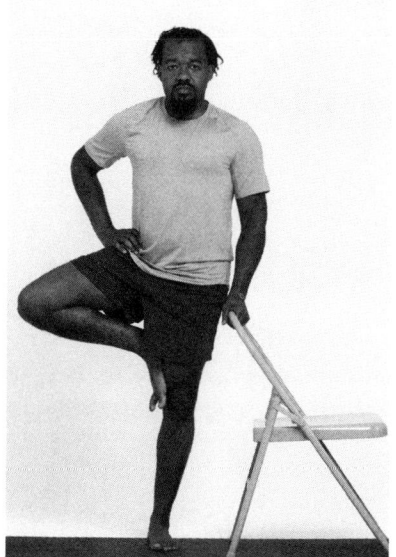

Tree Pose (Vrksasana)

Variation: Leg Lift

Request students try lifting their bent leg straight up in front of them for five breaths at the end of the posture. The height doesn't matter. Start with one inch off the ground and raise it higher as your students feel ready.

Variation: Tree Pose

Tree Pose and leg lifts can also be offered to those who are seated. For Tree Pose, students extend one leg straight in front with their foot flexed, then bend the opposite leg and press the sole of its foot along the side of their extended leg. Repeat on the other side.

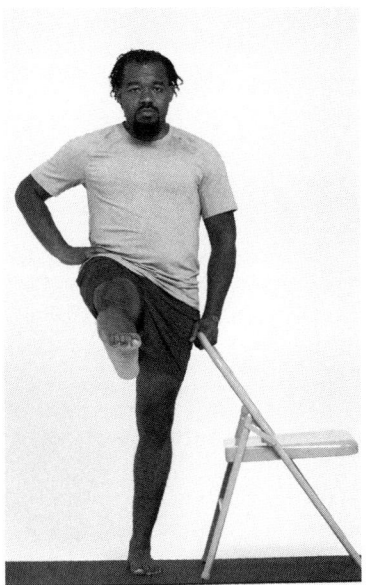

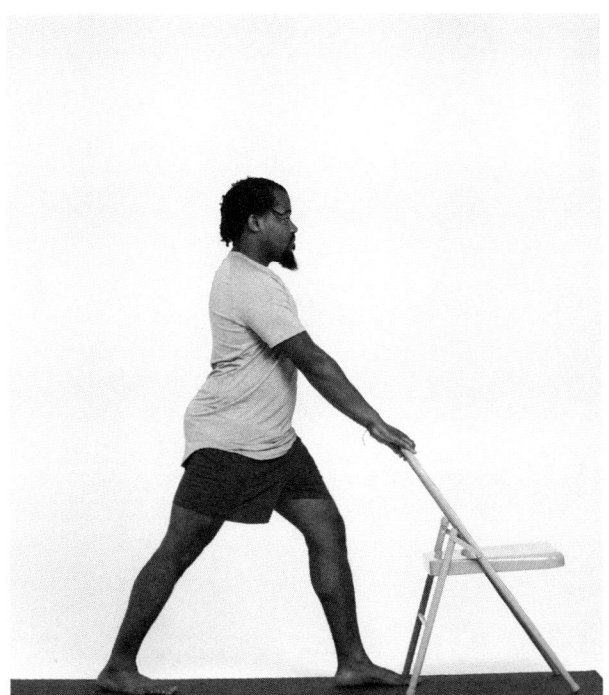
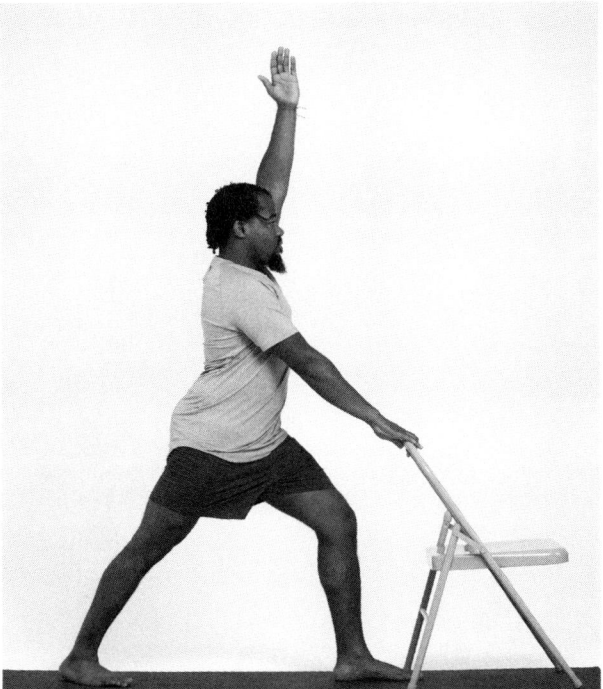

Warrior 1 (Virabhadrasana 1)

Warrior 1 (Virabhadrasana 1)

After Seated Warrior 1, you can introduce the standing version of the posture. Using a chair for support in Standing Warrior 1 helps anyone who many feel off-balance. Invite students who want to explore the standing variation to stand at the back of their chair. Ask that they step one foot back and turn that foot outward to a forty-five-degree angle. The front knee should be bent. Invite them to engage the muscles in their lower abdomen and waist, trying to feel where to find more stability. Ask: "How does the level of your engagement shape the experience?" Count five breaths in this posture.

After five breaths, give the option to lift one arm straight up. Ask them to notice how this one change affects the rest of their body. Has the quality or location of their presence been shifted? Can they still feel their legs and core while holding awareness of their arms and fingers?

Invite them to reach up the other arm, either to meet or switch with the first. Students can rest their gaze straight ahead, at their nose tip, or toward the ceiling. Ask students to recognize any changes they experience in body or mind. Count five breaths. Invite students to release their arm or arms to the back of their chair, switch leg positions, and repeat the variations on the other side.

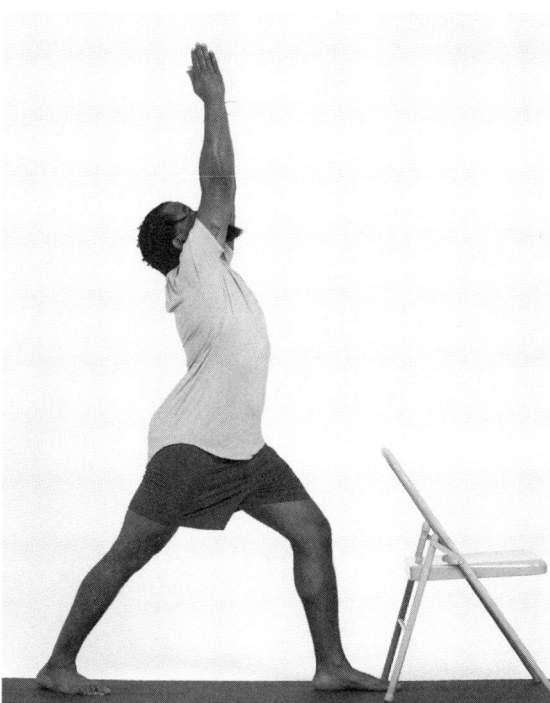

Staff Pose (Dandasana)

This posture is the first in the floor portion of the sequence. Those who prefer not to sit on the floor can do these poses from a chair. You may also skip seated postures and repeat the previous sequence or begin closing postures, depending on how long your class is.

Students who want to move to the floor can shift their chair aside and sit on their mat. Ask students to straighten their legs out in front of them, flexing their feet at their ankles. Encourage them to sit upright and tall. Let them experiment with leaning forward and back, similar to how they experimented with shifting weight in Seated Equal Standing Pose. Invite them to find stillness once they've found their center. Stay here for five breaths, bringing feeling awareness into the whole body and the space it takes up.

Seated Forward Fold (Paschimottanasana)

Ask students to walk their hands toward their feet and allow their torso to move into a forward fold. They can place a block or two under their forehead for support or let their head hang without strain. Guide students to send breath into any areas of tightness. Ask them to consider what their presence feels like. How has their awareness changed along the back of their body? Encourage students to stay here for ten breaths. They can remove a block to go deeper into the posture for the second half of the hold.

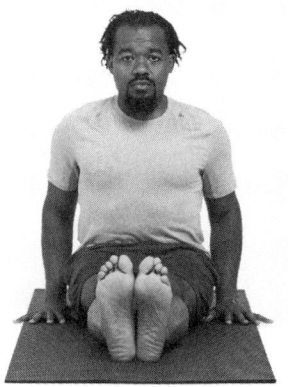

Staff Pose (Dandasana)

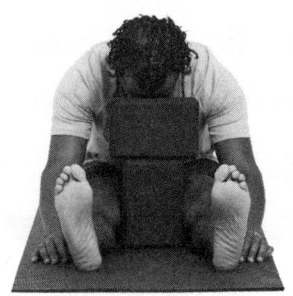

Seated Forward Fold
(Paschimottanasana)

Variation: Seated Forward Fold in a Chair
Folding forward while seated in a chair is possible and beneficial as well. Students can place blocks on the floor under their hands on either side of the chair for this variation.

Uprooting (Utpluthih)

Here we offer another powerful Utpluthih. In the floor version, those who choose to can use blocks beneath their hands to get more height. Adding Utpluthih between any poses of the seated sequence is always an option for students who like to stay active. Remind the practitioners not to hold their breath but instead to inhale as they lift up. (See page 108 for complete pose cues.)

Upward Plank Pose or Table Top (Purvottanasana)

This pose can be done with bent or straight legs. The bent-knee variation is easier. Both provide a great counterpose to forward bending. For the straight-legged version, students begin in Staff Pose. Invite them to bring their hands six to twelve inches behind them with their fingers pointing forward. On an inhale, cue students to press into their hands and lift up their body at the same time they press the front of their feet down. Just their hands and feet touch the floor. Students can drop their head backward, avoiding strain or discomfort. For the bent-legged version, offer the same instructions for the hands and arms but invite folks to take their feet hip-width apart and bend their knees to begin. Invite students

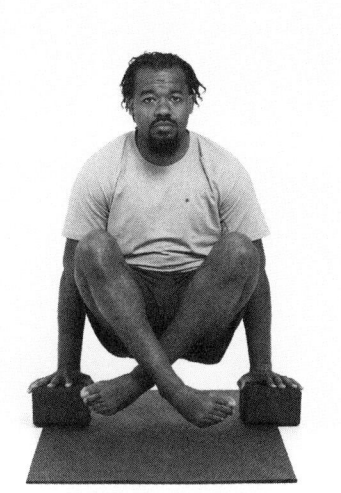

Uprooting (Utpluthih)

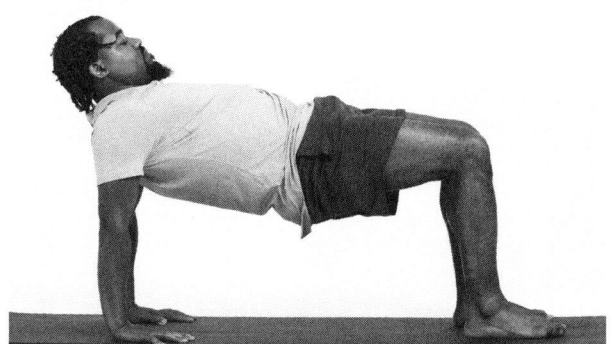
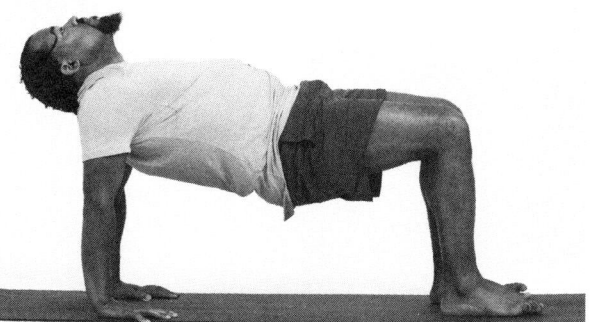

Upward Plank Pose or Table Top (Purvottanasana)

Purvottanasana exposes the front of the body, so it can be contra-indicated for some trauma survivors. Know your students and introduce poses like this only if and when they are comfortable with stretching the front of their body. You can offer a helpful pose variation by cuing that their head stay lifted. Dropping the head back can be hard on the neck and emotionally triggering as well.

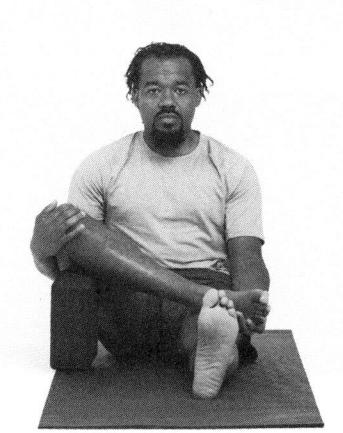

Half-Bound Lotus Forward Fold (Ardha Baddha Padma Paschimottanasana)

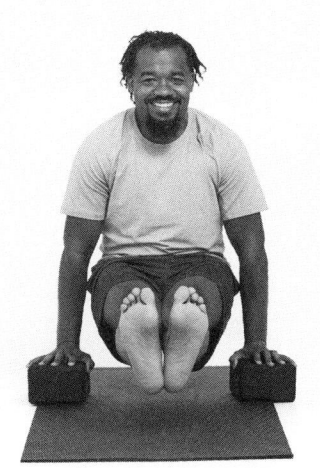

Uprooting (Utpluthih) variation

to match the energetic lifting up of their hips with a powerful inhale. After five breaths, invite students to bend their arms and lower down.

Most practitioners will start to drop their hips after a breath or two. Keep encouraging students to lift up and away from the floor, countering the downward energy by springing upward. This reinforces the healthy lesson that we don't have to go with the flow, especially if it's working against us. We can use our will and strength to push through and create something different. Students can keep their head lifted or drop it back and stay with this pose for five breaths.

Half-Bound Lotus Forward Fold (Ardha Baddha Padma Paschimottanasana)

We return now to Half Lotus, or Ankle-to-Knee Pose, this time on the floor (or in a chair as before, if students prefer). As cued during the first round, ask your students if they have knee pain or have had knee surgery before taking this posture. If yes, make sure they place a rolled-up towel in the crease of their right knee, deeply flex their right foot, or bring their foot inside their left thigh and take head to Knee Pose (Janu Sirsasana) instead.

Invite students to cradle their leg in the crook of their arm, rocking it side to side and releasing the muscles around their hip. Encourage them to feel the weight of the leg in their arms, letting it drop its weight and surrender, a sign it has released and the arm now controls its position. Then with a final rock, have them move their knee out to the side, lift their heel high, and bring their foot up toward their navel before placing it on the opposite hip crease. Ask that they stay there and slowly let their hip release and their knee drop. Invite students to use a block or other prop under their knee for support, if they'd prefer. Promote patience with this pose, and cue students to consciously send breath and awareness to areas of tightness. Stay for five breaths, straighten the legs, then repeat on the left side.

VARIATION: UPROOTING (UTPLUTHIH)
For those students who want to generate more heat and build strength, feel free to offer a straight-legged variation of Utpluthih between seated postures.

Ray of Light Pose/Sage Pose (Marichyasana A)

Now repeat Sage Pose, which appeared in the chair sequence. Students can take this posture while seated on the floor or remain in their chairs to revisit the earlier variation. (See page 104 for Seated Sage Pose.) Ask students to sit with their left leg extended and their right leg bent with their heel as close to the body as possible. Encourage them to leave some space between their right foot and their left thigh. On an inhale, invite students to extend their right arm out long, then wrap it around their right knee and toward their back as they exhale for a deep shoulder stretch. They can stay here or hinge forward. Stay for five breaths. Repeat the posture on the other side.

Repetition is a skillful way for folks to be in each asana longer and therefore reap more benefits from the pose. Many teachers seem to avoid repeating postures in a practice, concerned their students will feel bored. The opposite is often true: poses can feel new, refreshing, or vastly different based on where we put our emphasis or what part of the pose experience we choose to explore. The same pose can teach us different things based on where it comes in the sequence.

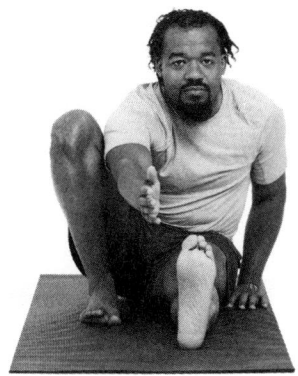 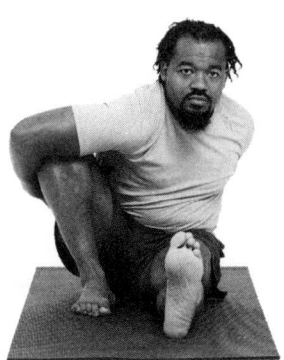

Ray of Light Pose/Sage Pose (Marichyasana A)

Cobbler's Pose (Baddha Konasana)

After all this hip opening, it would be neglectful not to bring in Cobbler's Pose. Invite students to bring the soles of their feet together and let their knees fall outward and sink down. Let them know that the closer the feet are to their body, the more intense the stretch will be. They can move their feet away from their body to lower the intensity. They can also place blocks or rolled towels under their knees for more comfort. Invite students to sit up tall in this position for five to ten breaths. Stay present with sensations that arise, ones that are not too hard to be with, and observe thoughts that pass through their mind.

Baddha Konasana can feel vulnerable and revealing. This feeling may shift for students after time spent in the pose and also between variations. You should know your students well before offering it, and even then, give an alternative pose, such as Hero Pose or even a squat. A small shift such as cupping the hands in the lap could make this posture feel safer. You may want to invite students to stay for one breath, then squat, then return to the pose again, to feel the sensations oscillate from vulnerable to grounded.

Next, invite practitioners to fold forward if that feels intriguing for them. You can suggest a flat or rounded back, or instruct for both. In both cases, make sure students know to stop folding when they feel discomfort. It's beneficial, if possible, to stay still and feel the discomfort and watch to see if it dissolves or changes. Students can place blocks under their forehead and/or knees to create more ease.

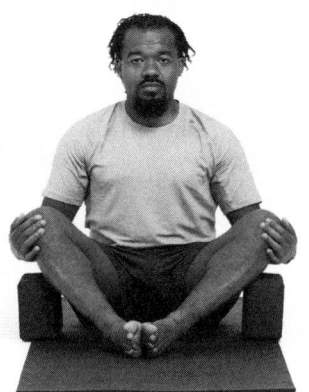
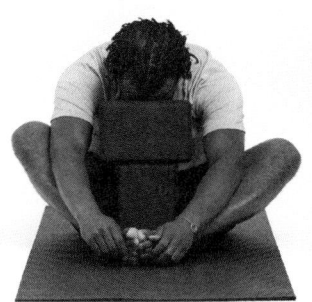

Cobbler's Pose (Baddha Konasana)

Garland Pose or Squat (Malasana)

Request that students remove their blocks and place their feet on the ground for their final deep hip and groin opener. Ask students to place their feet wide apart, with their toes turned out, which should help them to get deeper into the position. Let them know not to worry if their heels don't touch the ground. Invite students to bring their arms between their splayed knees and press the outsides of their arms firmly against their inner legs, with their legs pressing back against them. This tension causes the chest and hips to open. Let students feel that they are rising out of their squat as opposed to sinking in. Speak to them about pressing their palms firmly and relaxing their face. Count five breaths, directing the gaze toward the tip of the nose.

Crane/Crow Pose (Bakasana)

Your students may stay another five breaths in the squatting position or bring their hands to the ground and tilt their weight forward to prepare for Crow Pose.

To lift up into Crow, practitioners should keep their Malasana setup: engaging their outer arms and inner legs, head and chest lifted. Invite students to release their hands to the floor and bring their weight forward until their feet lift off the ground. For a greater challenge, invite

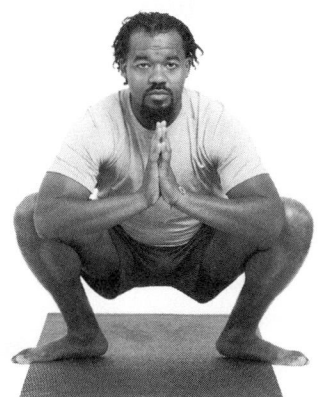

Squat (Malasana)

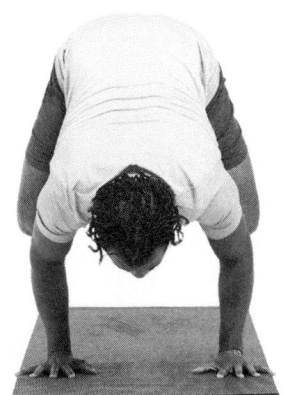

Crane/Crow Pose (Bakasana)

students to bring their feet together so toes and heels touch. Ask students to keep their eyes and breath steady and stay here for five breaths. Many students will laugh just hearing that request, and that laughter is a welcome part of the class and an element of healing. Feel free to laugh at yourself, too, and remind students to have fun with the practice.

Vinyasa (Dynamic Transition between Postures)

The following series of movements is called *taking a vinyasa*, and it can be done between any or all floor poses. Give practitioners the option of bringing their feet down to the floor or trying to walk or jump back into a push-up (Chaturanga) position. The trick to jumping back without the feet touching the floor is to make sure you dart your head and chest

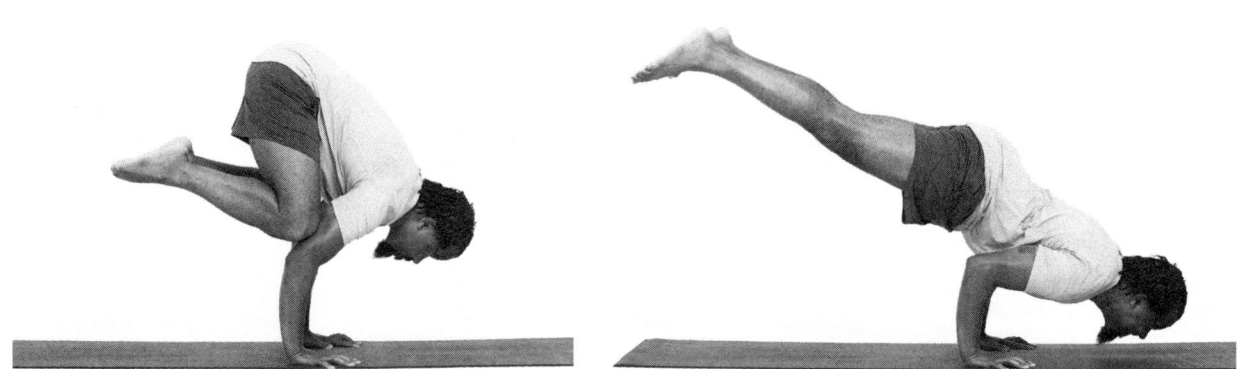

Vinyasa (dynamic transition between postures)

forward with equal and opposite force as the legs jump back landing in Chaturanga position.

From here, have students lower their legs and belly to the ground, shifting forward, straightening their arms, lifting their chest into Upward Dog. Press back with an exhale to Downward Dog. Then invite students to look forward between, but far beyond, their hands and step or jump forward to sit. It doesn't matter how far forward they can hop their feet; the benefits come from trying.

Students often want to lift their palms, but instead, encourage them to ground their hands down into the mat as they come forward. If their feet haven't gotten very far, they may need to shift their body forward on the mat to set up for the next position.

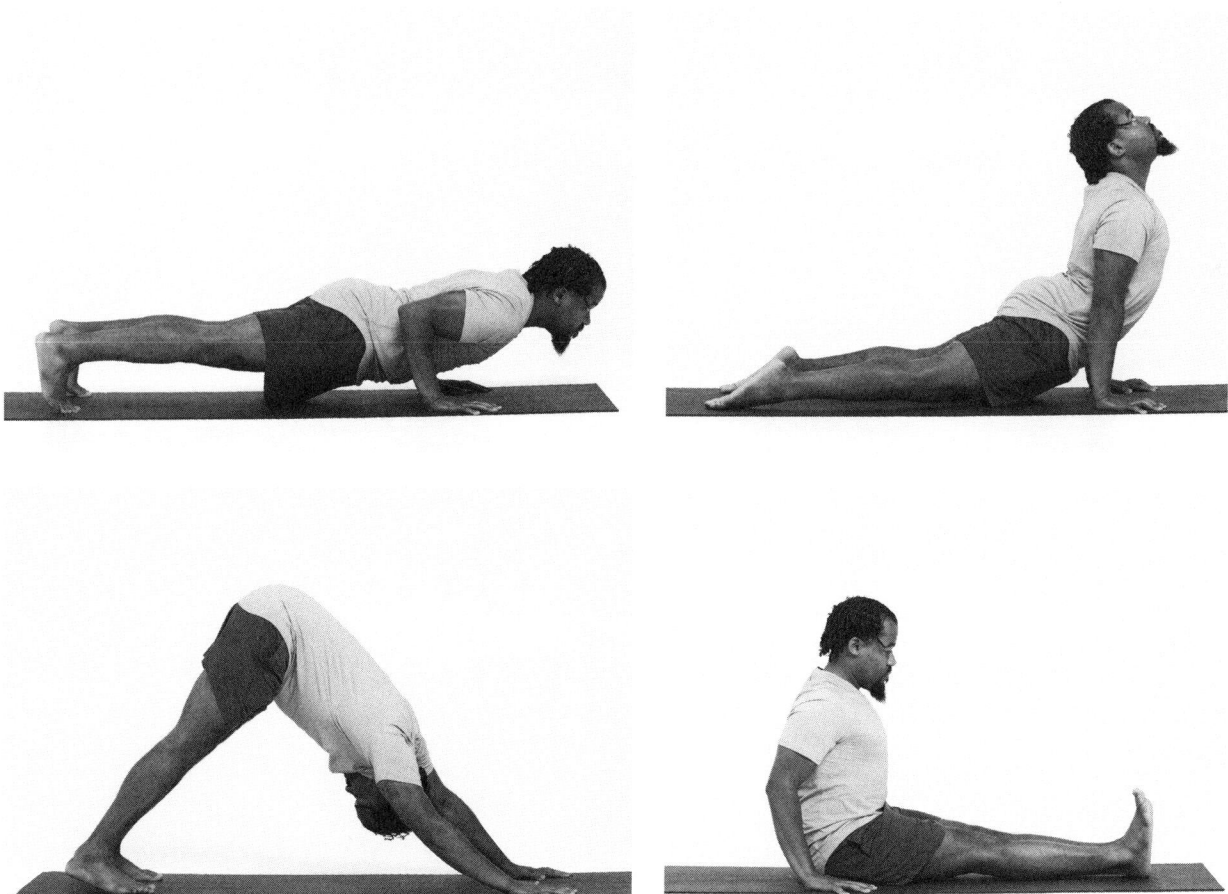

Boat Pose (Navasana)

The floor version of Boat Pose can be done with legs bent or straight. (See page 106 for cues for Boat Pose.) For more support, invite students to place their hands under their legs, holding them just below their knees. Make sure they keep lifting up their back so they don't fall backward. Stay here for five breaths.

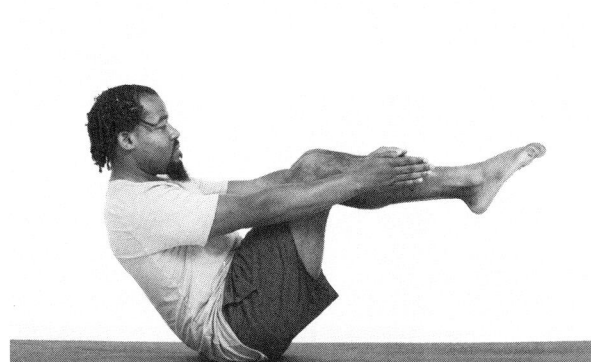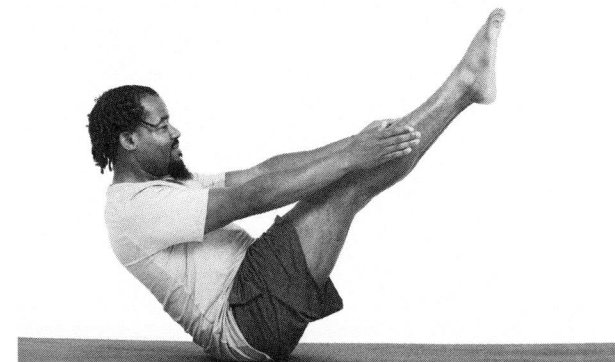

Boat Pose (Navasana)

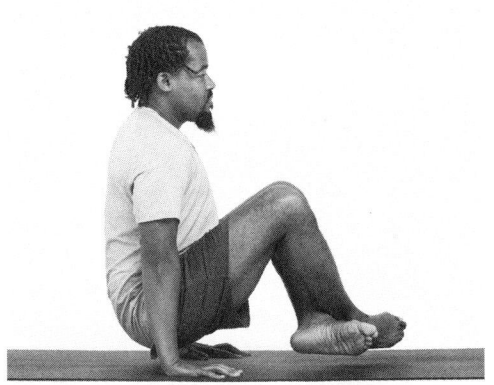

Utpluthih variation: Offer uprooting posture between Boat Poses (Navasanas).

Bridge Pose (Setu Bandha Sarvangasana)

Ask everyone to sit down, then lie down with the legs bent and feet hip-width apart (or more). Begin with their arms at their sides. Invite students to press their arms and feet firmly into the ground as they inhale and lift their back. Then instruct them to roll their spine to the ground as they exhale. Synchronizing each movement to its appropriate breath, lead five or more rounds of moving Bridge before pausing in the lifted position and staying there for five breaths. Bring awareness to the visible rise and fall of the chest as each student breathes, as this can increase the individual's breath capacity.

VARIATION 1: BRIDGE POSE (SETU BANDHA SARVANGASANA)
Students can remain in traditional Bridge Pose or roll their shoulders under their back, extend their arms toward their feet, and clasp their hands for another variation. Invite students to stay here for five breaths, watching their chest and noticing any differences in sensation this position elicits in their body. They can release their hands, roll their spine down, and take a breath here.

VARIATION 2: BRIDGE POSE (SETU BANDHA SARVANGASANA)
Invite students to explore Bridge Pose with their arms above their head on the floor, fingers interlaced, for more upper back and shoulder opening. Encourage folks to check in with any shifts in mind, body, and energy. Alternatively, they can repeat their preferred Bridge. Count them through five breaths before asking them to lower their back.

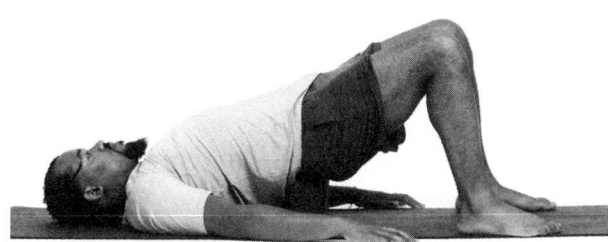

Bridge Pose (Setu Bandha Sarvangasana)

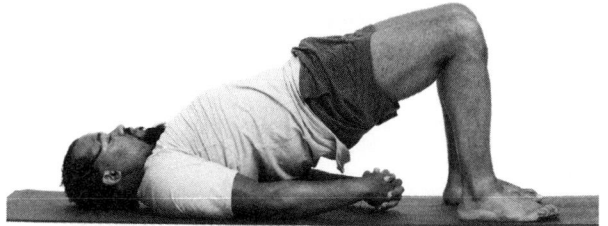

Bridge Pose (Setu Bandha Sarvangasana) variation 1

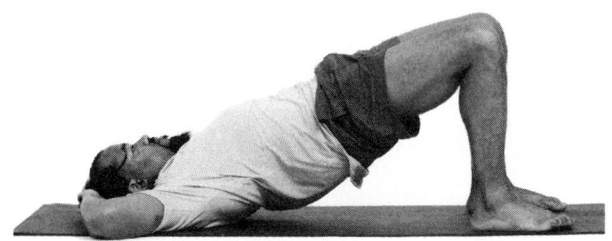

Bridge Pose (Setu Bandha Sarvangasana) variation 2

Wheel Pose (Urdhva Dhanurasana)

Wheel is an intense backbend variation usually reserved for physically advanced practitioners. Anyone may choose their favorite Bridge Pose variation in its place. Remind students to relax their mind and body, which can start to race in this posture, by taking deep even breaths. They may choose to come down at any time.

To set up for Wheel Pose, students lie on their back with their knees bent and their feet flat on the floor, hip-width apart (or more). Invite students to bring their hands by their ears with their fingers pointing toward their shoulders, then press into their feet and hands to lift up. Stay in the posture for up to five breaths, then lower to the ground slowly.

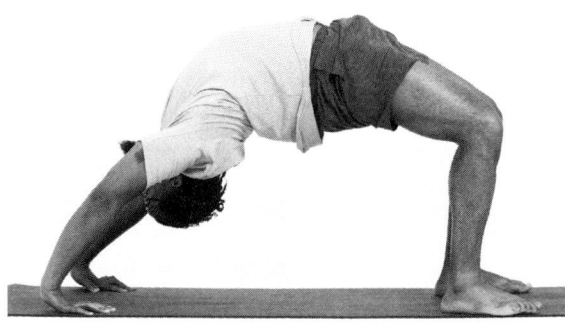

Wheel Pose (Urdhva Dhanurasana)

Wind-Relieving Pose (Pawanmuktasana)

After three backbends, invite students to lower themselves down to the mat, legs extended and arms at their sides. Students can hug their knees into their chest, a great counterpose to backbending. Aside from balancing out the flexion and extension of the back, this posture is an opportunity to return attention inward in a shape associated with safety and protection. Let students roll around on their back and explore what movements feel right in the shape.

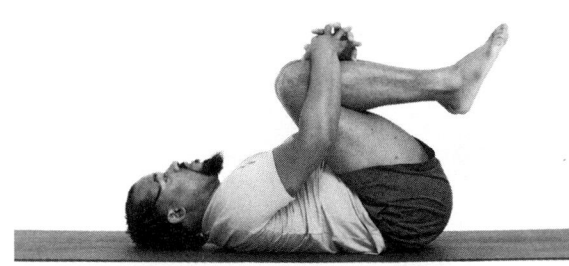

Wind-Relieving Pose (Pawanmuktasana)

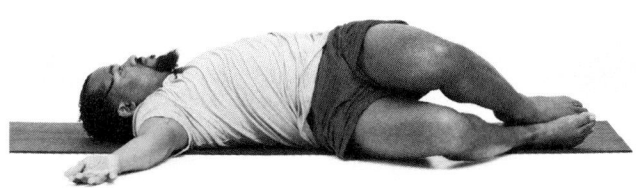

Supine Spinal Twist (Jathara Parivrtti)

Supine Spinal Twist (Jathara Parivrtti)

If it feels right, students can then reach their arms out wide on the floor in a T shape, letting their bent knees drop together to one side and turning their head to gaze in the opposite direction. Propose that they work toward keeping both shoulders on the floor. They can place a towel between their knees if that feels more comfortable. Stay for a full ten breaths. When the ten breaths are complete, they can bring their knees to center on an inhale. On an exhale, invite students to let their knees drop to the other side, staying there for ten breaths. As an alternative, offer a seated upright twist.

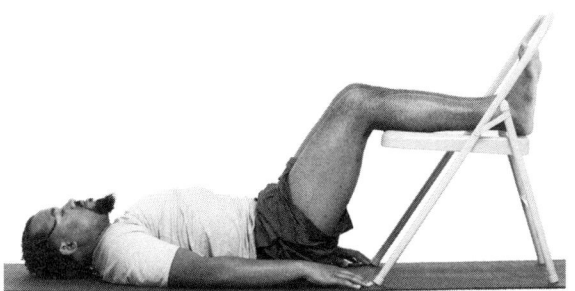

Supported Shoulderstand (Salamba Sarvangasana)

Bring the practitioners back to center and ask them to place their chair at the front of their mat, the seat facing back, for a supported leg elevation. This posture has many health benefits that stem from its activation of the parasympathetic nervous system: it reduces the body's stress response, creates calm, and helps with sleep. Offer students a chance to lie down with their arms at their sides and their legs up, resting on the seat of the chair. Alternatively, if a student does not want to lie on the ground, and you have enough chairs, they could sit in one chair and place another chair facing them, stretching their legs out to rest on the chair in front of them.

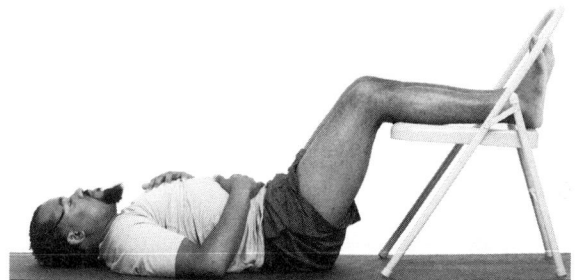

If possible, have students stay in this posture for twenty-five breaths. They can change their arm position, resting their hands on their belly and heart to encourage relaxation. They can turn their chair around, chairback facing them, then extend their legs and rest their feet at the top of their chair for a lengthened, straight-legged inversion. Make sure students come down slowly from Shoulderstand. They can roll to the side and stay there for a few breaths before coming to their knees for Headstand or take an uprooting posture and/or vinyasa.

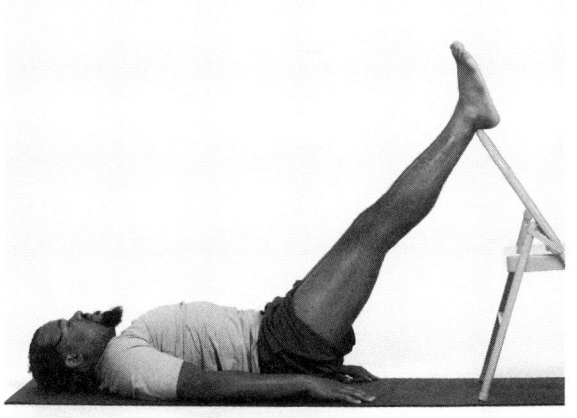

Supported Shoulderstand
(Salamba Sarvangasana) variations

Headstand (Sirsasana)

Shoulderstand and Headstand are often called the king and queen of asanas. They are said to help us hold on to vital energy, revitalizing youthfulness. A safe Headstand requires enough arm strength so the head barely touches the ground and there is no pressure on the neck. It also requires significant body awareness to align the spine and make the minute adjustments necessary to balance while upside down. Students are vulnerable in this position; they can be knocked over or lose balance, sometimes because of a passing thought. However, like many poses that are challenging to start, Headstand can become calming and empowering in its mastery.

Headstand is intimidating for many, so a longer Shoulderstand, a Dolphin Pose, or a Child's Pose can be offered instead. Teachers who

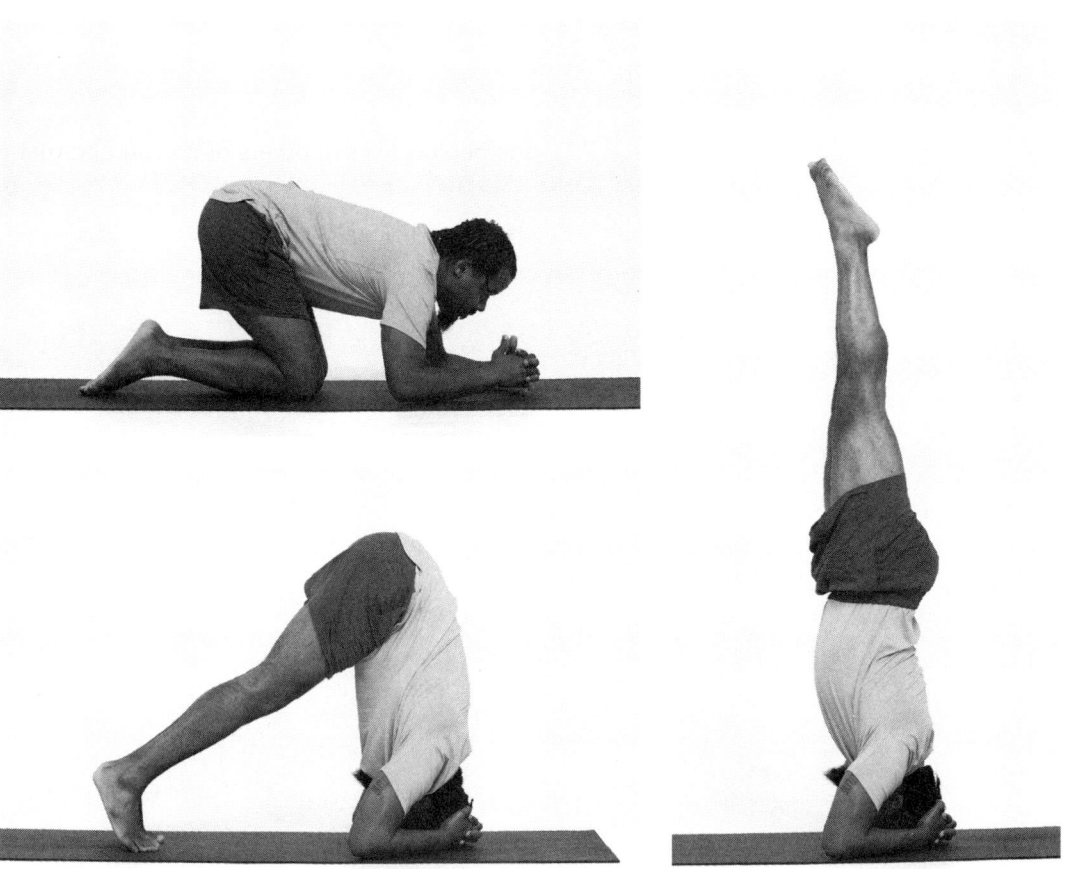

Headstand (Sirsasana)

are not ready to teach Headstand safely should not attempt it. You can become ready by apprenticing with more experienced teachers who have taught the posture to many bodies and who can use language to guide students safely.

The pike position is used to set up Headstand, and it is also a good preparation for the posture. Students can work on strengthening and building confidence in pike, engaging the muscles along their sides and lower waist, squeezing their legs together, and pulling their legs toward their head. Eventually they will be able to lift their legs off the ground as their hips move forward over their back, all while pressing their arms down and reducing the weight on their head. If you feel students need or desire to work on building arm strength, they can lift their head off the ground and move their chin forward and back over their clasped hands for Dolphin Pose.

Cue all students to bring their head and knees down to rest in Child's Pose.

Though it may seem hard to believe when they are first learning it, many people eventually find deep relaxation in Headstand. The experience of getting the feet off the ground often gives great relief. Some people report that this posture puts them in a new "zone" marked by calm and creativity. It seems that flipping ourselves on our heads may help us to flip our stories and perceptions on their heads as well, allowing for new possibilities and perspectives to arise. Ask your students when exploring this posture: "In what ways has shifting your physical position contributed to a shift in mental position? Are you easily able to hop into the perspectives of others or do you find that practice difficult and traitorous?"

Child's Pose (Balasana)

Never let anyone lift their head after Headstand: that message must be drilled into your brain. The head remains down so the blood can flow back into the body and a head rush or fainting spell can be avoided. After coming back to the ground after an inversion, always make sure students rest for a full minute or more with their head down in Child's Pose. To transition from Headstand into Child's Pose, they can slowly lower their toes to the ground, then bend their knees and drop them to the ground. They lower their hips toward their heels. Their hips do not have to touch their heels.

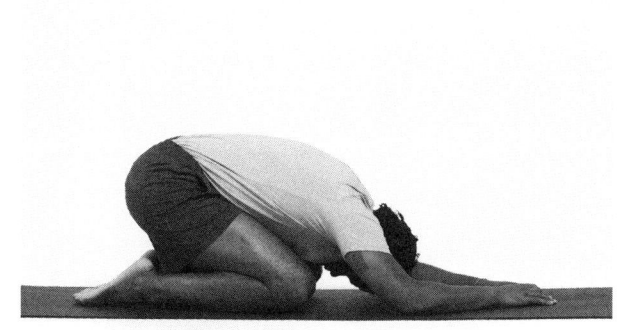

Child's Pose (Balasana)

Bound Lotus (Baddha Padmasana)

The closing poses of a yoga sequence are an opportunity for students to be with, feel fully, and gain the benefits of the yoga asanas they've just experienced. Invite students to cross their legs comfortably, sit on their heels, sit on a chair, or take a Lotus position. They can reach their arms behind their back and hold opposite elbows. Invite them to take a deep inhale, then exhale and fold forward.

Sealing the Practice (Yoga Mudra)

On the exhale, invite students to fold forward, bringing their head toward the ground. They should not strain to get there. The hope is that the posture is relaxing or at least approached from a standpoint of relaxation. Have the student rest with their head tipped forward for five to ten long, deep breaths—the deepest breaths of their practice.

Lotus (Padmasana)

After five to ten deep breaths, cue students to rise up to a seated position on the inhale, extending their arms straight and resting toward the outside of their knees. Their thumb and pointer finger are touching and their wrists faceup. The arm and wrist position allows for widening across the chest. Count ten breaths, encouraging them to rest their gaze at their nose tip.

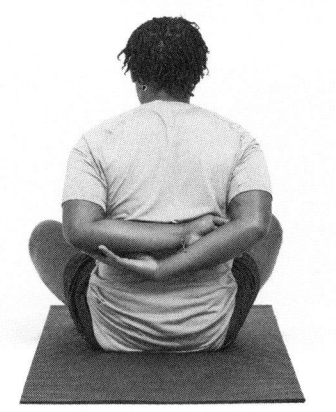

Bound Lotus (Baddha Padmasana)

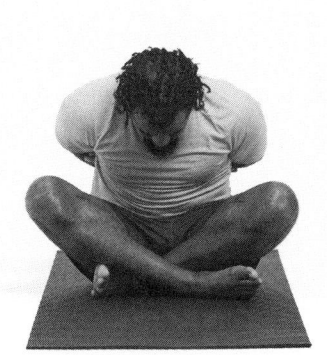

Sealing the practice (yoga mudra)

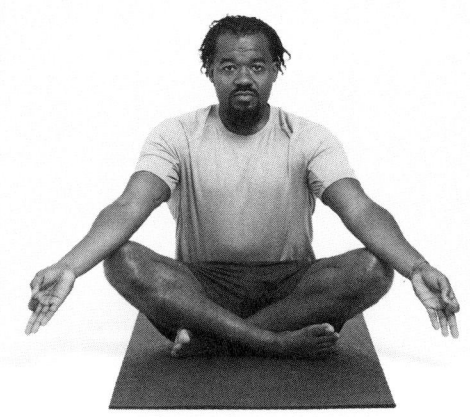

Lotus (Padmasana)

Uprooting (Utpluthih)

Cue a final uprooting pose, perhaps this time without blocks. Instruct students to cross their legs and squeeze their knees into their chest, which naturally lifts their feet off the ground. Invite them to bring their hands to their sides, just slightly in front of their hips, and press their palms into the ground. Inhaling, students should press down into their hands to lift up the body. Encourage them to keep pressing down and trying to lift for ten breaths.

Resting Position

To close the sequence, move students into a resting pose, either reclining in a chair or on the ground, with their legs bent or straight. Arms can be in any comfortable position. The important thing is to encourage stillness. Bring their attention inward and walk students through a body scan from their feet to the top of their head. Let them know that if there are any areas of their body they do not wish to focus on, they can ignore your instructions and bring their attention to a more neutral or positive-feeling part of their body. Encourage them to use their awareness to dispel any leftover tension or energy.

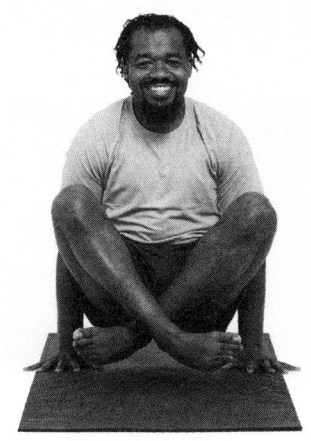

Uprooting (Utpluthih)

Spacious and Opening Sequence: Expansive Flow with Nikki

This sequence starts and ends with expansive postures that push the body to take up space. The postures and movements in Nikki's sequence are offered with the intention of feeling into the body and finding love and respect for what it can do, felt from the opening posture and through the hip circles, broad twists, and chest openers. Her poses are gentle yet powerful. They don't focus on any particular areas of the body but instead explore what the whole body can do.

This sequence flows in and between poses, which has a very different quality from holding static poses. Moving quickly from side to side disrupts the inclination to think too much and puts students directly into a felt experience. Coordination can be tricky for trauma survivors, who are often disconnected from their bodies due to disassociation, so don't be surprised (or judgmental of your teaching skills) if students interpret movements differently than you believe you are instructing them. Let them go with it. The important thing is that they move their bodies and start rebuilding the mind-body connection. This process requires support and a strong mental shift away from the binary of right and wrong.

This sequence also demonstrates how to use a chair for support in standing poses, when either sitting or standing, and for forward bending. It could be easily adapted to a chair-only sequence by adapting the Sun Salutation and final closing postures in a chair. The last part of the sequence is for those who choose to or need to practice in a bed, but it can also be done on a yoga mat on the floor. This is a gentle yet enlivening sequence, good for all levels. (It may not be suitable for folks who want to release energy via high-intensity postures.) The postures are empowering and fluid without demanding a ton of physical strength. It's also a sequence that translates well over a screen for streamed classes. Nikki works a lot with Three and a Half Acres programs that support folks with mental health and substance abuse struggles. She is also informed by her own MS diagnosis. This sequence supports students with similar challenges.

Five-Pointed Star Pose (Utthita Tadasana)

This pose can also be called Arms Up, and V for Victory Pose. Ask students to stand up if they can and separate their feet wider than hip-width apart. Encourage them to ground down into their mat and then pull their thighs upward without locking the knees. Give them time to drop their weight into their legs and feet. From that anchoring sensation, ask them to allow their spine to float upward. Invite them to lift their arms up and wide into a V position, dropping their shoulders down as they stretch through the elbows. They can turn their palms toward each other and feel the wide-open space between their hands. Their gaze can be upward or straight ahead. Invite them to relax their face.

Draw students' attention to all the space around their body and the space their body itself takes up. Ask them to note how this makes them feel. Invite them to find space for expansion of the breath into their chest and underneath their arms.

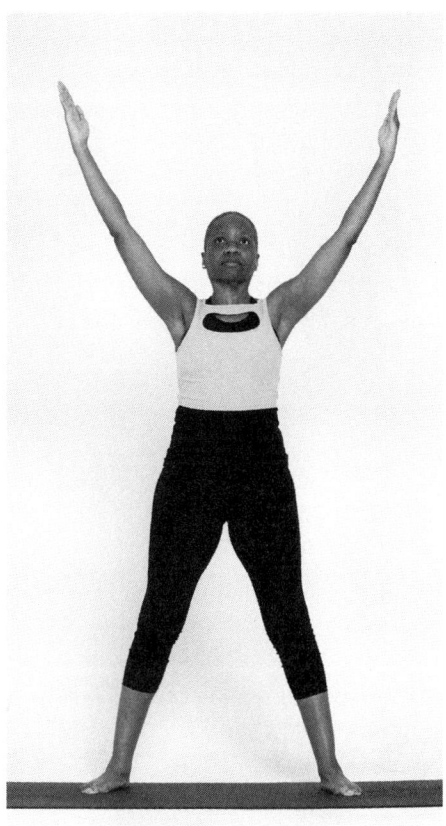

Five-Pointed Star Pose
(Utthita Tadasana)

Stay here for up to one minute, with slow and regular breath, reminding students they can take a break and return as needed.

Some students may not to want to or be able to do this posture because it feels too bold. They can try the seated version or bring their palms to Prayer Pose instead. Students can extend their arms only as straight as they are comfortable. This pose is great to begin with when students' energy level is low and you don't know how to change it.

VARIATION: SEATED FIVE-POINTED STAR POSE (UTTHITA TADASANA)

In the seated version of Star Pose, invite students to ground into the surfaces supporting their body. Suggest they lift all their toes, spread them, and then press them onto the ground. Propose they press all four corners of their feet into the floor and allow their thighs and bottom to release into the chair. Encourage students to use this grounding energy to anchor their body as they lift their spine for a straight but relaxed back. Release any tension in the neck or jaw.

Seated Prayer Pose (Anjali Mudra)

Prayer Pose can feel centering and protective, especially after the wide starfish stance. It calms the mind and brings the attention inward, and it is the perfect opportunity to move the focus toward the breath. After exploring boldness and vulnerability, students can take refuge in an equalizing posture that centers the energy inward.

Ask students to activate this pose by pressing evenly through their left and right palms and feeling the centerline of their body. Suggest that they notice if one side of the body feels more or less engaged than the other. Can they adjust their engagement to feel evenly balanced? Encourage students to stay here for ten breaths, gazing down at their nose tip and bringing in the three-pointed focus (see page 33).

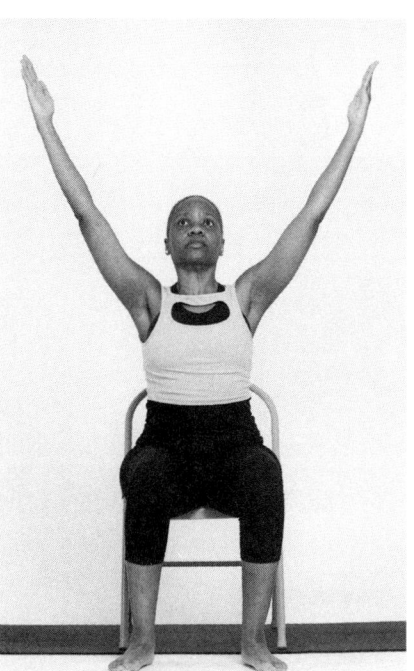

Seated Five-Pointed Star Pose
(Utthita Tadasana)

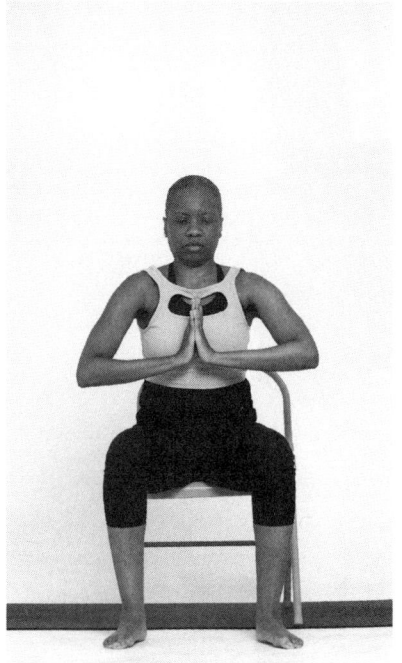

Seated Prayer Pose
(Anjali Mudra)

Seated Side Stretch (Parsva Sukhasana)

Ask students to release one arm toward the floor and bring the other arm up in the air, with the palm faceup. Invite students to reach their arm overhead so the side of the body gets a deep stretch. The other arm lengthens toward the ground. Invite them to notice when their seat lifts or tilts, and then ask them to reengage with their chair so only their side body stretches. Cue students to direct their gaze toward the extended hand or at the ground.

To create flow within this posture, invite students to switch between sides, back and forth, and pairing that movement with their breath. They can inhale as they raise one arm and exhale as they lower it before transitioning to an inhale as they raise the other arm. Rhythmic flow gives them an opportunity to explore breath, movement, and sensation in their body.

After several rounds of dynamic side stretching with palm upturned, ask them to turn their palm downward. What changes do they sense in their energy and in the spaces around their body with this shift?

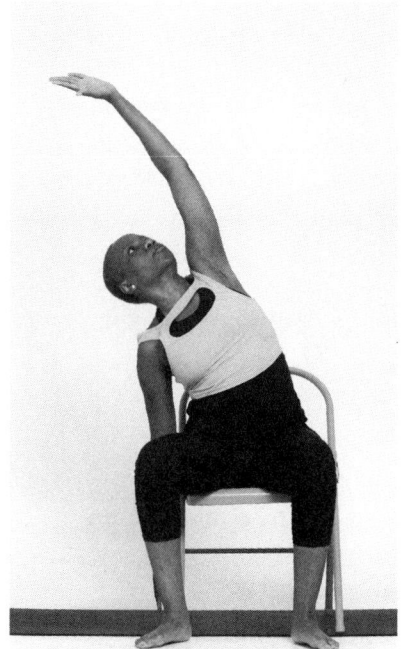 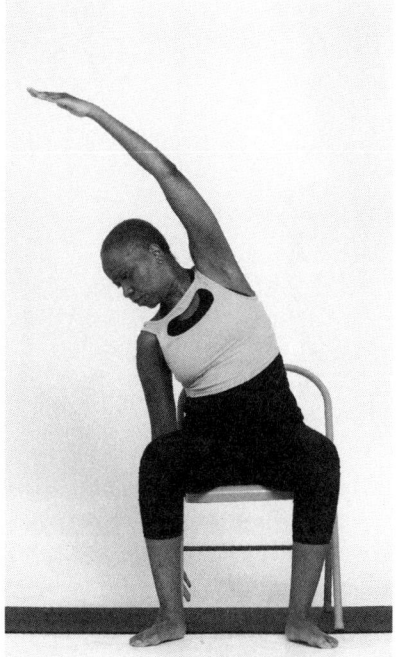 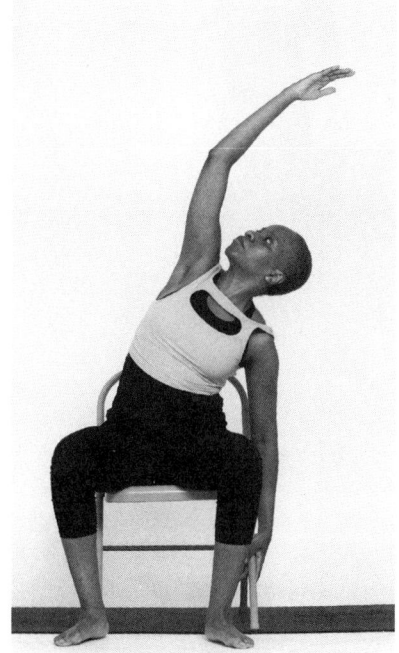

Seated Side Stretch (Parsva Sukhasana)

INTENSE SIDE STRETCH POSE

Give the option to intensify the side-body stretch by using the opposite arm to pull the body more deeply to the side. Students take their lower hand to the opposite, overhead wrist and pull gently, remaining grounded in the chair. Remind them not to pull too hard but rather use gravity to work with their intention to deepen the stretch. In this expression of side stretch, invite students into stillness, staying for five breaths on one side before switching to the other.

Seated Windmill Pose (Parivrtta Prasarita Padottanasana)

Invite students to take their feet and legs wider apart. On an inhale, they open their arms in a T shape. As they exhale, they bring their right arm to the ground near their left leg, across the body. The other arm reaches upward. On the next inhale, bring them back up to center in a T position. On the next exhale, cue them to switch sides, bringing the left hand down near the right leg. Invite them to flow, repeating the left and right sides five to ten times, pairing their movement to their breath. After five to ten rounds, cue students to stay in the posture for five breaths on each side.

While holding the pose, direct students to lengthen their spines all the way through the top of the head. Emphasize that the belly softens to allow for a deeper twist. Bring their minds to the widening of the chest as the arms reach in opposite directions. Then move attention to the back of the body, asking them to notice any sensations. Their gaze can be at their lifted hand or toward their foot. Ask them to reflect on what sensations arise in this position.

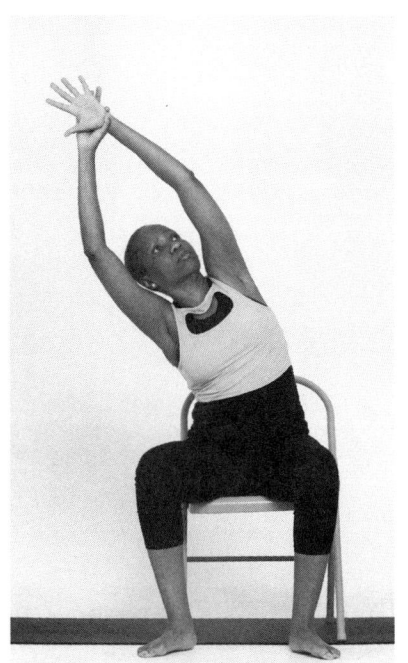

Intense Side Stretch Pose

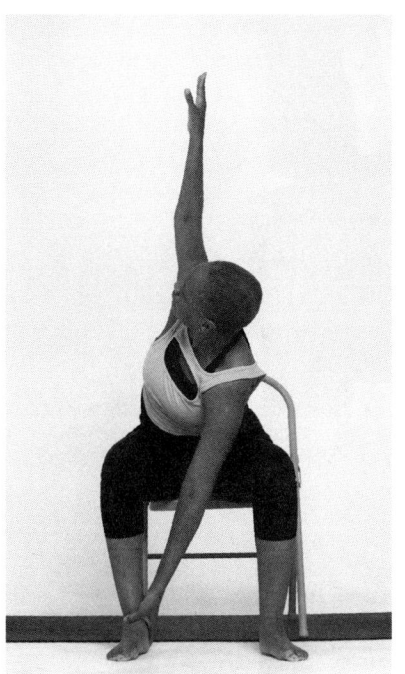

Seated Windmill Pose (Parivrtta Prasarita Padottanasana)

Torso Circles

Cue students to bend their left arm at the elbow, letting their torso lean toward that side. Guide students to continue to move their torso clockwise, pivoting at their waist with their chest leaning out forward between their legs, and then over their right knee, drawing an arc. The circle is completed as the arms straighten, hands still on the knees, with the back against the chair. Typically, the spine stays straight, but feel free to offer students the option to add a Cat/Cow movement in the spine as they rotate.

You can invite students to allow their hips to move as well, making the circle bigger and bigger. Have students experiment with small and large circles and at their own pace. Make sure to repeat the posture moving counterclockwise and leave equal time for each side.

Drawing circles with the torso involves complex, cascading movements. Let students play with it, allowing for feelings of confusion and fluster, and turn the movement into any flow they prefer. The goals are to awaken sensation and body connection and to feel into the body's ability to move and play. This can be scary for some. Encourage students to go slowly and take breaks when they need to, returning to Prayer Pose (Anjali Mudra) or another neutral position.

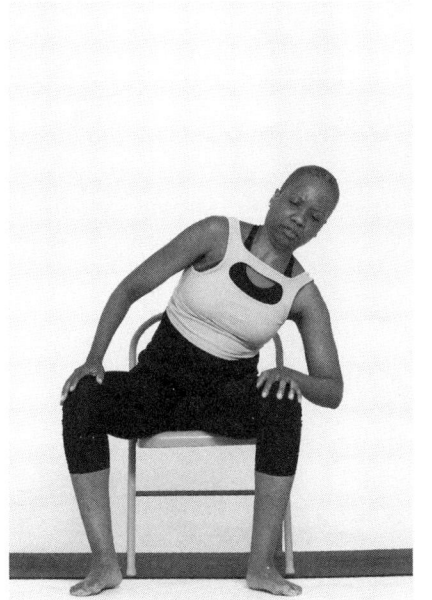 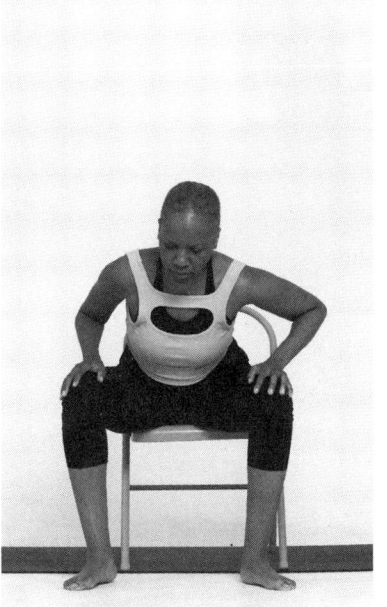 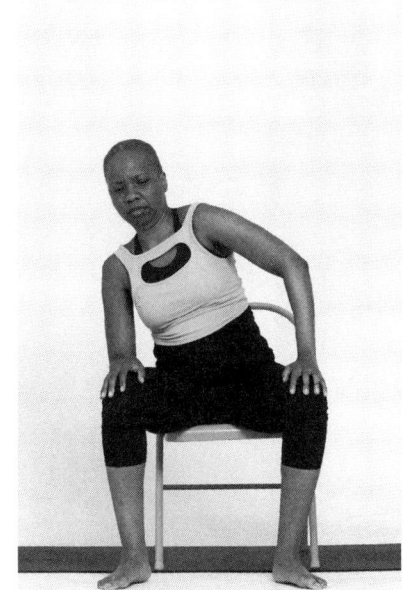

Torso circles

Seated Mini Sun Salutation (Surya Namaskar)

This seated version of Sun Salutation is similar to the one in Tim's Shoulders and Hips Sequence (page 100), but Nikki's Spacious and Opening Sequence includes a floating Chaturanga and Upward Dog. These positions can bring heat into the chair yoga practice, and I like to add them to sequences for that purpose. Healthy, appropriate challenge can get the mind focused on something outside the trauma.

Ask students to inhale and reach their arms up overhead, either shoulder-width apart or with their palms pressed together. They can use the entire length of the inhale to complete the motion. Pause here. Gaze can be toward their hands or the tip of their nose.

Ask students to fold forward as their exhale begins, bringing their hands to their thighs or down their legs. Remind them to release their head downward and allow the back to soften and fold.

On the inhale, instruct students to lift their torso part of the way up, stretching from the sternum and gazing forward. On the next exhale, they can fold forward more deeply. They can use their next inhale to come all the way back up to a seated posture with their elbows bent and their hands about two feet in front of them. Then on their next exhale,

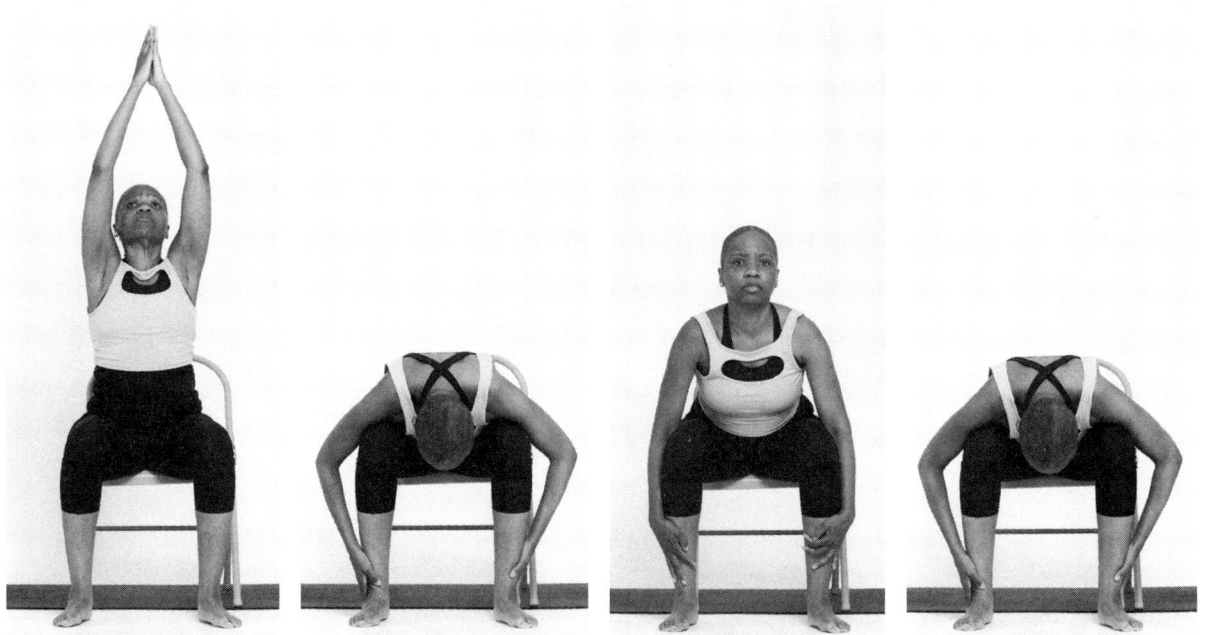

Seated Mini Sun Salutation (Surya Namaskar)

ask students to keep their elbows bent but bring their hands back toward their ears in a floating Chaturanga.

As they inhale, students try to keep their hands steady as their sternum leads the chest up and through the arms for a Seated Upward Dog. On the next exhale, they can fold forward once more. The next inhale brings them all the way up to a seated position with their arms overhead, either shoulder-width apart or with the palms pressed together. Gaze can be up toward their hands or down toward the tip of their nose. Finally, an exhale brings them back to their starting position, palms pressed together.

Repeat the Seated Mini Sun Salutation two to three times as a group and then invite students to take two to three Seated Mini Sun Salutations on their own, turning close attention to pairing their movements to their breath.

Invite students to take a few breaths in stillness after completing all their Sun Salutations. Acknowledge the inclination that may be present to adjust clothing or to move in some way. Encourage students to see what happens when they override that temptation and retain the energy they've created. Is there a power in not giving in to the mind's cravings? Do they become stronger or fade when they choose not to respond?

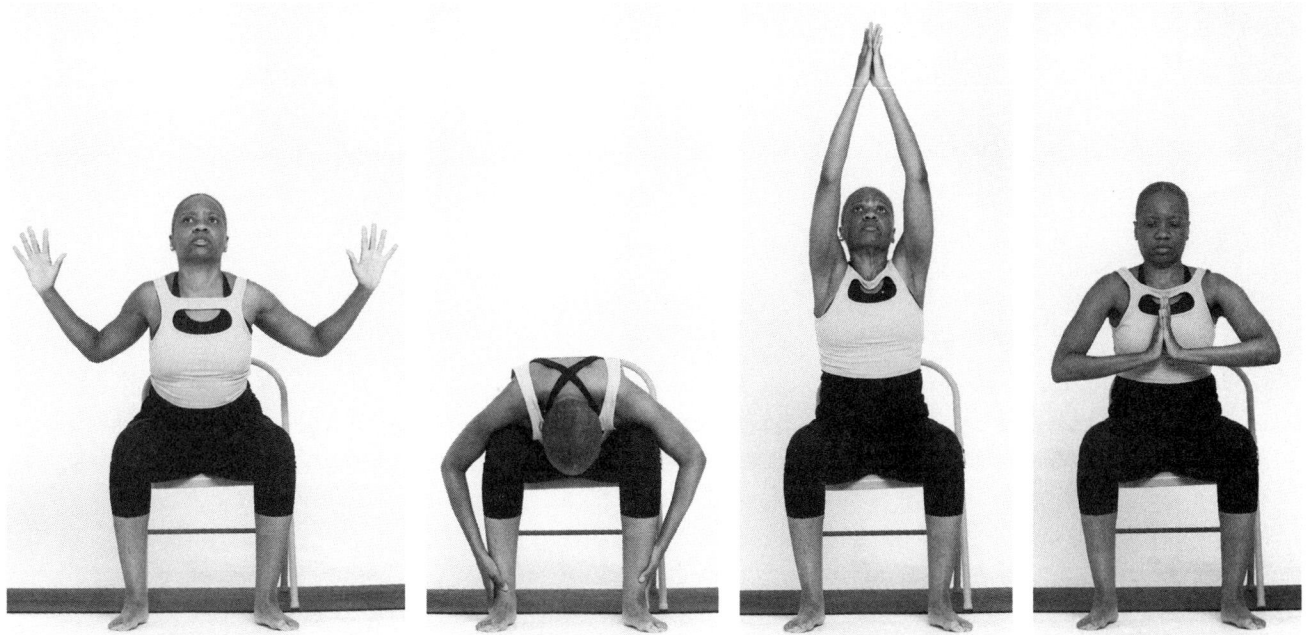

Seated Triangle Pose A (Trikonasana A)

To transition into Seated Triangle Pose, students can adjust in their seats slightly so they are facing toward the right rear corner of their mat. Encourage them to bring their legs into a wider stance and point their right foot out toward the back of the mat. On the inhale, invite them to open their arms wide like a T, and as they exhale, they elongate through their right hand and fingers, stretching their whole body to the right before reaching their right arm down their right leg. Ask them to actively press their right arm against the inside of their right leg to open their chest.

They can place their left hand on their waist or reach it straight up overhead. The gaze can be at their left hand if it's lifted, at the ceiling if it's not, or down toward their right big toe.

Encourage them to take five breaths in stillness in this position, noticing the feeling of being in the shape. On the following inhale, bring them up to center and invite them to switch their legs to face the other side before exhaling into the left side of the pose.

Seated Extended Side Angle A (Parsvakonasana A)

Ask students to extend their left leg long and straight. They can keep their right leg bent and toes pointing to the side. Invite students to come into the pose by opening their arms wide on an inhale, then on an exhale, dropping their right forearm to their right thigh and bringing their left hand to their side waist. Their left arm can also reach overhead, extending over their ear, creating a long diagonal line from the outer edge of their left foot all the way up to their left middle fingertip. Their gaze is up at their hand or the ceiling or down at their right

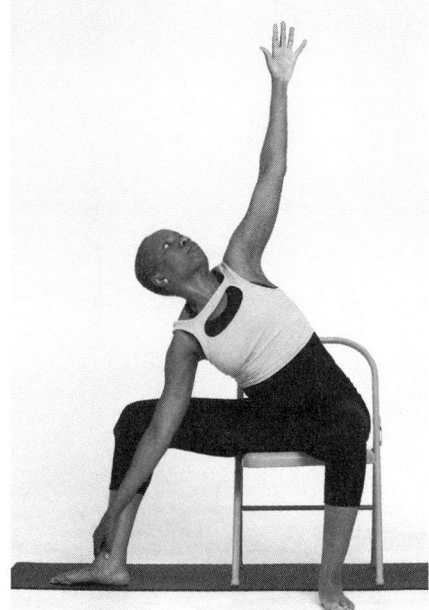

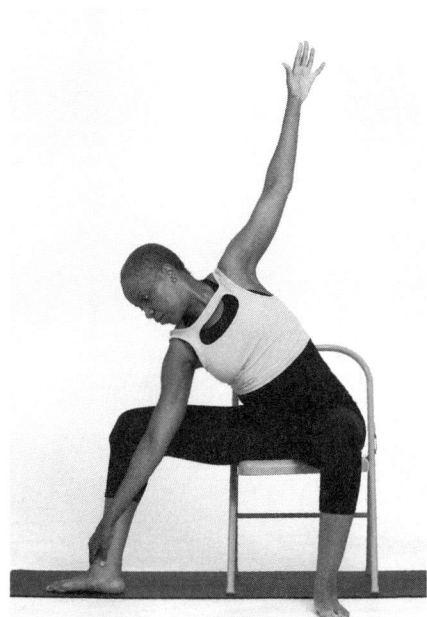
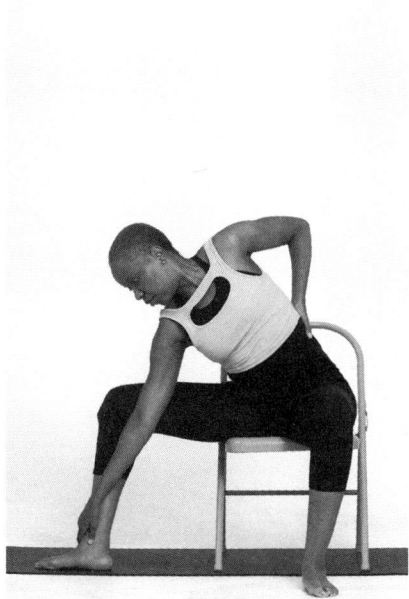

Seated Triangle Pose A (Trikonasana A)

big toe. Invite students to actively open their chest toward the ceiling and to feel into the long line from the outer edge of their left leg and up through their left fingertips before settling into stillness for five deep breaths. Instruct students to use the next inhale to lift up off their right thigh. On the exhale, guide them to switch their leg positions to set up for the left side of the posture. Settle into stillness for five breaths.

At the next inhale, guide students up and into the center.

Wide-Legged Seated Forward Fold (Prasarita Padottanasana) with or without Blocks

Guide students into a wide-seated stance and cue an inhale. On the exhale, invite them to fold forward between their legs, bringing their hands to the ground, shoulder-width apart. Students may use stacked blocks to support their head or hands if the full forward fold feels too deep.

When set up properly, this posture should feel supported and encourage a sense of surrender. Instruct students to bring awareness to muscular release and use the breath to aid in softening muscle tension. Stay in this pose for five breaths, and rise up slowly on the next inhale. It's common for students to feel a little light-headed when coming out of this posture. If dizziness occurs, encourage a few slow, calming breaths in a still, upright seated position before moving to the next pose.

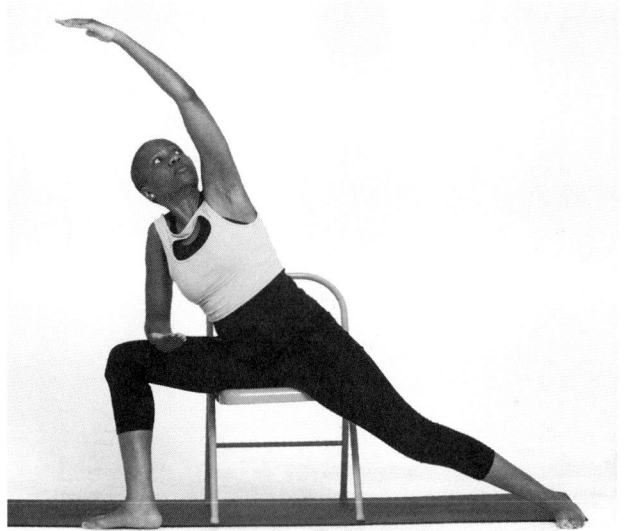

Seated Extended Side Angle A (Parsvakonasana A)

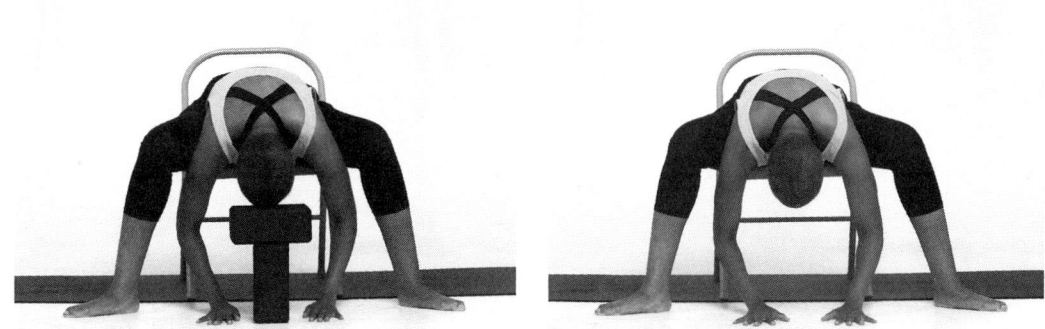

Wide-Legged Seated Forward Fold (Prasarita Padottanasana) with or without blocks

Seated Warrior 1 (Virabhadrasana 1)

Invite students to turn sideways to the right so they are sitting with their right buttock on the edge of their chair, wherever is most comfortable. Their left knee is bent and resting on a block, folded blanket, or the ground. The top of their left foot can be flat on the ground or their toes can be flexed with their heel pointing upward, which may lift the back knee up, where it can remain. Give students a chance to try all options and choose which one feels best. Their arms can be in several different variations, too. Hands can grip the edges of the chair, press in Prayer Pose in front of the chest, or reach up into the air shoulder-width apart or with palms pressed together.

The intensity of this posture is determined by these many discrete choices within it. Take time when teaching this to explore how different choices change the feeling in the body. This mindful exploration is at the essence of trauma-informed yoga, and the information gained by this exploration can be applied in all areas of life.

Seated Warrior 2 (Virabhadrasana 2)

Invite students to transition from Warrior 1 to Warrior 2 by straightening their back leg, pressing into the outer edge of their back foot, and reorienting their hips so they face the side of the mat instead of forward. They can orient

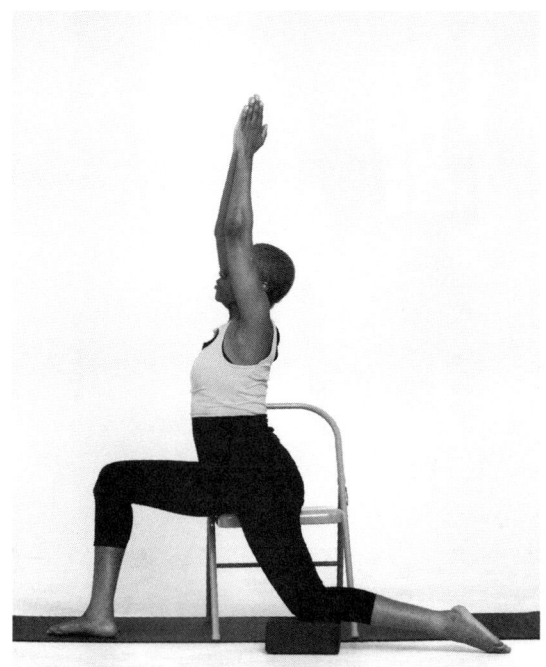

Seated Warrior 1 (Virabhadrasana 1)

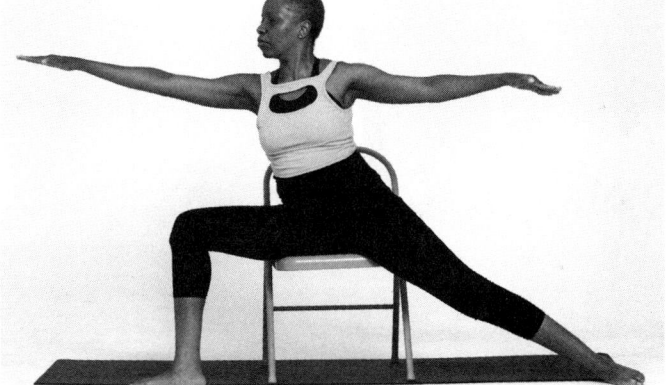

Seated Warrior 2 (Virabhadrasana 2)

their chest to the side as well. Encourage them to stretch their arms wide, keep their fingers together, and gaze over and beyond their front middle fingertip.

Stay in this pose for five breaths. Explore the gaze point in this posture by inviting your students to bring most of their three-pointed awareness there. Ask them to sense how the gaze is supporting any feelings in the pose.

Students can now flip their feet and bend their back leg to set up for Seated Warrior 1 on the left side, using the chair for support if needed. Repeat Warrior 1 and 2 on the left side.

Sun Salutation (Surya Namaskar)

Invite those students who wish to stand now to do so. Remind others of the Seated Sun Salutation they were introduced to earlier (page 136). Cuing both a Seated and Standing Sun Salutation at the same time can be extremely challenging! Make sure if you choose to offer both that you still watch and address the needs of your seated students. Overlooking the seated group may feel neglectful for the student and out of alignment with the intention to celebrate all choices students make in the classroom.

EQUAL STANDING POSE (SAMASTHITI)

Those who wish to now have the option of standing in Samasthiti. Guide students to feel the body in this shape, bringing their awareness to the entire space they embody. Ask them to tune in to their effort in this standing posture. Is it strained? Sloppy? What would a balanced amount of effort and awareness feel like? Is it possible to feel both alert and at ease? Remind students of the three-pointed focus and encourage them to deepen their sounded breath as they begin.

On the next inhale, ask them to reach up their arms, matching their breath to their movement. Palms can press together or remain shoulder-width apart. Invite students to gaze toward their hands if that feels right for their body. On the exhale, invite them to fold forward, bringing their hands to the ground, even if they bend their knees to get there. Encourage them to release their head down so their chin tucks toward their chest and their head drops heavily.

As they inhale, they can hinge at the waist halfway up, keeping their hands where they are or allowing them to slide up the legs for support. The gaze is at the nose tip. On the exhale, invite students to hop or step

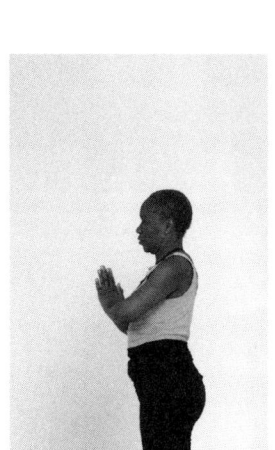
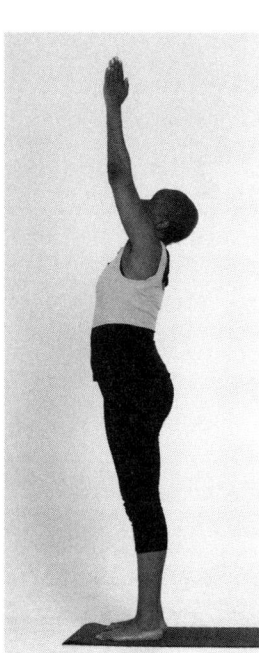

Sun Salutation (Surya Namaskar)

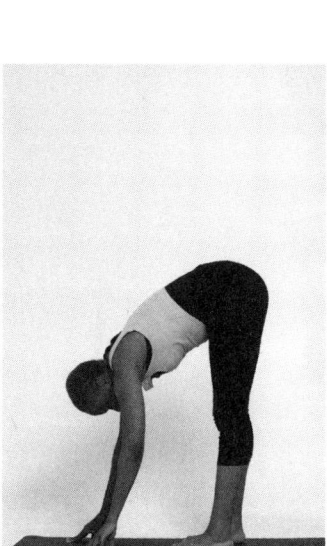
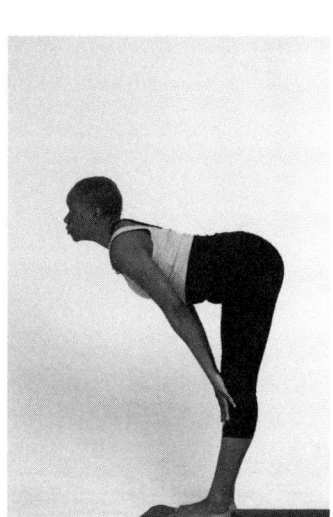

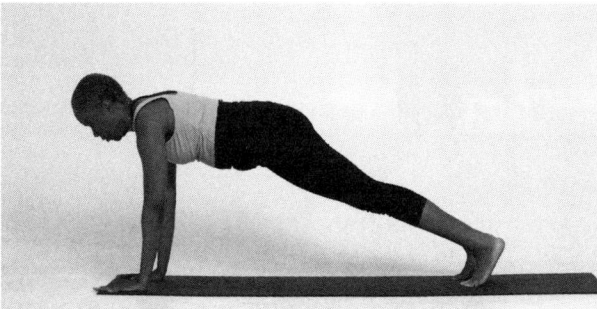
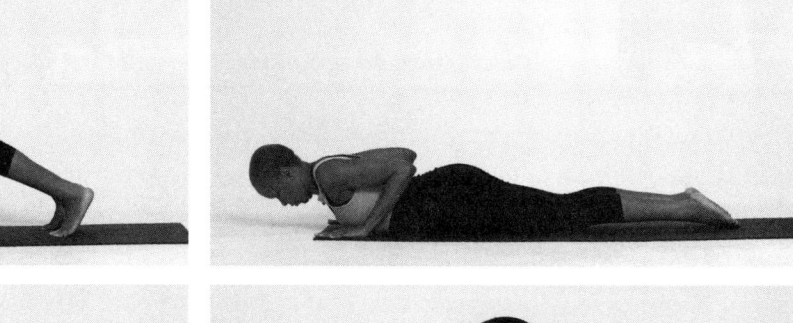

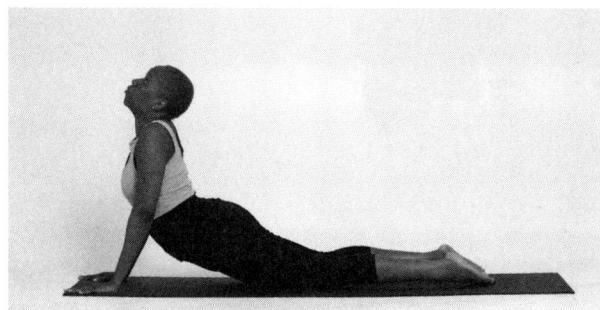
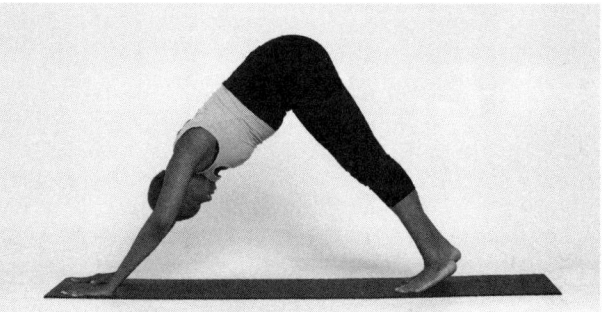

back into a plank position, with their shoulders aligned over their wrists and their feet hip-width apart. Continuing to exhale, they bend their elbows to lower their body to the floor. Knees can touch the ground, if needed for support.

Instruct students to inhale and move their hips forward, allowing their chest to move forward between their arms. The gaze can remain at their nose tip. If they would like, they can also allow their feet to roll or flip so the tops of their feet press down into the ground. In this position, the thighs can activate and lift off the ground.

On the next exhale, students transition from Upward Dog into Downward Dog. Students press their hands into the ground, flip their feet so the toes are flexed, and push their hips up and back. Invite them to spread their fingers wide and ground their palms. They can release any tension in their ankles before settling into stillness with their gaze toward their navel. Count five even breaths, cuing the Tristana and offering students the option to bring their knees down and take Child's Pose.

After the fifth exhale in Downward Dog, ask students to hop or step their feet forward and together at the front of the mat as they inhale and lift their torso and head up and gaze at their nose tip. Encourage them to fold deeply, hands to the floor and knees bent if needed, with the next exhale. On the next inhale, they can rise all the way upright with their arms overhead.

Finally, ask them to exhale and return to Samasthiti. You can talk them through this Sun Salutation three to five times, then invite them to try one on their own.

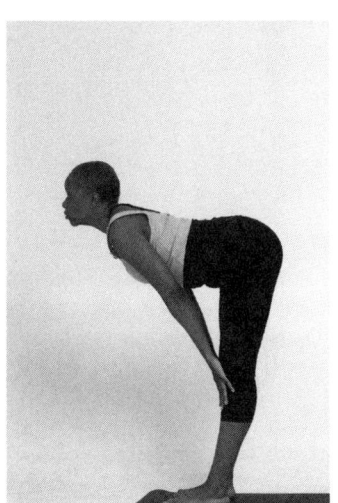 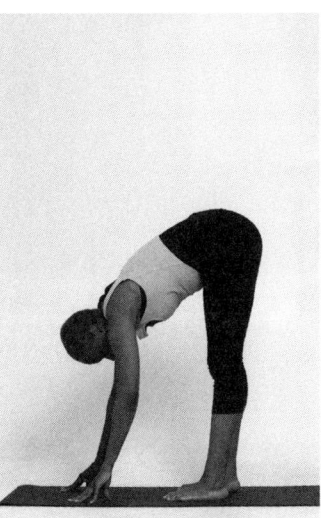 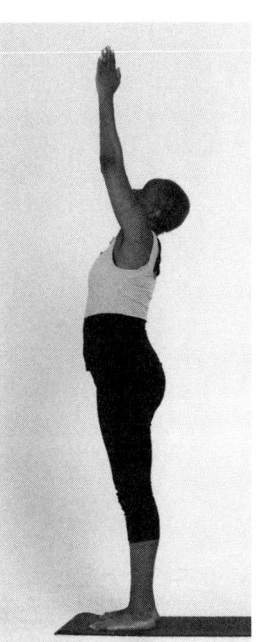 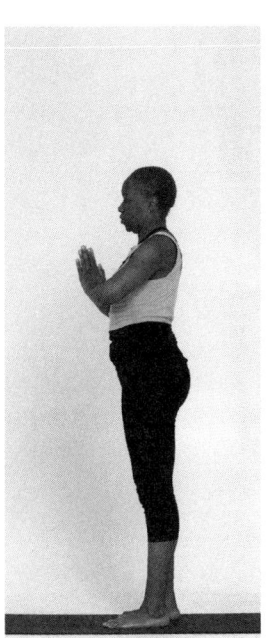

Downward Dog (Adho Mukha Svanasana) with Chair

All students may now enjoy the feeling of a supported Downward Dog. Invite students to bring their chair to the front of their mat, seat facing forward. They can begin by standing behind the chair with their hands placed firmly on the top. Guide students to walk back their feet until they are able to hinge at the waist and elongate their entire back. Advise that students press down with their hands to keep their chair grounded. Encourage them to send breath into their upper back and shoulder blades. Count five even breaths.

Supported Forward Fold (Paschimottanasana)

Next, have students turn their chair around and give them the opportunity to walk their feet forward and place their elbows and forearms on the seat. Invite them to fold forward. Encourage students to let their head hang heavily. If they prefer support, they can rest it on the seat or on a block or blanket on top of the seat. Count five breaths here, inviting students to bring deep focus to their breathing and how they might consciously release muscle tension. If you want, you might cue an audible sigh or a blowing of the air through the lips for further tension release.

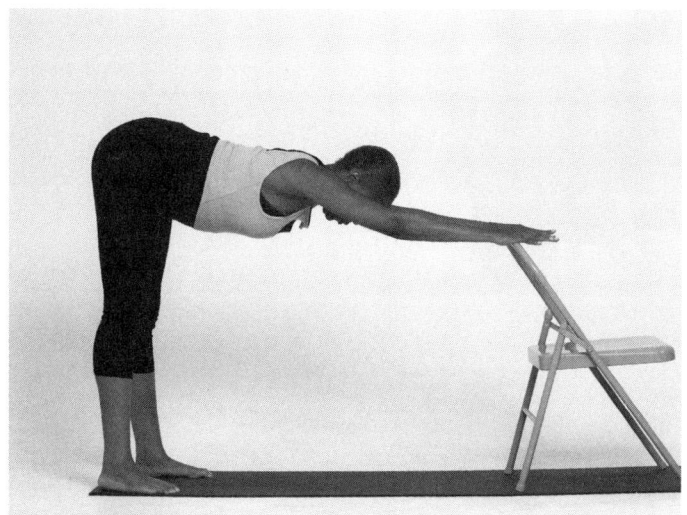

Downward Dog (Adho Mukha Svanasana) with chair

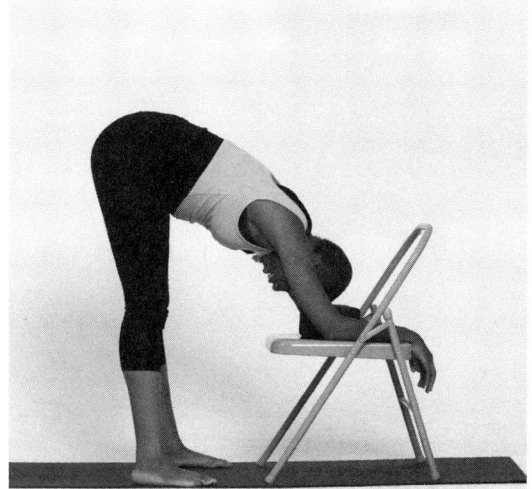

Supported Forward Fold
(Paschimottanasana)

Triangle Pose (Trikonasana A) with Chair A

From supported forward fold, students should rise slowly and leave one hand on the seat of the chair to transition into Triangle Pose. Students can take the other hand to their waist or reach it upward as they step that same-side foot back and turn its toes out. Their gaze can be down at their supported hand or up at their raised hand or the ceiling. Count them through five breaths, encouraging awareness of the three-pointed focus. It is also an option to do this pose from a seated position (see page 138).

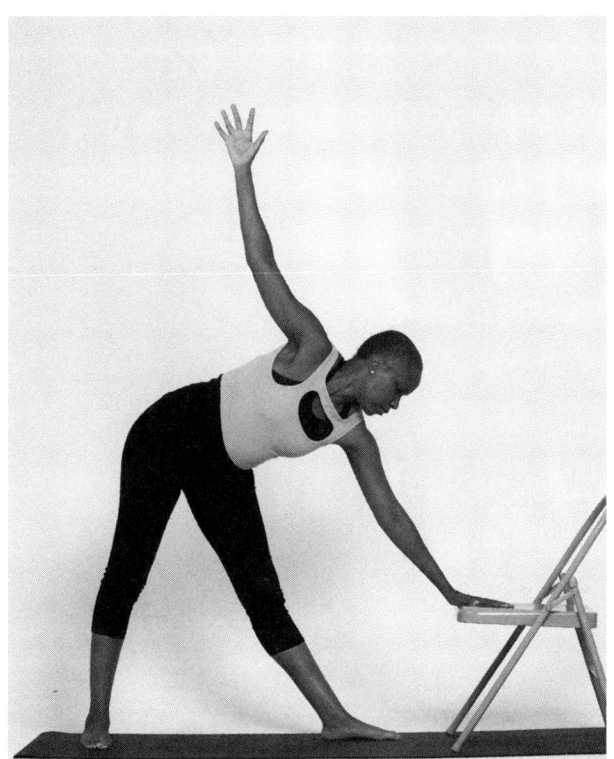 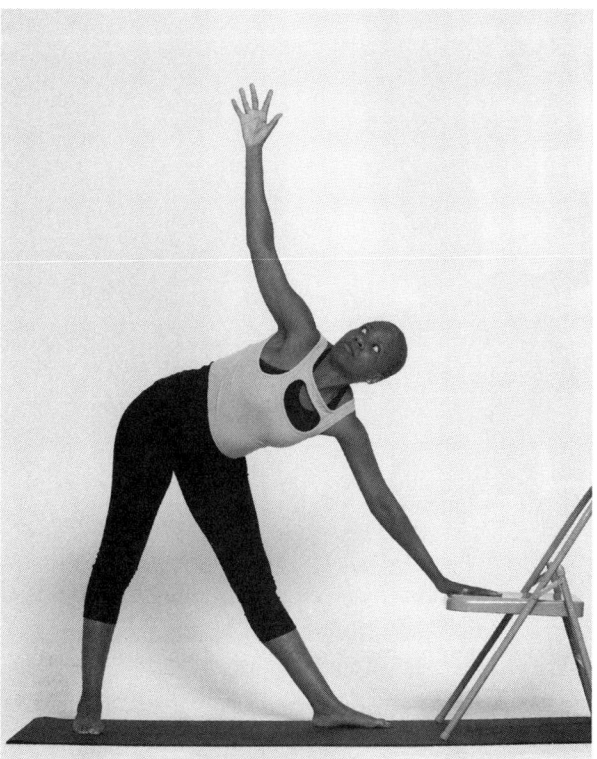

Triangle Pose (Trikonasana A) with chair A

Revolved Triangle (Trikonasana B)

Invite students to turn their back toes a bit toward their chair so they can square their hips forward. Have them see that there is at least hip-width space between their legs (more if the student feels off-balance) and that their heels are not crossing a midline. Ask practitioners to switch their hands so the side with the leg back has the hand on the chair and they are twisting toward the side with the leg forward. Their other arm can take the waist or reach upward.

Focus students on engaging their legs by pressing their feet into the ground for stability and using that stability to help move their hips forward. They can actively press their hand into the chair as well. On the inhale, steer them toward finding equal length on both sides of their spine. On the exhale, they can twist their torso to the side, softening their belly. Count five breaths here. Ask students to take a deep inhale as they come back up to stand. On their exhale, students switch their legs and repeat Triangle A and Revolved Triangle on the opposite side.

Seated Windmill Pose (see page 134) is a great seated alternative to this pose for those who feel too unstable in Revolved Triangle.

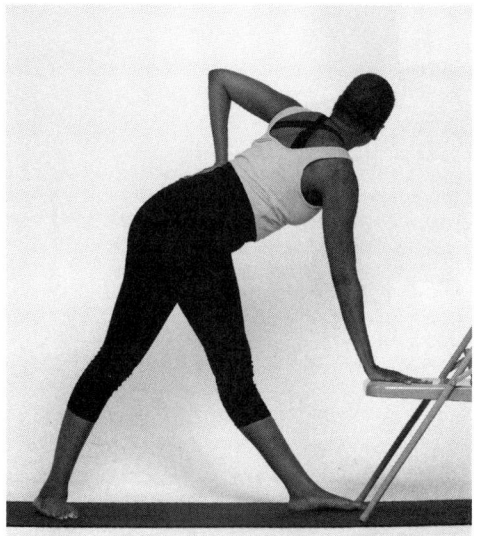

Revolved Triangle (Trikonasana B)

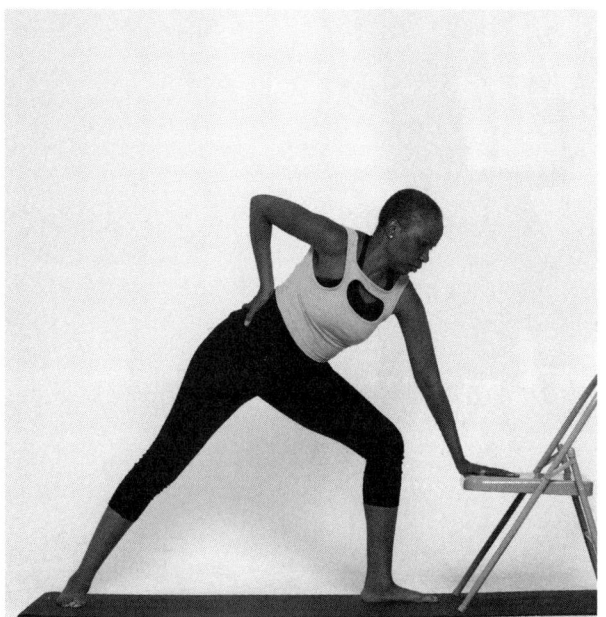
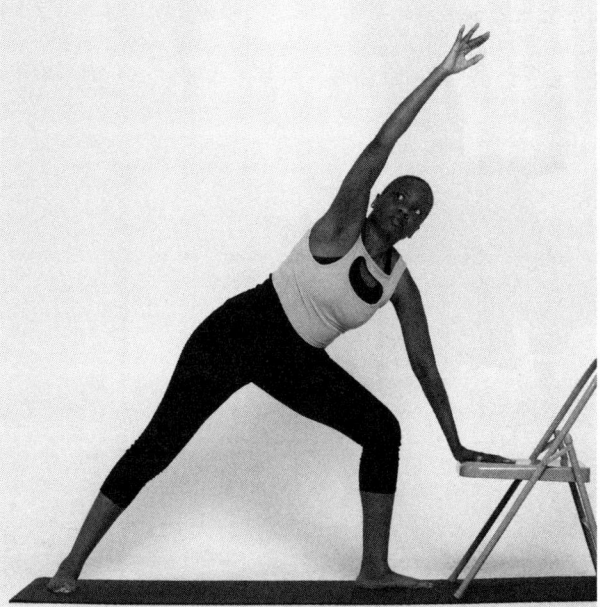

Extended Side Angle A (Parsvakonasana A)

Extended Side Angle A (Parsvakonasana A)

Invite students to take a wider stance to the side so their feet are about five feet apart with front toes pointed toward the chair or placed under it. The back foot is perpendicular to the front. Heels are aligned. Ask students to bend their front leg so their knee comes over their ankle. Place that side's hand on the chair for support. They can take their other hand to their waist or reach it up and over their head so it forms a long diagonal line from the outer edge of their back foot through their fingertips. Ask students to stay here for five breaths. After their last breath, cue students to straighten their legs and stand up on a strong inhale. Exhaling, they switch legs to set up for the other side of the posture.

Students can also take this posture seated in the chair (page 138).

Intense Side Stretch Pose (Parsvottanasana)

Ask students to turn to face their chair again and bring their back leg closer in for a shorter stance. As they grip the edges of the chair, cue students to hinge at their hips and fold forward for a strong back-of-leg stretch. Remind students that they determine much of the intensity by how deeply they choose to fold and to listen to the signals their body is giving them. Cue five breath cycles in this posture. Talk them through lifting up and switching legs to repeat the posture on the other side.

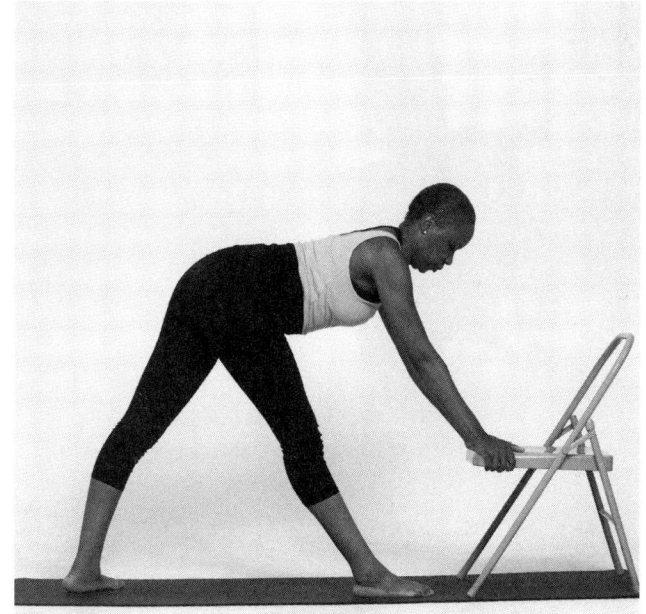

Intense Side Stretch Pose (Parsvottanasana)

Supported Wide-Legged Forward Fold (Prasarita Padottanasana)

Ask students to place their chair at the center of their mat. Invite them to place their feet wide and lean forward so their elbows and forearms rest on the seat of the chair. They can release their head forward, letting it hang heavily or placing it on the chair or on a block or blanket on the chair for support.

Encourage them to concentrate on their legs, making them firm and strong. Direct them toward exploring the feeling of their leg muscles engaging as the muscles in their neck and back release. How does one influence the other?

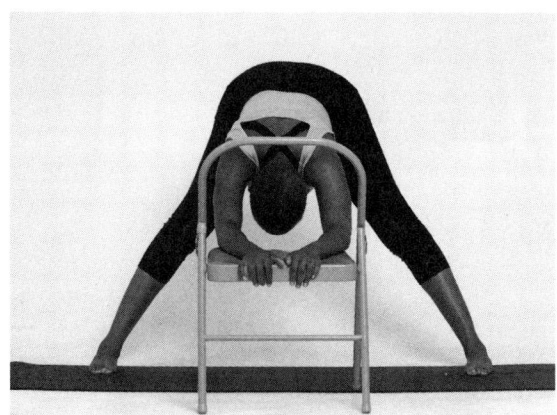

Supported Wide-Legged Forward Fold
(Prasarita Padottanasana)

Standing Big-Toe Hold (Utthita Hasta Padangusthasana)

Though it's called Standing Big-Toe Hold, I rarely teach the yogic toe bind in this posture. The focus is exploration of the internal network that keeps the body in balance. Ask students to position their chair so that it's at their right side. Students can stand to the outside of their chair;

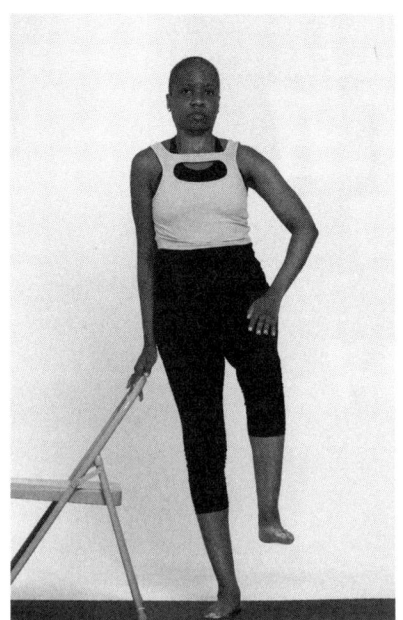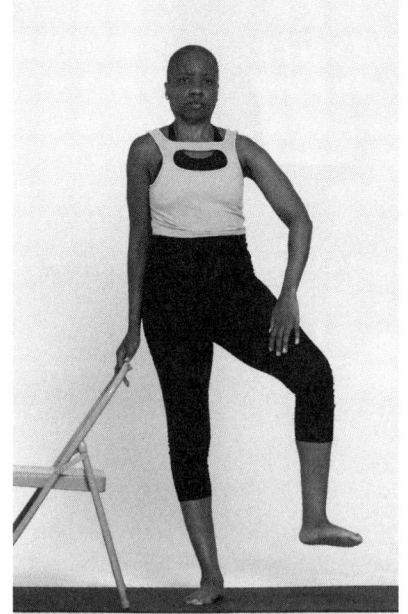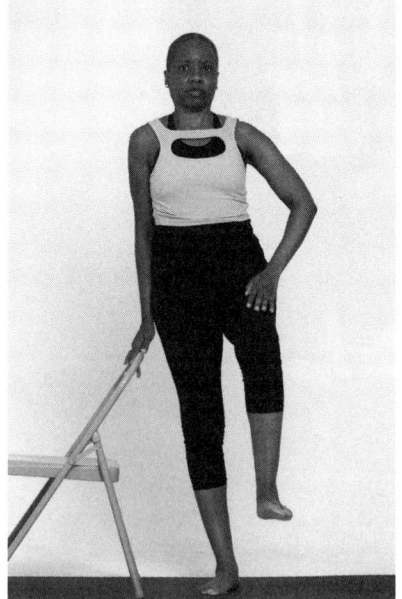

Standing Big-Toe Hold (Utthita Hasta Padangusthasana)

encourage them to use the chairback for support. Ask students to gaze at one spot straight ahead, lift their chest, and ground down so much through the leg closest to the chair that, like a pulley, the other leg can't help but lift up, with knee bent. They can also allow their foot to come up just a bit off the ground, perhaps resting their hand gently on their thigh or knee.

Ask students to stop here and reconnect to their three-pointed focus, noticing what it feels like to be in this balancing position. If they are stable and they want to increase the intensity, they can lift their leg a little more. Challenge students to stay here for five breaths with the same gentle focus they've held since the beginning of class.

Those who want to can then bring their leg out to the side, adding a hip opener. The gaze can remain forward, or they can turn their head away from the lifted leg and look to the side. Count five breaths here. Ask students to stay with the breath, noticing any sensations arising.

Guide students to bring their lifted leg to center, then lengthen and try to straighten it. Challenge them to keep their toes off the ground, even just an inch. Talk them through five breaths here before guiding them to bring their foot to the ground. Invite them to take a breath and feel into standing on two feet after balancing on one. Students can move to the other side of their chair to take the posture on the opposite side.

This pose usually elicits a lot of laughter. If it does, go with it. Give time for folks to let all that energy out before gently coaxing them back to concentration and stillness.

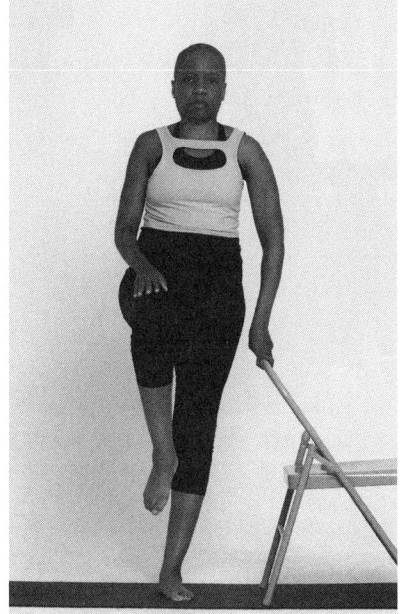
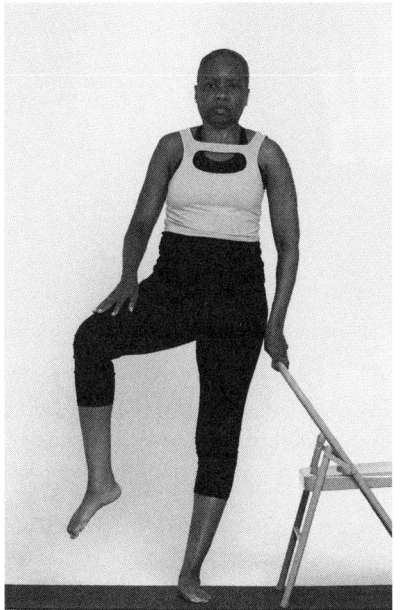
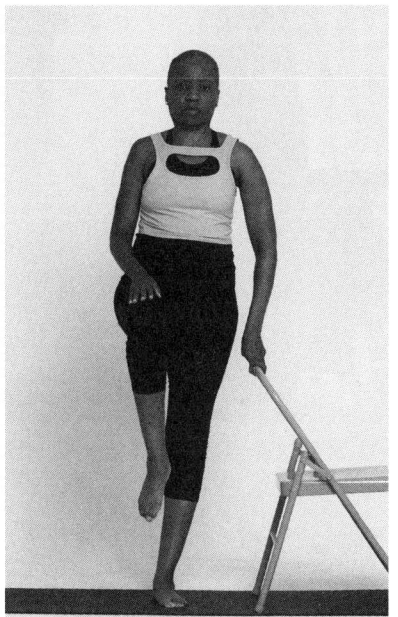

Staff Pose (Dandasana)

Invite students to return to a seated position in their chair. They can hold the sides of their chair and stretch their legs out in front. Invite them to flex their feet so their heels are on the ground and their toes come toward their body, stretching the back of their legs. Remind them to lift up through the sternum so there is some opening across the chest and shoulders. This is an important cue to offer, as it counters shoulder rounding, often seen after trauma and more broadly in our culture. They can gaze softly down the tip of their nose as they breathe in this position. Feel free to stay here longer than five breaths if you feel the class needs some time for grounding and centering.

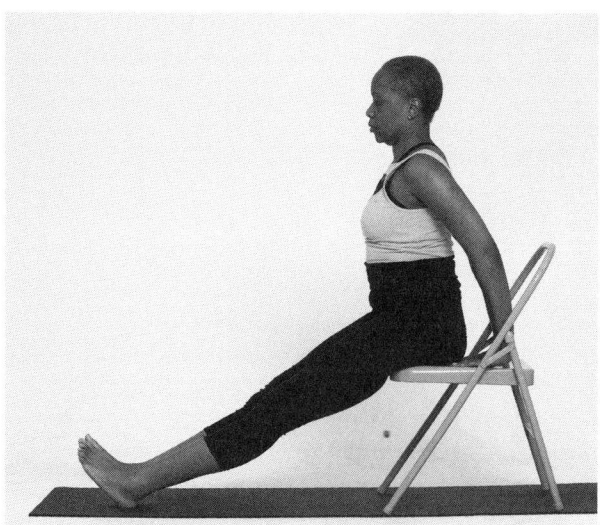

Staff Pose (Dandasana)

Seated Forward Fold (Paschimottanasana)

Remind students to keep their feet flexed and cue them to fold forward over their extended legs. When sensations arise, they should pause and focus on the breath count, waiting for the sensations to pass before folding more deeply. They can place their hands on blocks on the floor first, then bring their fingertips to the ground if needed. Let students know that uncomfortable sensations are normal in this posture. Invite them to be as still as possible and breathe into any

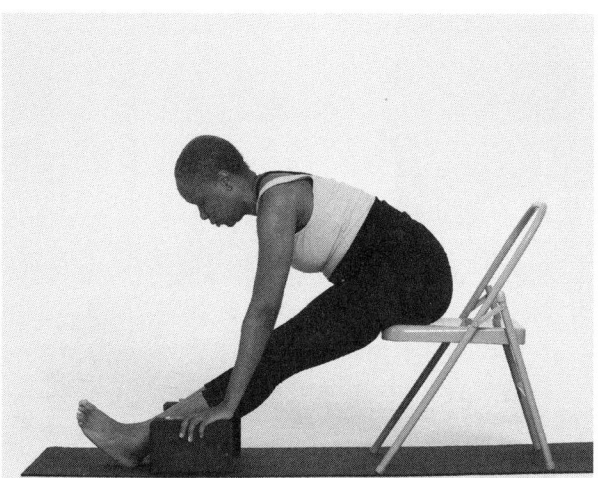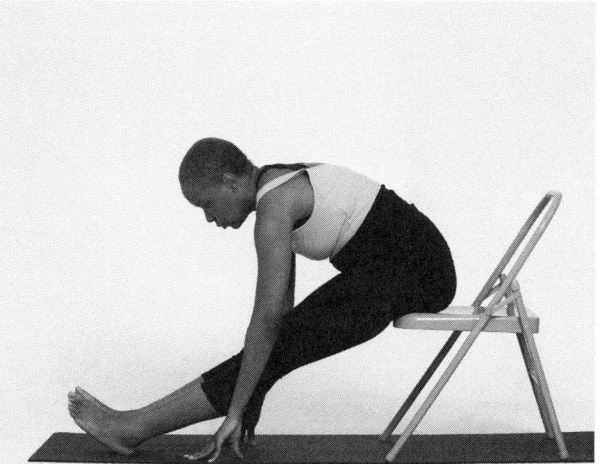

Seated Forward Fold (Paschimottanasana)

areas of discomfort while reminding them that if that discomfort grows, they can choose to disengage. Rest in this posture for five to ten breaths before slowly rising up to sit.

Upward Plank Pose/East-Facing Stretch (Purvottanasana)

Upward Plank Pose is a counterpose to the forward fold, a stretch for the front of the body. Still seated, students extend their legs in front with feet pointed, touching their toes to the ground. Ask students to grip and push into the sides of their chair to lift their body out of the seat. This lift works the muscles of the arms. Have students tune in to how they feel in this posture and how they can maintain steady strength in their arms to keep the body lifting throughout the five breaths. On an exhale, sit down on the chair.

This posture is contraindicated for some trauma survivors, so do not teach it to your beginners or until you know your group's needs.

Half-Bound Lotus or Ankle-to-Shin Forward Fold (Ardha Baddha Padma Paschimottanasana)

Cue students to keep one leg extended in front of them and bend their opposite knee, rotating their leg in the hip, and cradle the other leg up and in to place ankle on shin. The foot of the extended leg can be pointed or flexed, but the bent leg's foot must flex. If students have more flexibility, they can bring their foot up higher on the leg as long as they avoid placing their foot directly on their knee. Students can hold the chair as they hinge forward from the waist with a flat back. Encourage them to stop folding and find stillness as soon their chest starts to curl. Talk them through five breaths before guiding them to switch sides. (Alternatively, you may instruct the next pose, Easy Twist, first and then repeat both on the second side.)

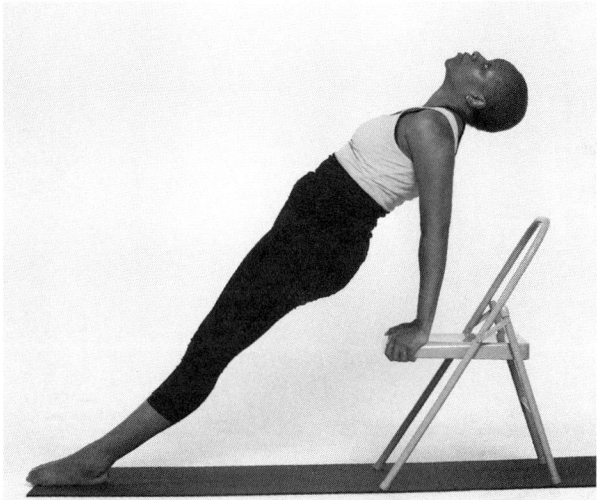

Upward Plank Pose/East-Facing Stretch
(Purvottanasana)

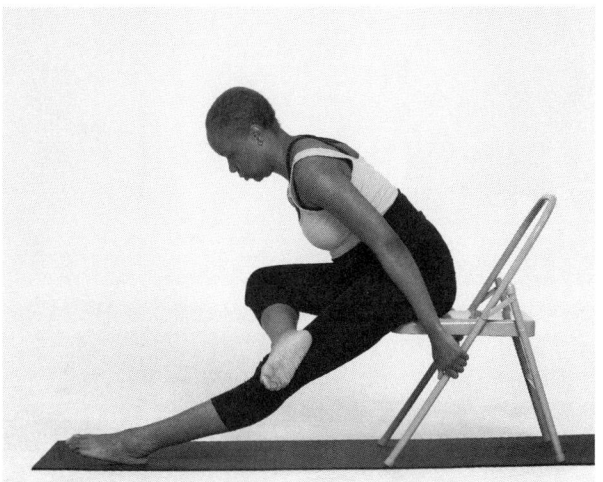

Half-Bound Lotus or Ankle-to-Shin Forward Fold
(Ardha Baddha Padma Paschimottanasana)

Easy Twist (Parivrtta Sukhasana)

It's a smooth transition from Ankle-to-Shin Forward Fold into a cross-legged twist. Students can bend their extended leg, placing the sole of the foot flat on the floor, and use that movement to slide the other leg into a cross-legged position. For those who can't cross at their thighs, their legs can be crossed at the ankles. The twist is the focal point. Ask students to take the hand on the same side of the body as the top leg to the back of the chair and their other hand to the outer side of their top knee. Encourage students to allow the weight of their body to drop more deeply into the support of the chair. Invite them to inhale and lift their spine gently, softening their belly as they do so, and on their exhale, twist. You can guide them to use their next few exhales to deepen the twist. As they do so, they can stretch their gaze behind them as far as they

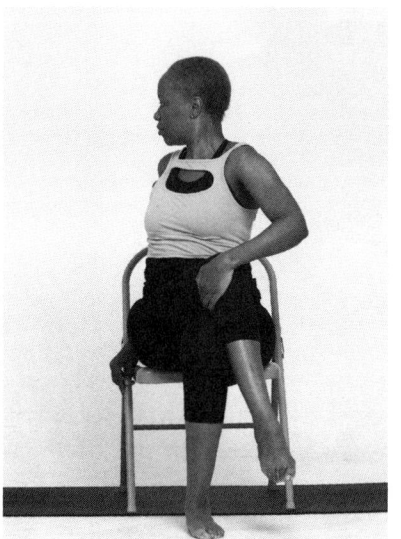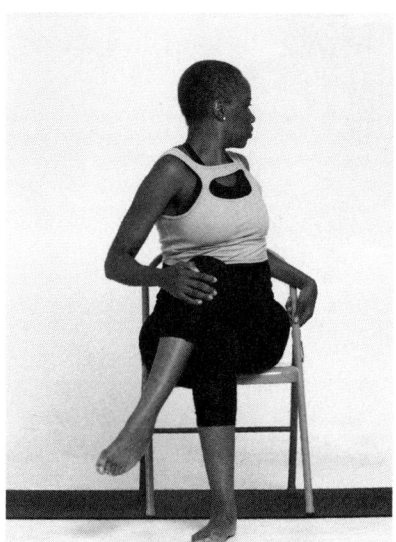

Easy Twist (Parivrtta Sukhasana)

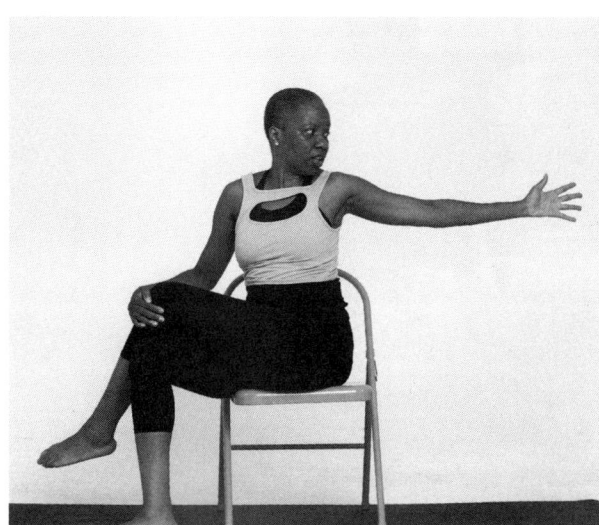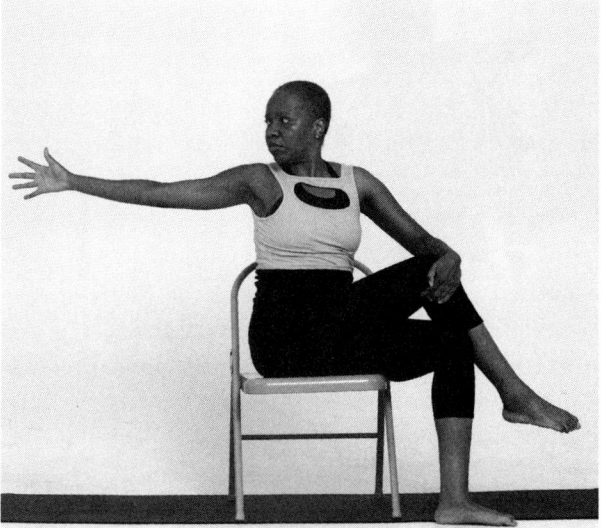

Easy Twist (Parivrtta Sukhasana) variation

can. After five breaths, instruct them to return to center, then switch legs and repeat on the other side.

VARIATION: EASY TWIST (PARIVRTTA SUKHASANA)

Students can stay with the previous posture, or if it feels possible, they can start exploring a more heart-opening version of this twist. This extended-arm variation stretches the muscles across the chest in a way that can feel unusual and sometimes uncomfortable. It offers students an opportunity to get more comfortable with their discomfort and also with their decision to stay in or come out of it. If concentration on the feeling of the body in this shape is too triggering, invite students instead to focus on their eyes as they gaze at their extended hand. If the pose is still too open, offer the opportunity for students to bend their arm at the elbow and place their hand to their heart. Breathe into that shape before extending the arm out again. Bring students back to a neutral position, facing forward on their chair before switching the crossed legs and repeating on the other side.

Seated Cat and Cow (Bitilasana Marjaryasana)

Bring students back to center and encourage them to feel both feet on the floor as the sequence shifts into the closing postures. Ask students to place their hands on their knees. Exhaling, invite them to push their knees gently away from their body as they draw their belly button toward their spine. This movement allows the chest to cave in and the shoulders to round. Inhaling, invite students to move their chest forward between their shoulders, allowing their shoulders to draw back and the back to arch. Ask students to repeat these Cat/Cow movements five to ten times, flowing with their breath. The final few cycles can be subtle and slow before coming to stillness.

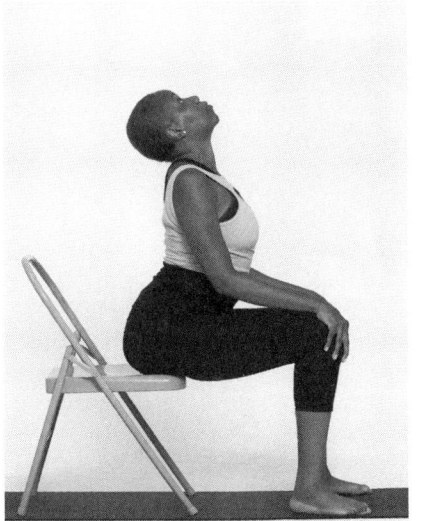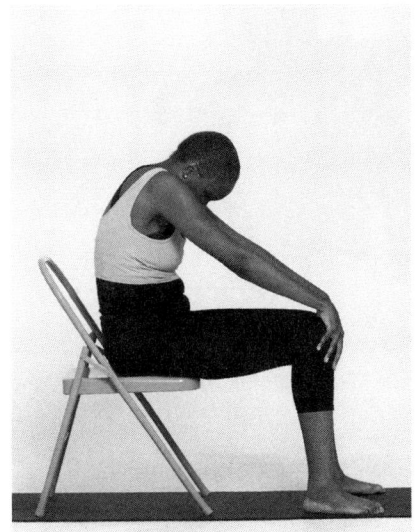

Seated Cat and Cow (Bitilasana Marjaryasana)

Final Rest (Savasana)

Final Rest looks different in a trauma-informed class and different in each body. Savasana can be taken while seated in a chair or lying on a mat with arms in any position that feels comfortable for the practitioner. The invitation is to be still in a way that feels right for the person's body. The gaze can rest softly at a spot on the floor, or the eyes can close. Hands can rest on the knees, chest, or belly, or rest cupped or nested in the lap. Encourage students to once again tune in to the parts of their body engaging with the chair and ground, allowing those parts to accept support. Guide them through a body scan, from their feet to the top of their head, prompting them to bring their attention into each part, but skip parts that feel triggering. The body scan builds awareness until they have a complete image of their body in their mind's eye, present and vital. When students finish their scan, offer them thirty seconds to a minute to be in quiet awareness before opening up the group for questions.

Special Consideration: Hospital or Bed Sequence

One of the biggest barriers to yoga practice is the idea that it has to be done in a certain kind of place (such as a yoga studio) with special props

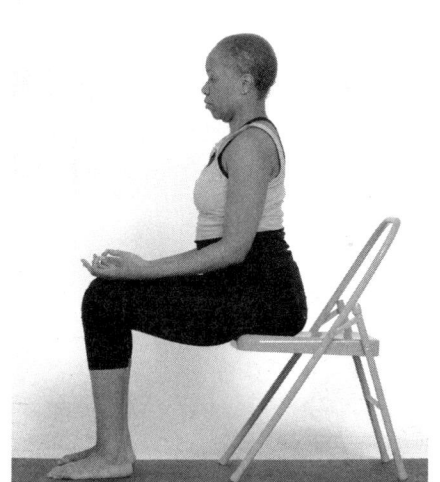 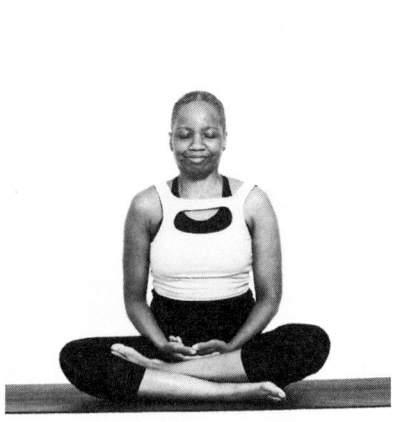 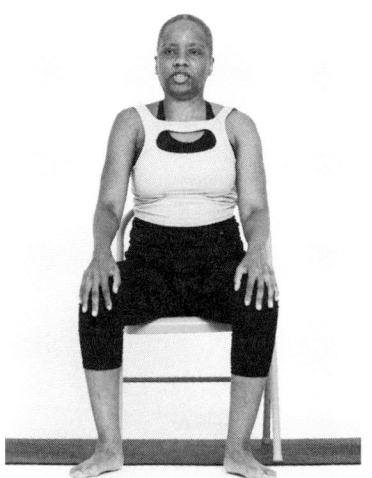

Final Rest (Savasana) variations

and clothing. The truth is that the practices are designed to support us throughout our lives, including during our most challenging times. We never have to wait for the ideal circumstances to practice.

The following poses demonstrate just that: they can be done on the floor, on a mat, or on a bed. They can be incorporated into the previous sequence before Savasana, or they can be done as a stand-alone sequence in the morning, evening, or anytime one is confined to or in bed. You can offer these postures to students to practice on their mat in class or invite them to experiment with these poses at home. And if you are fortunate enough to have the opportunity to share yoga with someone who is hospitalized, you can offer these there as well.

One-Legged Wind-Relieving Posture (Apanasana)

Invite students to lie on their back, then hug one knee into their chest. Remind them not to push or squeeze too hard but instead to hug only as deeply as they are comfortable. When they feel resistance, they can stay there, breathing into any tension and feeling for muscles signaling release. They may begin to feel where things want to shift. Encourage them to stay as present as possible with sensations and allow their knee to come in closer naturally without force. Stay with this posture ten or more breaths before switching sides. Ask students to recognize how each side feels different without having judgments around this.

Supine Spinal Twist (Supta Matsyendrasana)

Ask students to bring the first knee back into their chest, then, with an exhale, let it sink in closer to their chest. Cue a deep inhale and, as students exhale, instruct them to let their knee drop across their body, moving their spine into a gentle twist. Invite students to stretch the opposite arm away from their body and look away from their knee, aiming to keep both shoulders down as much as possible. Challenge students to take ten or more breaths here, then with an inhale, lift their knee and return to center. With an exhale, repeat posture on the other side.

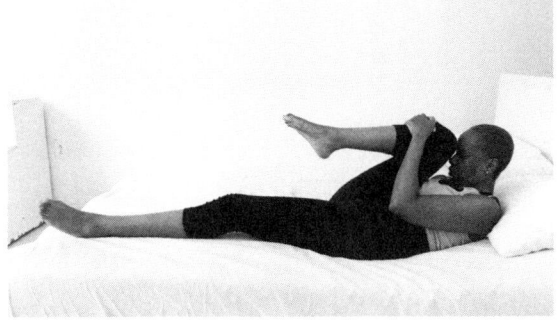

One-Legged Wind-Relieving Posture (Apanasana)

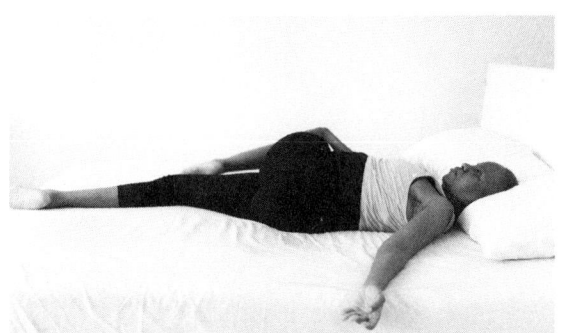

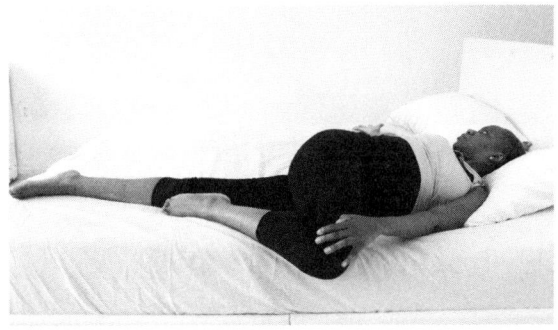

Supine Spinal Twist (Supta Matsyendrasana)

Reclined Extended Hand-to-Big-Toe Pose (Supta Utthita Hasta Padangusthasana)

With students lying flat and centered, cue them to lift one leg up and wrap their first two fingers around their big toe. It's okay if the knee is bent. You can invite students to straighten only as much as they can. Bring their attention to their breath and remind them to allow their leg to release with each exhale. The unbound hand can be used to encourage their leg closer or to press their opposite thigh to keep it grounded.

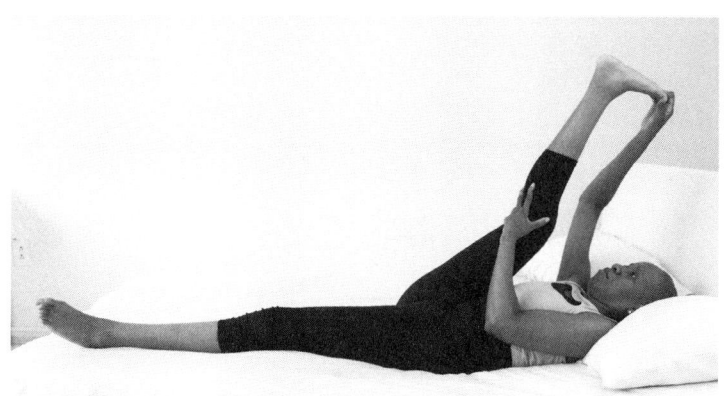

Reclined Extended Hand-to-Big-Toe Pose
(Supta Utthita Hasta Padangusthasana)

Two-Legged Wind-Relieving Pose (Apanasana)

Invite students to hug both legs into their chest and rock up and down on their spine for a gentle spinal massage. This should feel good on the back. Let students know they should stop immediately if it doesn't. As a challenge, they can try to roll all the way up to a seated or squatting position. Their ability to do so may be impacted by the firmness of the bed.

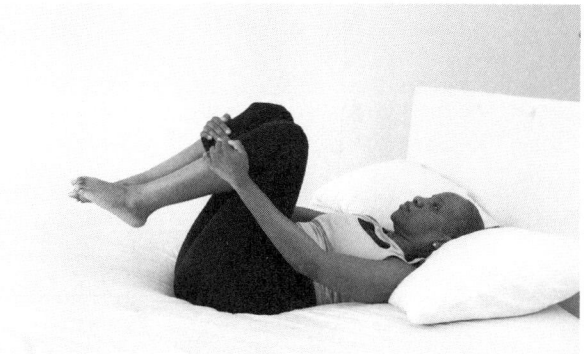 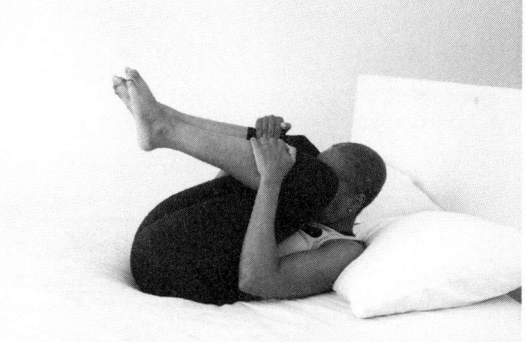

Two-Legged Wind-Relieving Pose (Apanasana)

Upward Plank Pose/East-Facing Stretch (Purvottanasana)

Sitting on the bed, invite students to cross their legs and reach their hands behind them, palms grounded. On an inhale, cue them to press into their hands and lift their back and chest for a final heart-opening posture. Encourage them to soften their throat and the muscles of their face to allow for more breath to flow in. As with all heart openers, always give the option to skip this pose or to come down at any time.

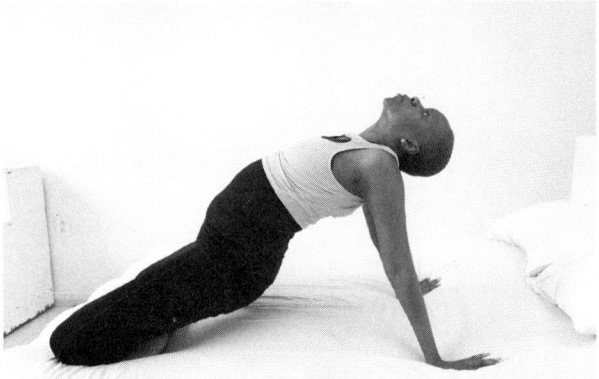

Upward Plank Pose/East-Facing Stretch
(Purvottanasana)

Seated Forward Fold (Paschimottanasana)

Follow the heart-opening asana with a long forward fold, which can help bring the energy more inward. Invite students to be in this shape in stillness and awareness for ten breaths, allowing sensations to come and go without reaction.

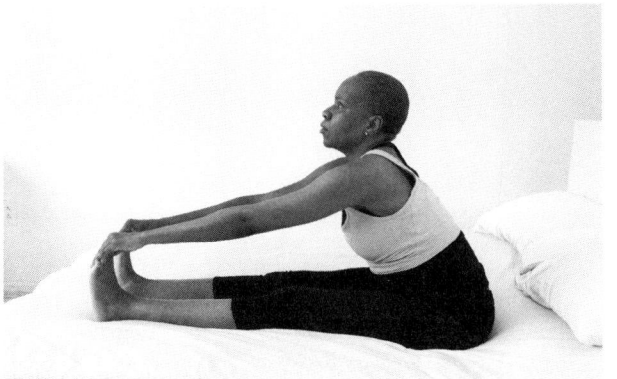
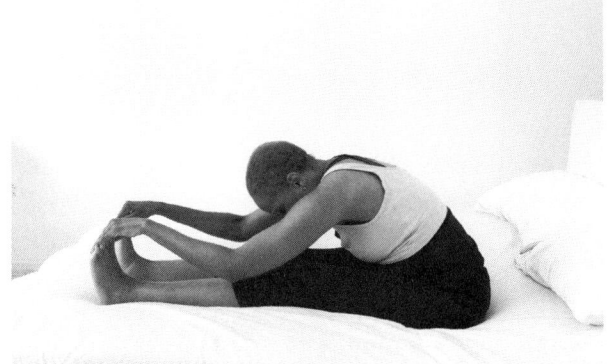

Seated Forward Fold (Paschimottanasana)

Legs Up the Wall (Viparita Karani)

For a final closing pose, guide students to extend their legs up the wall and place their hands on their belly and chest. Encourage them to stay present in this asana and to work their way up to ten to twenty minutes in this restorative position. Let them know they can bend their knees slightly if they start feeling achy. If practicing this posture at night, students can transition to sleep afterward.

Seated Five-Pointed Star or V for Victory Pose (Utthita Tadasana)

If students are just starting their day, help them give their energy a boost by closing their practice with their arms held up high and wide in a V. Challenge them to stay in this shape for one minute before concluding their practice.

Honing the Trauma Sensitive Teaching Voice

I suggest the teacher practice this sequence while cuing themselves the way they would a trauma sensitive class. Notice what comes naturally and which parts are harder to cue. Practice those sections again on yourself and eventually with a willing friend or practice partner. Take notes to better remember what you want to change or work on.

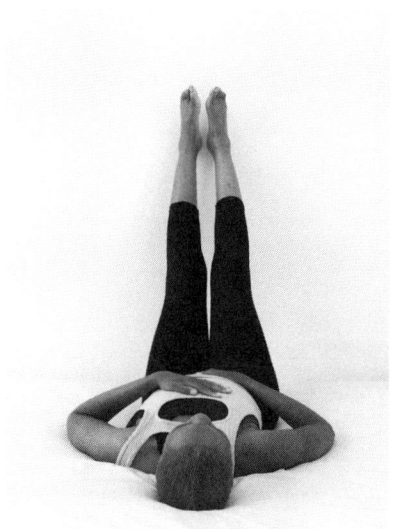

Legs Up the Wall
(Viparita Karani)

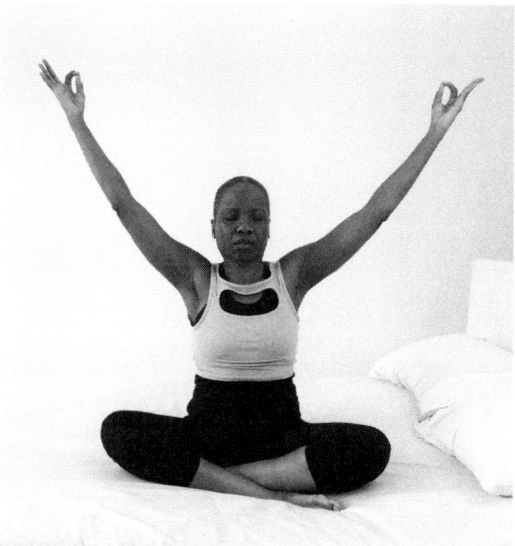

Seated Five-Pointed Star or V for Victory Pose
(Utthita Tadasana)

Healing and Awakening Sequence: Modified Ashtanga Flow with Samantha

In some ways, Sam's sequence is classical Ashtanga modified for her amputation, but it veers off in interesting ways to address subtle emotional trauma that manifests as tightening in backbending and hip-opening postures. Teachers should note when working with this sequence that it is quite advanced. Omit postures or substitute more accessible postures from other sequences if you'd prefer to modify this. It's also important to note that the inversions are intended to be held as long as possible to counter overly stimulating heart-opening postures such as Camel Pose (Ustrasana) and Pigeon Pose (Kapotasana). These poses often leave students bubbly and excited, a result teachers can mistake for progress. Though your students may feel good after backbending, this is more of a fleeting feeling brought on by nerve activation than a long-term shift toward more happiness and balanced emotions. Teachers should be aware of this and focus on long-term emotional regulation. Forward folds and inversions offer balance and calm the nervous system. This sequence is appropriate for experienced practitioners who have matured in their focus and crave a full-body asana experience with special attention on working the spine.

Sun Salutation A (Surya Namaskar A)

Equal Standing Pose (Samasthiti)

Starting students in a standing position helps them build discipline and confidence and dispels the myth that one has to warm up to practice or to do other life tasks. It's important when you do start your class in Samasthiti, however, that you allow some time for finding the three-pointed focus. Encourage practitioners to come to stillness and steady their eyes on one spot. Remind them to feel the shape of their body in space, guiding them to take special care to recognize the top, back, and sides of their body and other areas that can often go unnoticed. Tune them in to their breathing and ask them to bring some energy into their breath. Remind them to listen to and hear each of their inhales and exhales. Only when you feel they've captured this three-pointed focus should you guide them into movement.

Invite students to inhale and reach their arms up overhead, allowing their gaze to follow. Guide them to exhale and fold forward, letting their head hang heavily, touching the ground with their hands even if they must bend their knees to do so. On the next inhale, ask them to rise from the waist halfway, lifting their head, while trying to keep their hands on the floor. On their exhale, cue them to keep their chest forward, head up, and shoulders aligned over their wrists as they hop or step back their feet into a plank position. Ask students to bend at their elbows to lower down to

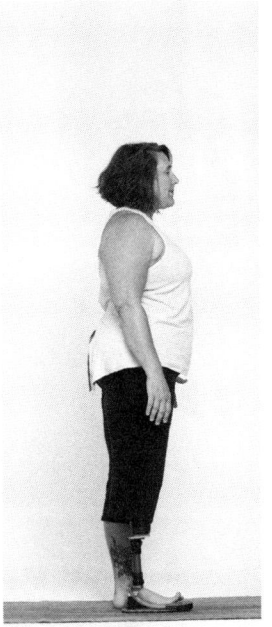
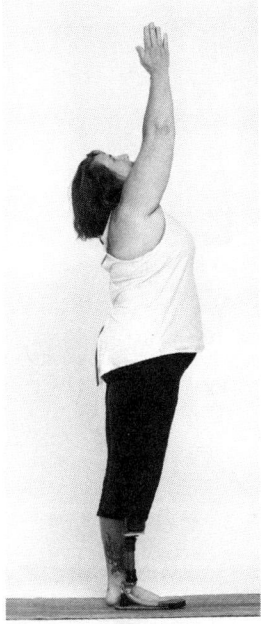
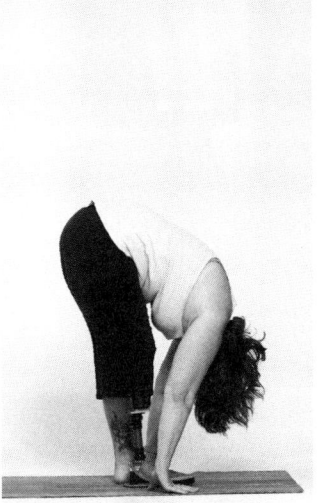
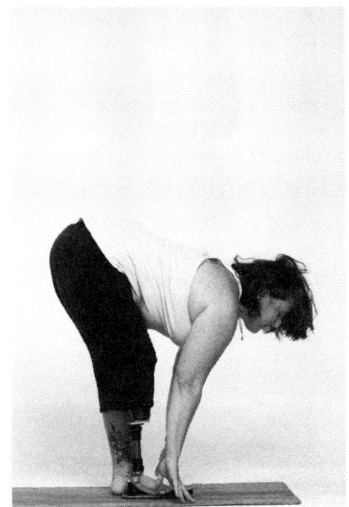

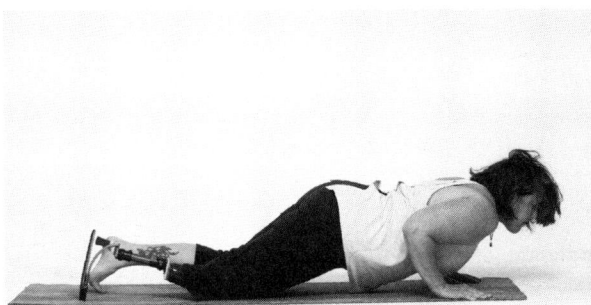
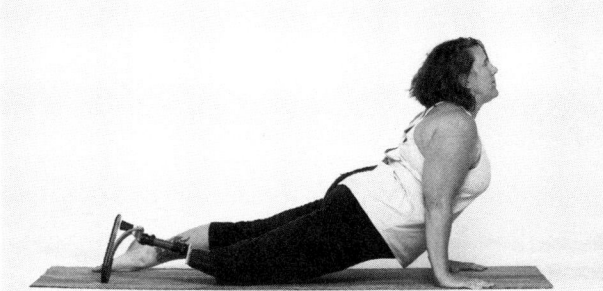

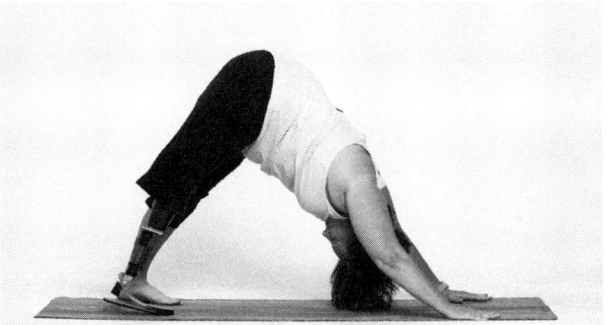

Sun Salutation A (Surya Namaskar A)

the ground, either with bent knees or with straight legs for increased intensity.

On the next inhale, students can roll their hips forward and lift their chest up, letting their sternum lead, for Upward Dog, keeping their gaze on their nose tip. Then exhaling, they can press back into Downward Dog, bringing their gaze toward their navel. Stay in this posture for five full breath cycles, trying to remain aware of each breath.

After the fifth exhale in Downward Dog, instruct students to step their feet forward and together. With an inhale, they can lift their head up with hands or fingers touching the floor.

As they exhale, cue them to fold forward deeply, dropping their head toward the floor.

On the next inhale, they rise all the way up to standing, sweeping their arms overhead. On the next exhale, ask students to return their arms to their sides and into Samasthiti. Invite them to repeat this sequence three to five times, cultivating focus and inward attention with each breath.

Sun Salutation B (Surya Namaskar B)

Practitioners should now be in Samasthiti. Encourage them to remain in stillness as they take a breath or two before starting Sun Salutation B. To begin Sun Salutation B, on an inhale, ask students to bend their knees as they reach their arms upward at a diagonal, keeping their gaze at their fingertips. Exhaling, students can fold forward and straighten their legs as much as possible, as in Sun Salutation A.

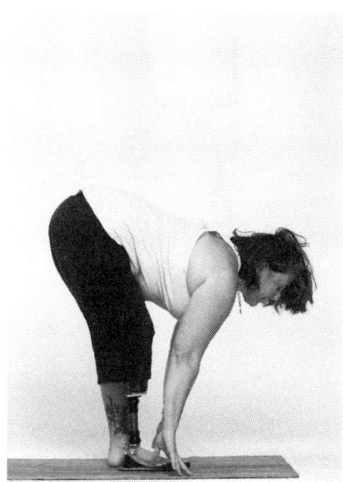
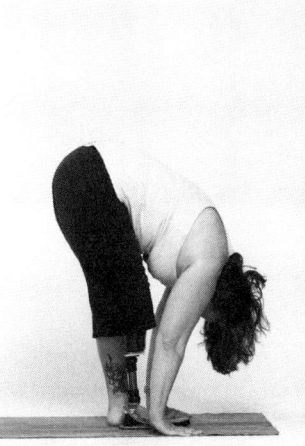
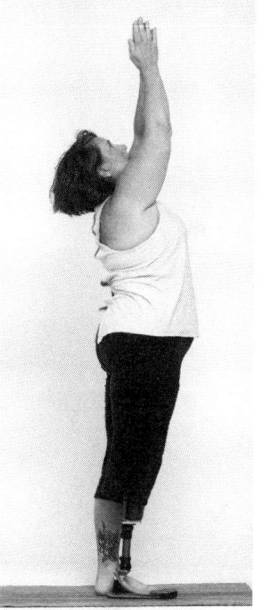
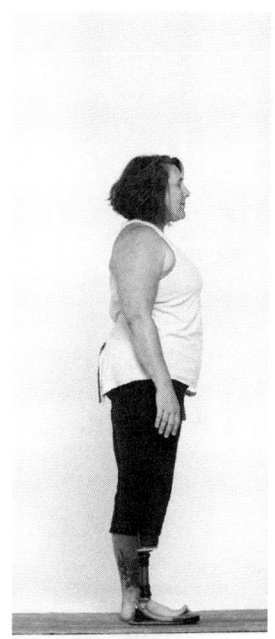

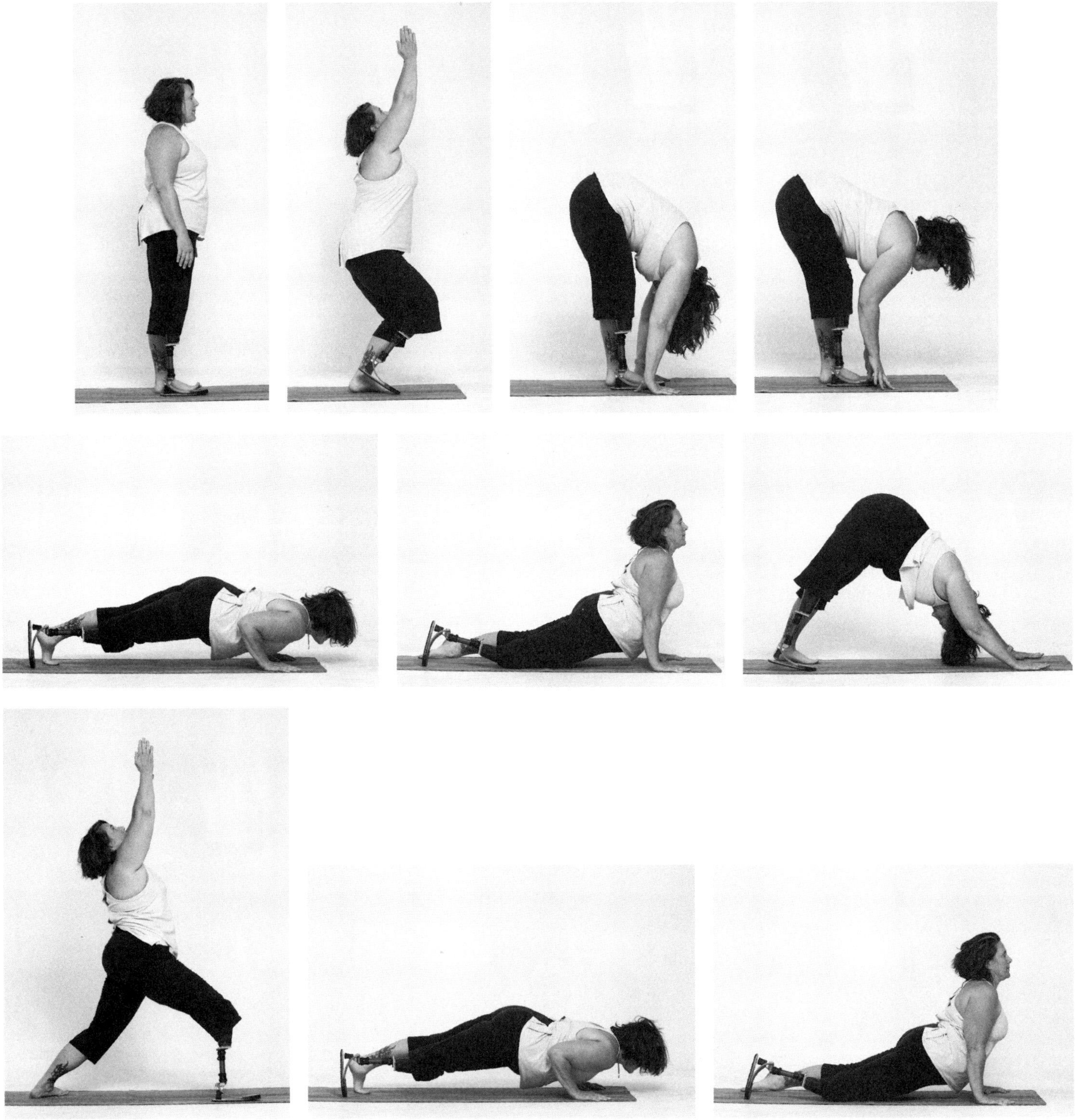

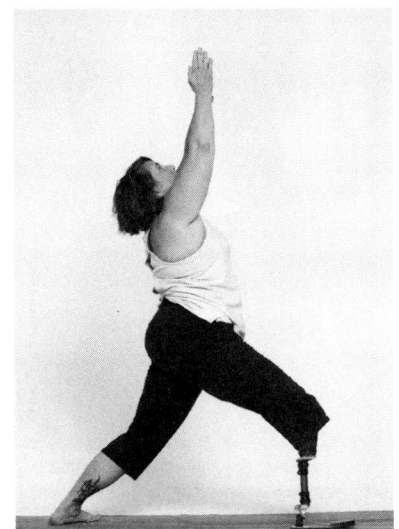
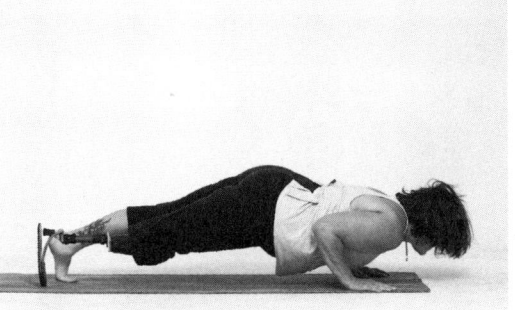
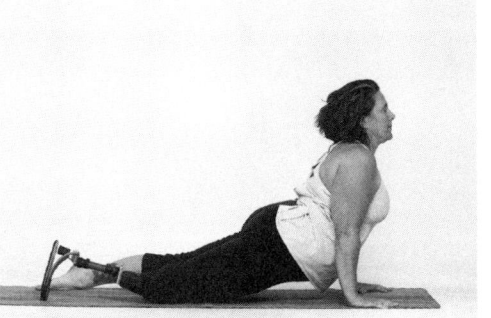

Sun Salutation B
(Surya Namaskar B)

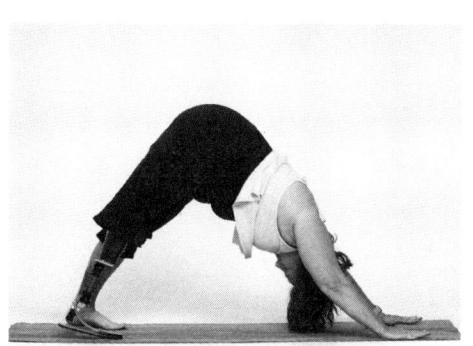

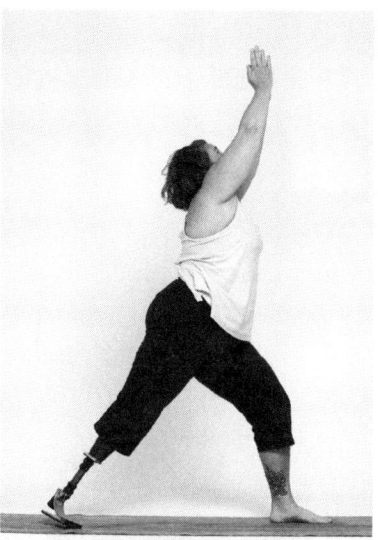

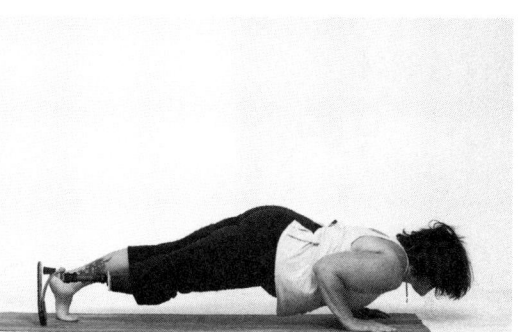

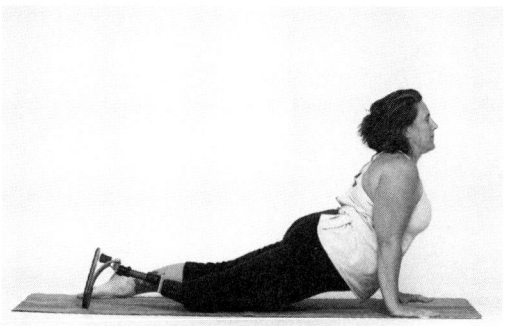

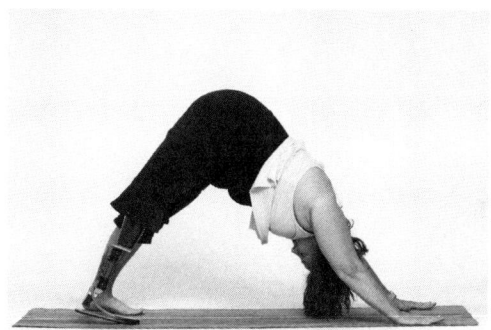

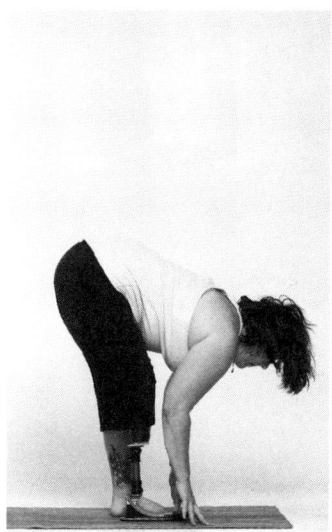

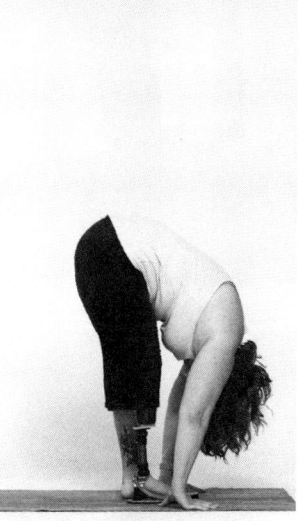

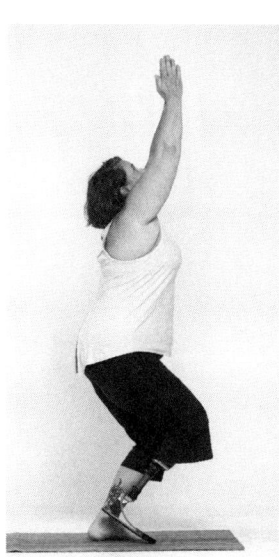

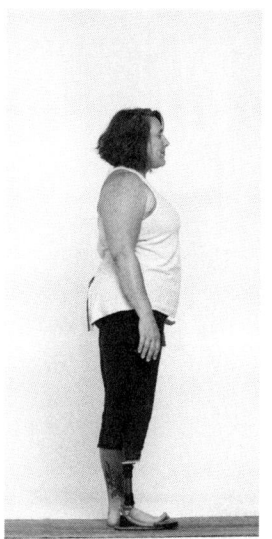

On the inhale, students can lift their head up, aligning their shoulders over their wrists. With the exhale, they can hop or step back into a plank position, bending at their elbows to lower their body down with bent knees or with straight legs for more intensity.

Invite students to roll forward, lifting their thighs, hips, and chest for Upward Dog. Their inner thighs are engaged to ensure their lower back and the rest of their body are supported. Exhaling, cue them to push back into Downward Dog.

On the next inhale, students can step their right foot forward and pivot their left heel to the ground, heels aligned, reaching arms up and touching palms to rise into Warrior 1. If they can't step their foot forward from standing, they can use their arms to help, or bring their back knee to the ground first and step forward from there.

Next, cue students to come all the way down from Warrior I into Chaturanga, using one exhale if possible. To do so, they should bring their hands to the ground, shoulder-width apart, at the front of their mat. Keeping their chest forward and shoulders over their wrists, they step their right foot back to meet their left as they bend their elbows (and knees if they want to) and lower down. If holding Chaturanga is too challenging, students should feel welcome to lie all the way down on the ground. Then ask them to inhale, roll forward, and lift their chest for Upward Dog. On the exhale, they push back into Downward Dog.

On the next inhale, students step their left foot forward and pivot their right heel to the ground, heels aligned for Warrior 1 on the other side. The same modifications can be taken here as on the first leg, if needed. Challenge students to use one exhale to come all the way down into Chaturanga, using the same modifications as described on the first side.

On their inhale, students can roll forward into Upward Dog. On their next exhale, they can come into Downward Dog or take a Child's Pose. In either position, they should stay for five breaths and cultivate the three-pointed focus. After five breaths, those in Child's Pose lift into Downward Dog.

Instruct students to step forward, bringing their feet together, inhaling, and looking up with their fingers touching the ground. On the next exhale, they can fold forward. Then, with an inhale, ask them to bend their knees as they lift their chest and arms, palms together, keeping their gaze is at their fingertips.

The next exhale brings them into Samasthiti. Invite students to pause for a few breaths before repeating this salutation two or three times. If students have memorized this flow, they can do these repetitions on their own count, matching the movements to their own breath pace.

Triangle Pose A (Trikonasana A)

From Samasthiti, have students inhale and step out to the side of the mat with their feet three feet apart and parallel to each other. Direct them to reach their arms wide and stretch out through their right fingertips so their whole torso moves to the right. When they can't stretch any further to the side, they should reach downward, placing their right hand on their right leg or a block, or to take their big toe. They can stretch their left arm up into the air or bring their hand to their waist. Their gaze is up at their fingertips or down at their toes if there are issues with balance or neck pain.

After getting into the pose, encourage students to take a moment to press into their feet and engage a feeling of lift. Guide them toward lengthening their spine in both directions, up through the middle of their head down through their tailbone. Stretch both vertically and horizontally in opposite directions. Then, with continued attention on those actions, ask them to turn most of their attention to the feeling of the whole, embodied shape. Invite them to imagine themselves as a structure in space—the front, back, top, bottom, and sides all one collective unit. Remind them to keep their eyes steady and listen as they breathe five breaths in and out. How does this experience differ from one in which the focus is on each individual body part?

Instruct them to inhale to come up, pivoting their feet parallel with their arms wide. On their exhale, repeat the posture on the left side.

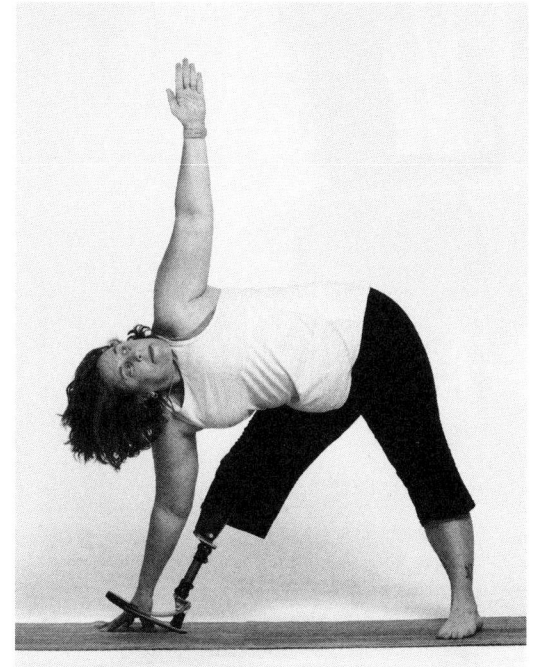

Triangle Pose A (Trikonasana A)

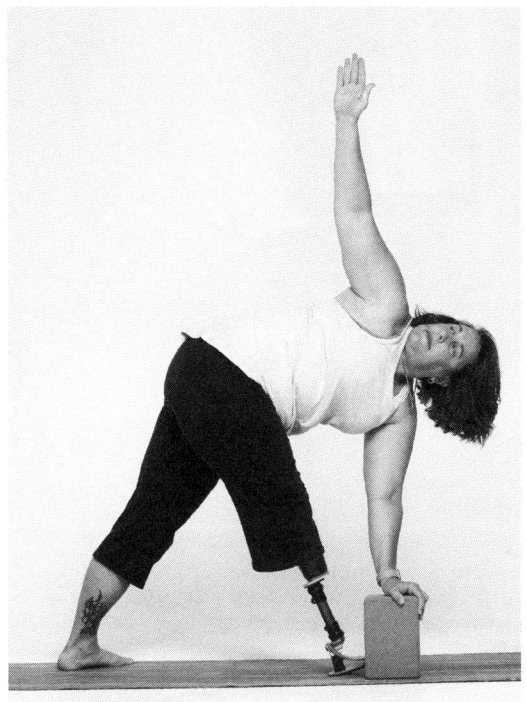

Revolved Triangle (Trikonasana B)

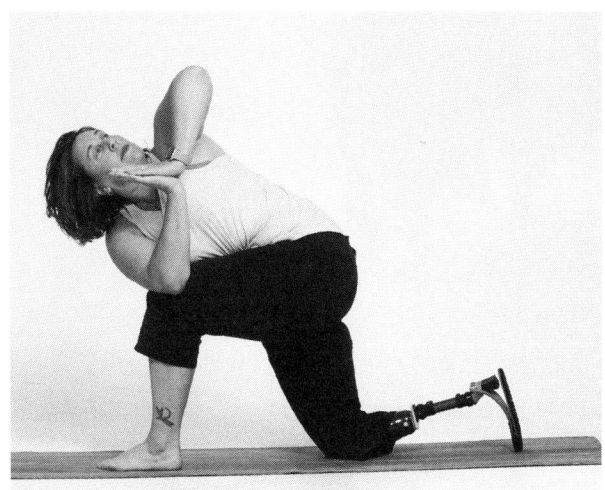

Revolved Side Angle (Parsvakonasana B)

Revolved Triangle (Trikonasana B)

After Trikonasana A, lead students through an inhale to come up through center, then ask them to pivot their feet so their right foot faces out again and their left toes turn so their hips can square forward. Then request they reach downward and take their left hand to the outside of their right foot for the twisting version of triangle. Remind them that it is normal to feel instability in this posture. They can turn their attention to the reactions this posture is causing in their inner world. Can they work with the pace and intensity of the breath to shift that reaction?

If students need more stability, suggest they take their feet wider apart from each other horizontally so their heels or arches are no longer aligned. They can also place their left hand on the floor to the inside of their right foot when twisting. Whatever variation they take, remind them to breathe and soften their belly to deepen the twist.

Cue them through an inhale to come back up through the center position, pivoting their feet as they turn, and an exhale to take the left side. Take students through five breaths there and then through an inhale to rise up before bringing them back with an exhale to Samasthiti.

Revolved Side Angle (Parsvakonasana B)

Ask students to step their right foot to face the back of their mat and drop their back knee to the ground. Invite them to lift their arms up high and stretch through the sides of their body as they press into their feet.

Then have them take their left elbow to the outside of their right knee so their knee is tucked near their armpit. Encourage them to bring their palms together and pull them toward their heart to deepen the twist, making sure their top elbow points up at the ceiling. Invite them to find ways to soften and open to deeper breaths even in a constricted position. Stay here for five breaths before switching legs and repeating Revolved Side Angle on the other side.

Wide-Legged Forward Fold A (Prasarita Padottanasana A)

Before including this posture in the sequence, make sure your classroom space allows for students to be staggered with enough space to fold forward to the side of their mats. If they have the space, invite them to take the widest stance they can while still feeling grounded. Their feet can be parallel to each other or slightly pigeon-toed (toes facing in). Welcome students to bring their hands to the ground, shoulder-width apart, with fingertips and toes aligned. On their inhale, request that they lift their head up and gaze at their nose tip.

On their exhale they should bring the crown of their head toward the ground and breathe five breaths there with their gaze resting at their nose tip. Encourage them to engage and use the power of their legs to increase their stability in this posture.

To come out, cue them to inhale and lift halfway up from their waist. They can stay and exhale there. Then on the next inhale, lead them the rest of the way up to stand and bring them back to the front of their mat to Samasthiti.

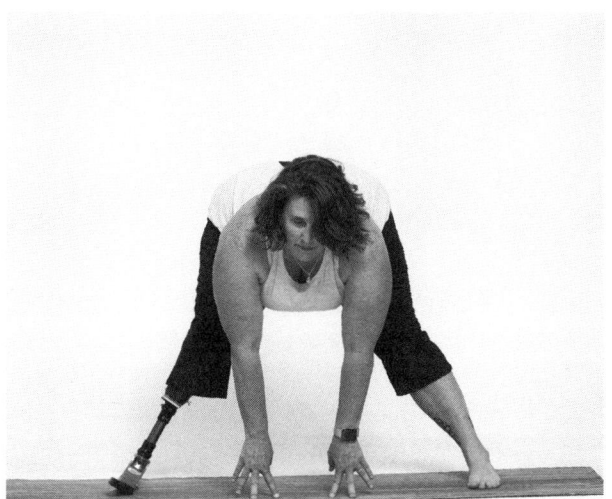 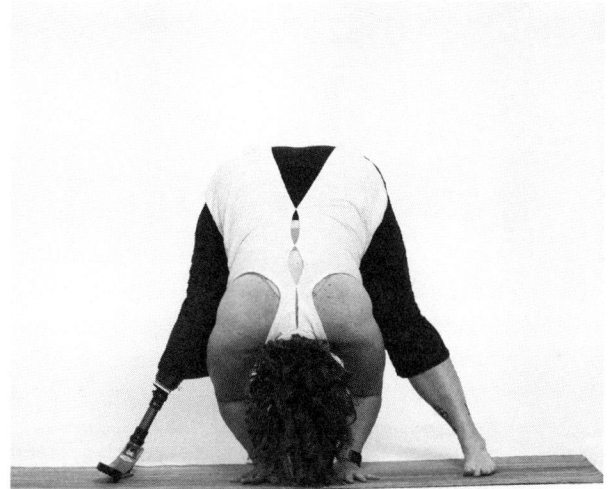

Wide-Legged Forward Fold A (Prasarita Padottanasana A)

Intense Side Stretch Pose (Parsvottanasana)

Students can continue to strengthen, stretch, and stabilize their legs in this last fundamental standing asana of the sequence. On an inhale, guide students to take a small step and pivot to face the back of their mat. Cue them to bring their arms behind the back to hold opposite elbows or slide hands into Reverse Prayer Pose. On their exhale, they can fold forward over their extended leg. They should drop their head, letting their neck curl, and gaze at their nose tip. If their chest can lie flat on their extended leg, they can place their chin on their leg and look down at their big toe. Cue them to breathe five conscious breaths in this position. Then bring them through an inhale to come up and an exhale to pivot and fold over the other leg. Cue them through five breaths on that side before inviting them back up to stand and step to the front of their mat for Samasthiti.

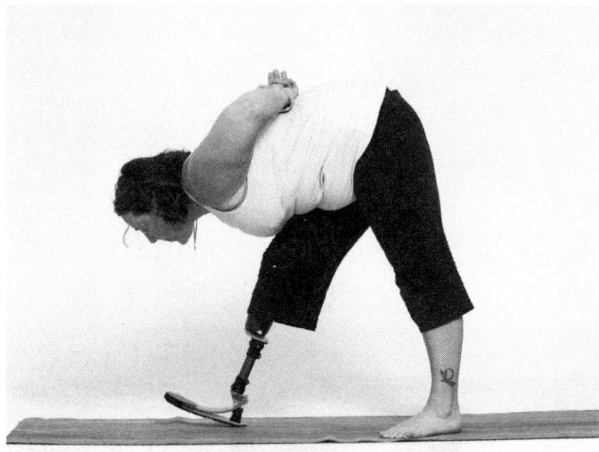

Intense Side Stretch Pose (Parsvottanasana)

Standing Big-Toe Hold (Utthita Hasta Padangusthasana)

For this powerful standing balance pose, students can use a chair for support or balance hands-free. Remind students that the focus is on finding power in the legs and exploring feelings of opposition within the body. Ask students to press down through their left leg so much that the right leg can't help but lift off the ground. They can touch the top of their right knee or take their big toe with their right hand. Students can straighten their right leg if they want to. Even as the leg extends, the shoulder pulls back in, creating friction and opposition, which aids in balance. Students can gaze at their foot or at a spot in front of them. Count five breaths.

Then invite students to take their leg out to the side and shift their gaze over the opposite shoulder. They can stay here for five breaths.

Close the pose by directing students to bring their leg back to center and take their hand to their waist. They can hold their leg aloft, at any height, for five breaths. Repeat this sequence on the other side.

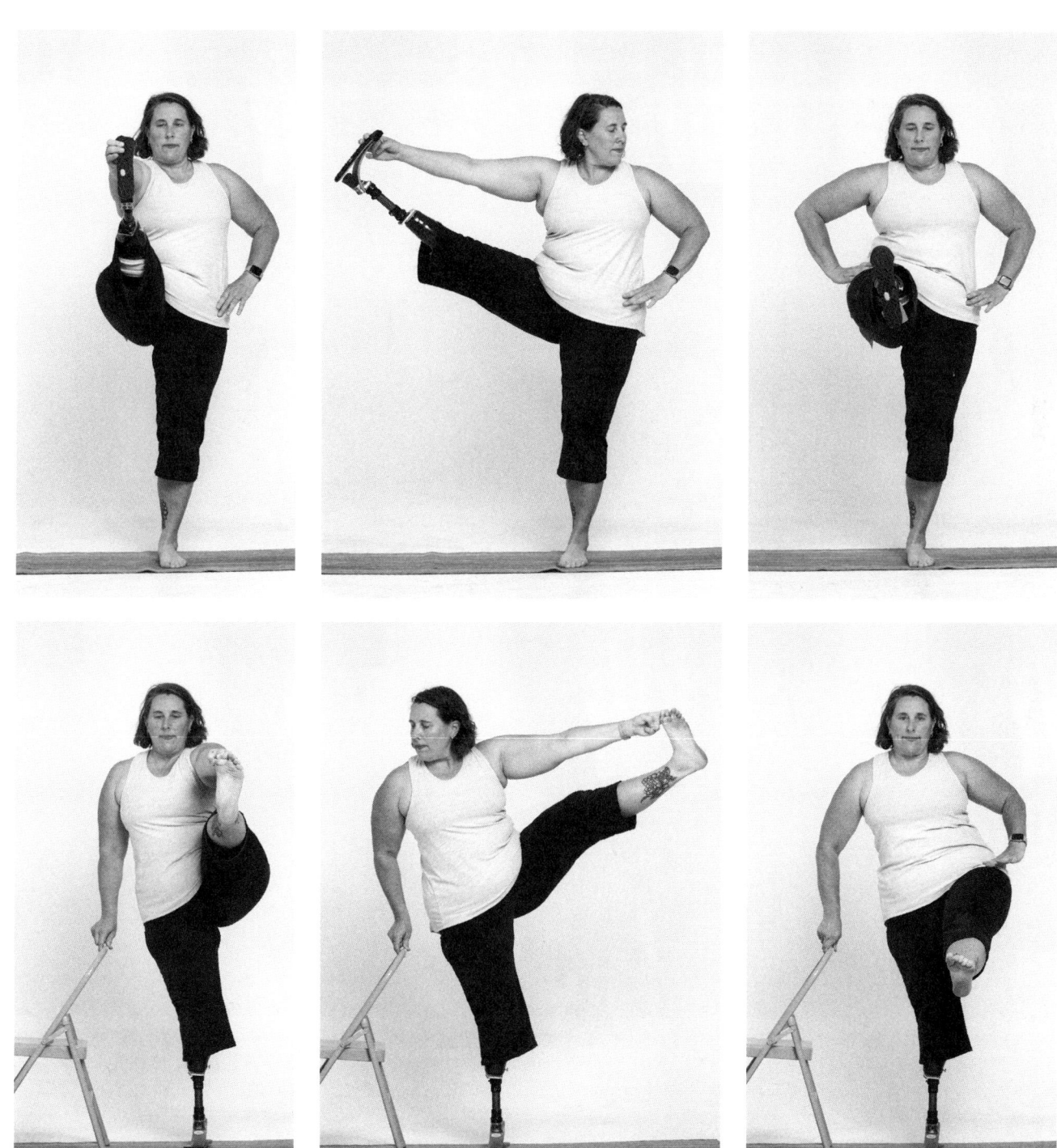

Standing Big-Toe Hold (Utthita Hasta Padangusthasana) and variations

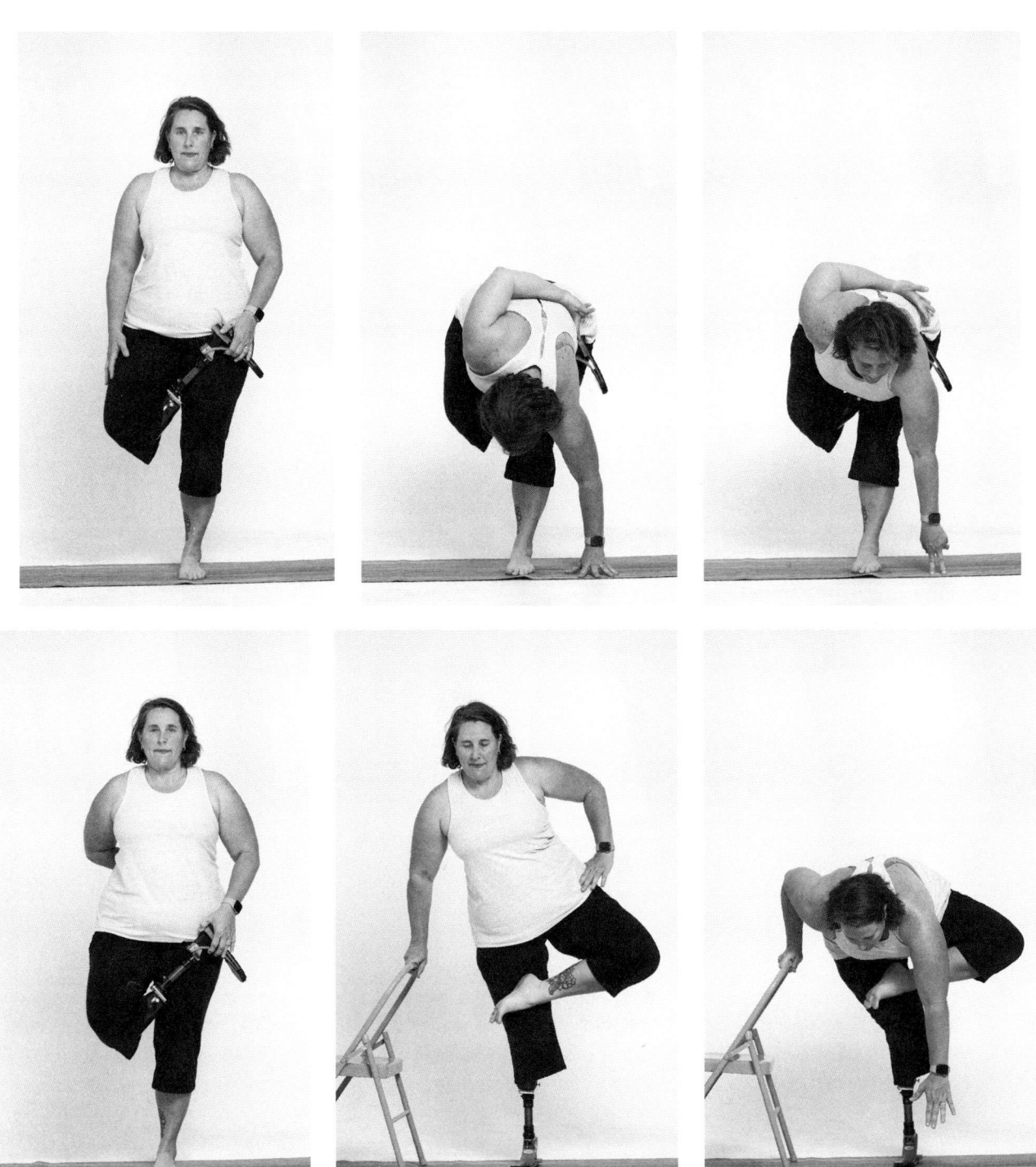

Half-Bound Lotus (Ardha Baddha Padmottanasana) and variations

Half-Bound Lotus (Ardha Baddha Padmottanasana)

In this pose, students can also play with friction and opposition. Have them lift up their right leg, rotating their knee outward and turning it down, bringing their heel toward their belly button and turning their toes out. Their foot rests near the hip crease. They can press their foot into their thigh and press their thigh back into their foot to keep their foot in place and create balance.

Ahead of attempting this asana, make sure to alert students to be careful if they have any knee problems or injuries. If so, they can cross their right foot over their left so that their right toes are on the ground and either remain here or fold forward. They may also use a rolled-up towel under their bent knee, taking the right foot to their left thigh in a flexed ankle-to-knee position, or taking Tree Pose (see page 111).

Those who want to may reach their right hand behind their back to reach toward or take their big toe and fold forward in this posture. Have students stay in this position or the upright standing version for five breaths. If they aren't binding their toe from behind their back, they can reach both hands to the ground.

On an inhale, have them rise halfway from their waist to come out of the pose, stop there and exhale. On the next inhale, ask them to rise all the way to standing, trying to keep their foot in position. On an exhale, release the bind into Samasthiti. Repeat the posture on the other side.

Seated Warrior 1 (Virabhadrasana 1)

Invite students to set up their chairs for a Seated Warrior 1. They can sit sideways in their chair with their pelvis fully supported for this version. Both hips face toward their front leg as their back leg stretches back straight and strong, their back foot grounded with toes turned slightly inward. Encourage students to let go and release into the chair's support in this posture. The more they drop down into their seat, the more they can use that energy to propel their arms upward. They can look forward or up and breathe here for five breaths.

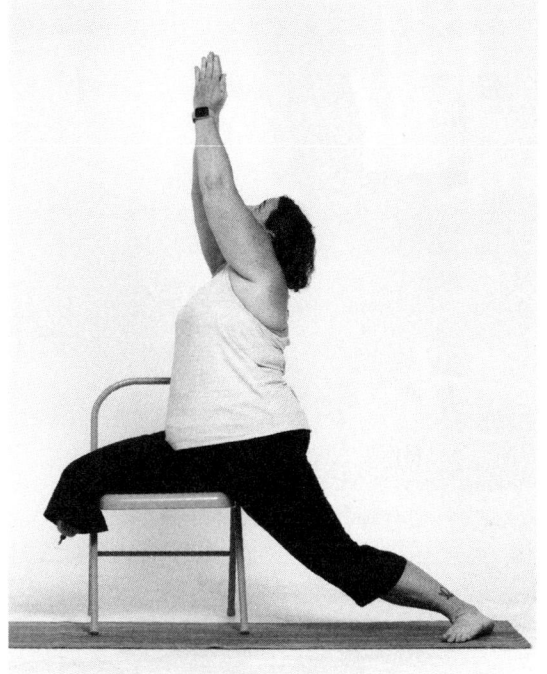

Seated Warrior 1 (Virabhadrasana 1)

Seated Warrior 2 (Virabhadrasana 2)

Transition students into Seated Warrior 2 by directing their arms to stretch out wide and their hips to reorient to the side. Tune students in to the feeling in their fingers as they reach forward and back. Cue them through five breaths, then guide them through Seated Warrior 1 and 2 on the other side.

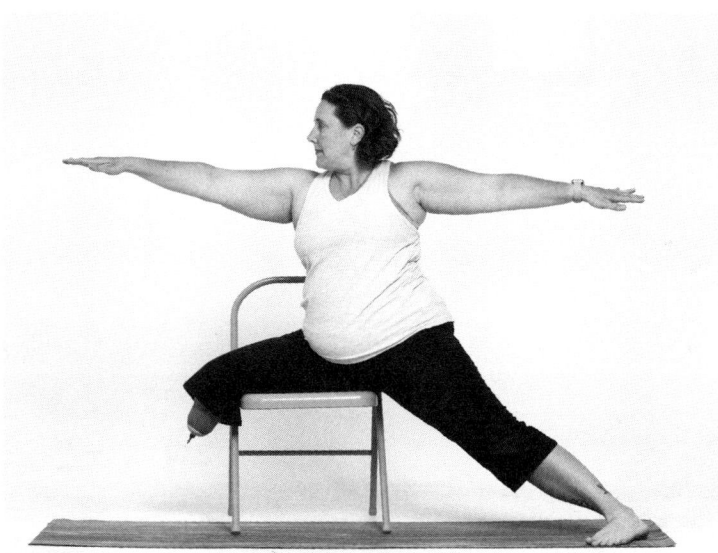

Seated Warrior 2 (Virabhadrasana 2)

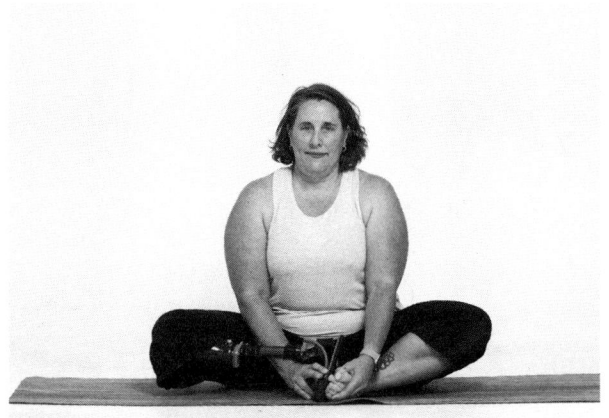
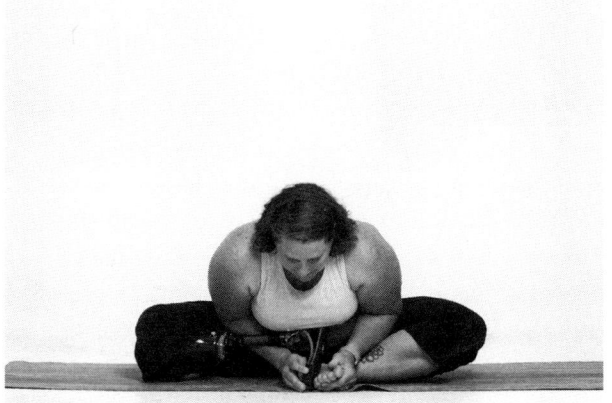

Cobbler's Pose (Baddha Konasana)

Cobbler's Pose (Baddha Konasana)

Invite students to move the chair aside and find a comfortable seated position on the floor. For Cobbler's Pose, they should take their feet together, allowing their knees to splay out to the sides. Encourage them to play with how close their feet are to their body. Farther away will feel less intense. Close in can be more of a challenge. Ask them to bring their hands to their feet, peeling them away from each other like opening a book. Ask students how that changes the experience of the posture. Invite them to breathe here five times.

On an exhale they can fold forward, leading with the crown of their head and maintaining a flat back. Invite them to bring their chin toward the ground, stopping when they feel their back start to curl. They can breathe five breaths here and then inhale to sit upright.

Students who find this position too triggering might consider a Squat (Malasana) a good alternative (see page 119). It has similar benefits but may feel more empowering because the soles of the feet are on the ground, making it easy to change position. The head is upright for easy access to visual cues of danger.

Ray of Light Pose/Sage Pose (Marichyasana A)

Suggest students now extend their left leg straight in front of them and bend their right knee so their foot is grounded close to their seat. On an inhale, have students stretch their right arm forward and wrap it around the inside of their knee to find the other hand extended behind them, or reach toward it with that intention. Then, on the exhale, they can fold forward over their extended leg. They can extend their spine to find a flat back or curl their spine to bring their nose toward their knee. Offer some extra time for students to get into this asana and to try each variation, allowing them to choose which works best in their body.

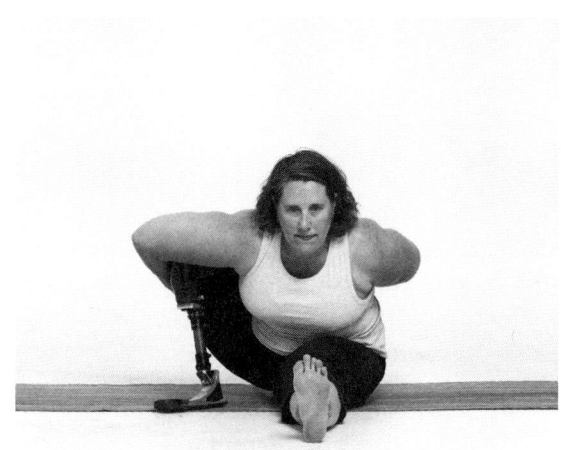

Ray of Light Pose/Sage Pose (Marichyasana A)

Ray of Light Pose/Sage Pose (Marichyasana B)

For Marichyasana B, have students bend their extended leg and turn their knee out so their leg lies flat. They can place it in a Lotus Pose (foot tucked into hip crease) or keep it tucked under the Marichyasana leg. Students can take five breaths here or they can wrap their arm around their bent leg (as in Marichyasana A) and then fold forward. Encourage them to pay attention to their breath and send breath and awareness to any areas of tightness during this posture.

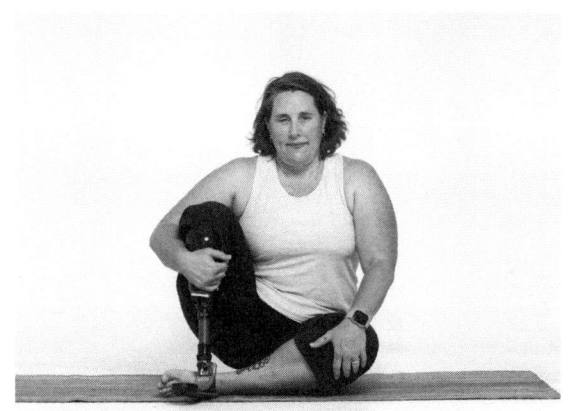

Ray of Light Pose/Sage Pose
(Marichyasana B)

Ray of Light Pose/Sage Pose (Marichyasana C)

In Marichyasana C, the legs are set up as in Marichyasana A, with one leg extended and the other leg bent, with foot on the floor in Marichyasana position. Ask students to release their Lotus leg and extend it straight. Then have them take their opposite arm to the outside of their bent leg and use their other arm behind them to brace themselves to come into a twist. Emphasize that they extend their gaze behind them, being conscious to look as far away as possible to give them a good stretch.

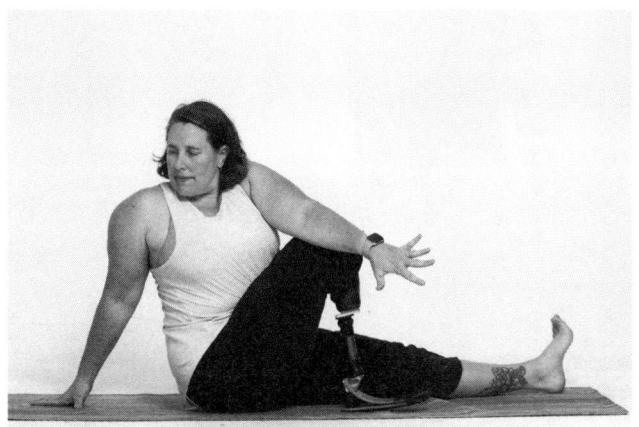

Ray of Light Pose/Sage Pose (Marichyasana C)

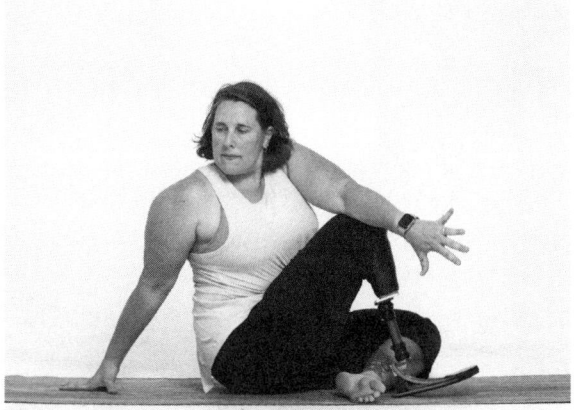

Ray of Light Pose/Sage Pose (Marichyasana D)

Ray of Light Pose/Sage Pose (Marichyasana D)

For Marichyasana D, ask students to bend their extended leg once again in Half Lotus or a more accessible bent position, as in Marichyasana B. They can bring their left arm outside their right leg and bring their other arm behind to brace themselves while they work on a deep twist, stretching their eyes behind them to see one spot at the farthest edge of their peripheral vision. Remember that these constricted positions can be emotionally triggering. Cue students to look for areas of spaciousness in their body and mind. Invite in whimsical curiosity as they look back around the room. Invite them to stay here for five breaths. Lead students through Marichyasana A, B, C, and D on the other side.

Boat Pose (Navasana)

Bring students back to center now to prepare for Boat Pose. Invite them to bring both feet flat on the floor and engage their lower abdomen as they pull their knees in close, lean back slightly and begin to lift their feet up off the ground. Their legs can be bent or extended straight. Students can use their hands to support their legs or reach their arms forward and parallel to the floor. Ask students to repeat this pose three to five times, breathing five breaths each time they are in the asana. Between repetitions, invite them to squeeze their knees in and give themselves a hug.

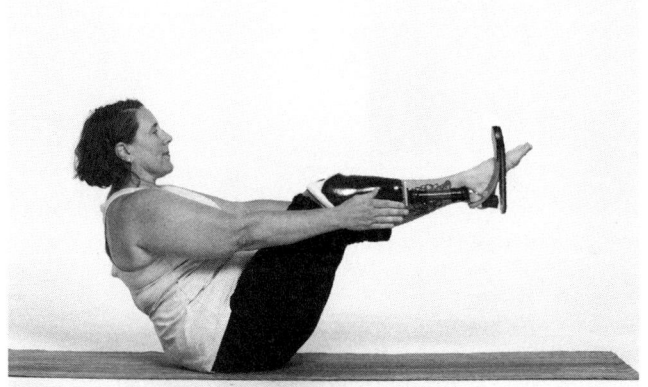 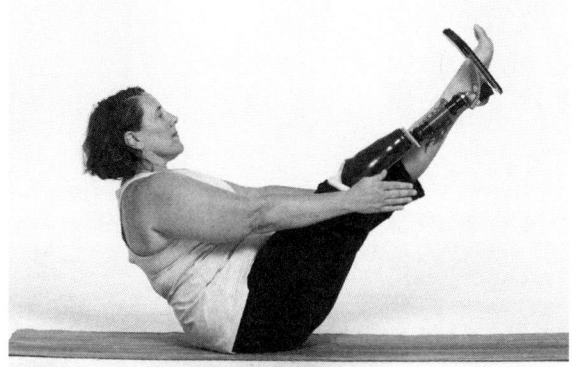

Boat Pose (Navasana)

Garland Pose or Squat (Malasana)

Bring students into a squat position, feet planted as wide as necessary, with toes turned out. They may want to swivel around in this position, stretching their ankles, legs, hips, and groin before settling into stillness. Allow time for this and encourage movements to be exploratory. Let students know they should spend time stretching areas that feel good to stretch into. Invite them to notice how it feels to be low to the ground but still on their feet. Can they find a source of power in their connection to the earth?

Crane/Crow Pose (Bakasana)

Remind students that they are free to stay in the squat position during this pose. Those who want to add an arm-strengthening challenge to the hip-opening challenge can bring their hands to the floor, lean forward, and lift up into Crow Pose. The important detail is that they keep their chest and head lifted as they try to balance on their hands. Many folks feel more inspired to attempt this pose if they have a blanket or folded towel on the floor below their head to cushion any fall. Challenge them to stay for five full breaths.

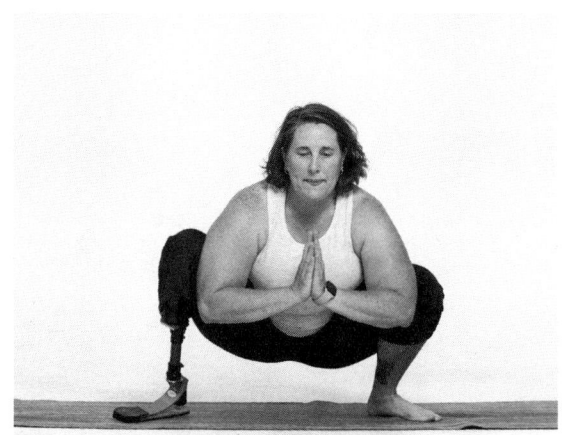

Garland Pose or Squat (Malasana)

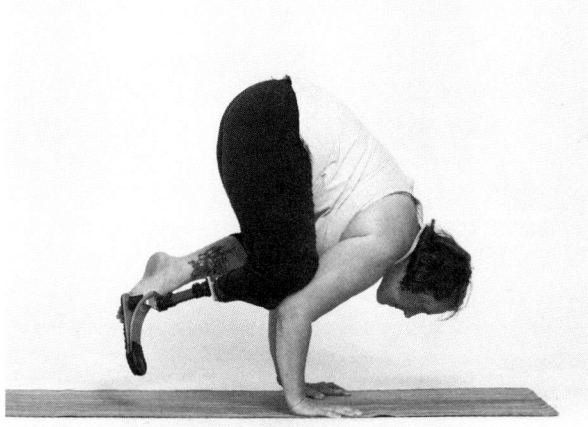

Crane/Crow Pose (Bakasana)

Locust Pose (Shalabhasana)

As they come down from Crow Pose, invite students to lay on the floor on their belly and rest their head to one side. Many of us are not used to this feeling of gentle pressure on the front of the body. The invitation is to stay with the strangeness for as much of five breaths as one feels able and see how it evolves. When ready, students can lay their arms at their sides with their palms turned up. Then with an inhale, they can press their hips deeply into the ground to lift their chest and legs. They can also press the backs of their hands down to lift up higher while keeping the main action at their hips. Remind them to keep their gaze on their nose tip, especially in this pose, to avoid neck strain. Count them through five breaths. On the final exhale, cue them down, inviting them to turn their head to the other side for rest.

VARIATION: LOCUST POSE (SHALABHASANA)

Instruct a variation where hands come forward on either side of the rib cage with the palms facedown. All other actions are the same. In this variation, the palms can help actively draw the shoulders back and down. Students can be cued not to use their hands too much. Their hips and back should do most of the work. You can offer students a test if they are really using their body to create the upward action: invite them to lift their palms off the ground completely. Encourage them to reflect on the effect this has on their spine and on how they manage their effort in this shape.

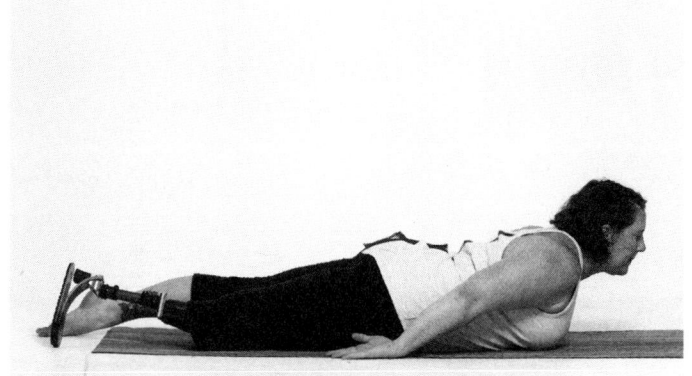

Locust Pose (Shalabhasana)

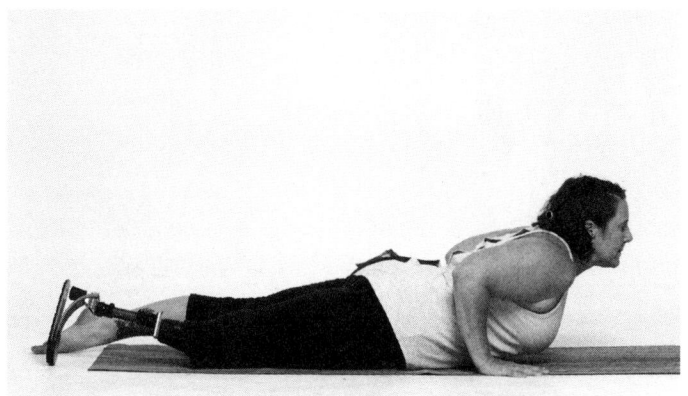

Locust Pose (Shalabhasana) variation

Camel Pose (Ustrasana)

Camel Pose is a natural pose to take after Locust Pose because of all the feedback, safety, and support the body gets from the ground. In Camel Pose, students will need to arch their backs without that reassurance. Cue students to kneel with knees hip-width apart. Have students push their hips forward so much that they almost tip forward. At the last moment they should lift up their chest and spine before stretching back with their hands on their lower back. Ask them to stay for five breaths.

Encourage students to bring forth the memory of the hips pressing into the floor in Locust Pose to help inform this posture. If students can learn to pull forward the feeling of safety and support in the body during times of fear and anxiety, this can serve as a daily resource.

Variation: Camel Pose (Ustrasana)

Have those who are ready prepare for a Camel variation. Invite students to reach their arms down to take their heels or to rest their hands on blocks. They continue to press their hips forward. Suggest students start with the blocks on their highest level and work over time to lower them. To come back up, suggest students bring one hand at a time to the waist, as they tuck their chin and roll back forward through their spine to the starting position. The inner thighs remain engaged and the hips press forward the whole time. I recommend taking a vinyasa (linked Chaturanga, Upward Dog, and Downward Dog; see page 120) between Camel and the next pose to loosen the body and keep it warm. More active practitioners may insert a vinyasa between any poses in this sequence.

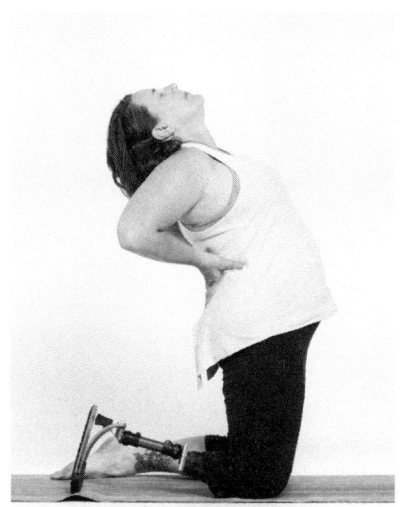

Camel Pose (Ustrasana)

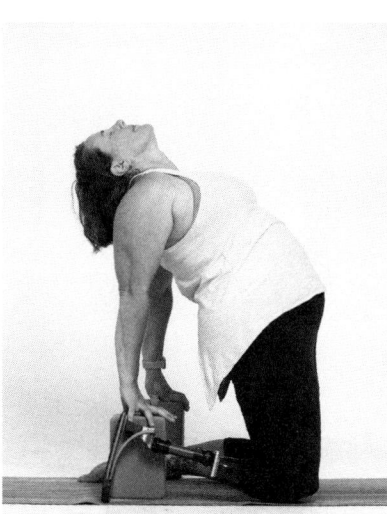

Camel Pose (Ustrasana) variation

Pigeon Pose (Kapotasana)

Pigeon Pose is known to intimidate even the most fearless practitioner, causing many to skip it altogether (which is a totally valid decision). As always, all poses are optional. For those who want some experience of the deep chest opening it provides without being in its extreme expression, ours is a good pose variation.

Starting on their knees, students press their hips forward until they feel their body about to fall forward. At the last moment before they fall, they should lift their torso up and back, concentrating on finding more space in the rib cage with each breath. They can reach their arms up with their palms pressed together and their elbows moving inward so they don't flare out. Ask students to inhale and exhale here, trying to lift their arms up and back more deeply as they counterbalance and press their hips forward.

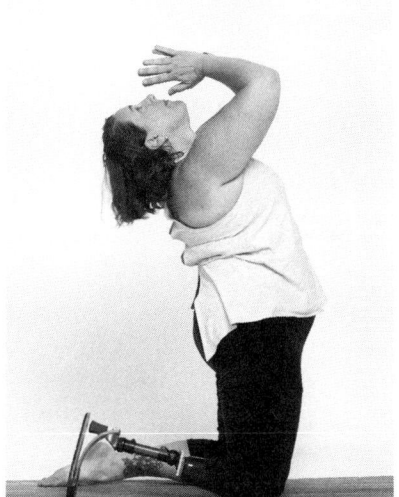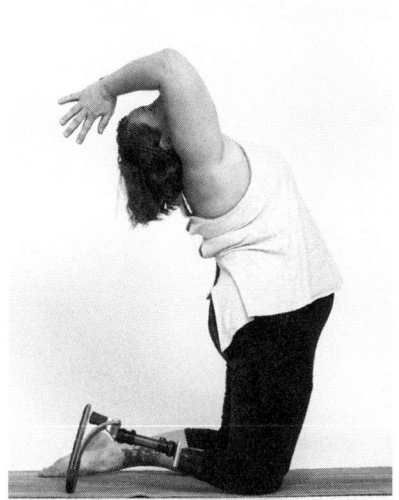

Pigeon Pose (Kapotasana)

Child's Pose (Balasana)

Students can take Child's Pose after Pigeon Pose to draw their energy inward.

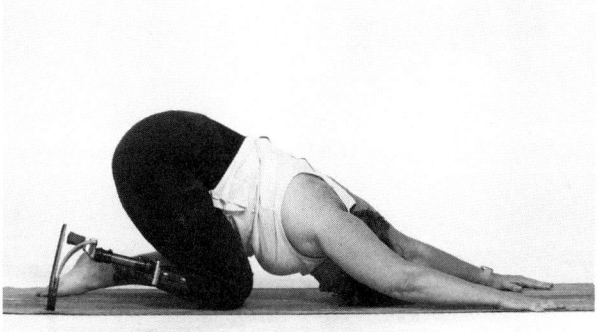

Child's Pose (Balasana)

Bridge Pose (Setu Bandha Sarvangasana)

Cue students to recline on the ground with their knees bent and their feet flat on the floor. Legs should be hip-width apart or wider. Invite students to press into their feet and lift their back off the floor for Bridge Pose. Cue students to position their arms at their sides with their hands reaching toward their toes, or they can roll their shoulders under and clasp their hands under their back. A third option is to press more intensely into one leg and allow the other to lift up. Regardless of the pose adaptation, students should press into all parts of the body that are interacting with the ground and lift their hips as high as they can. They can try three variations, each for five breaths, coming down in between for a one breath rest.

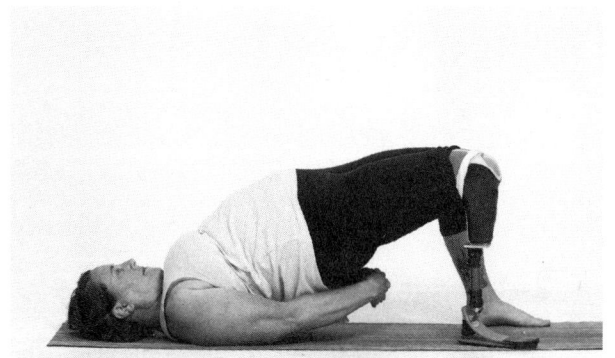 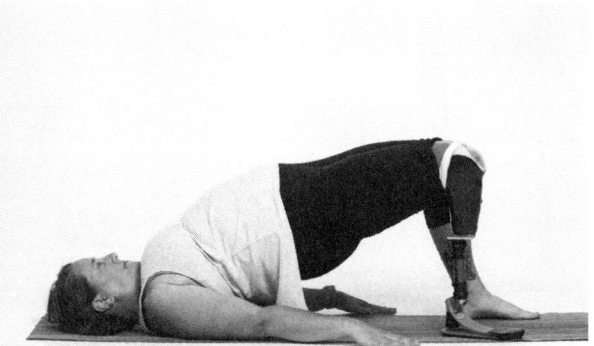

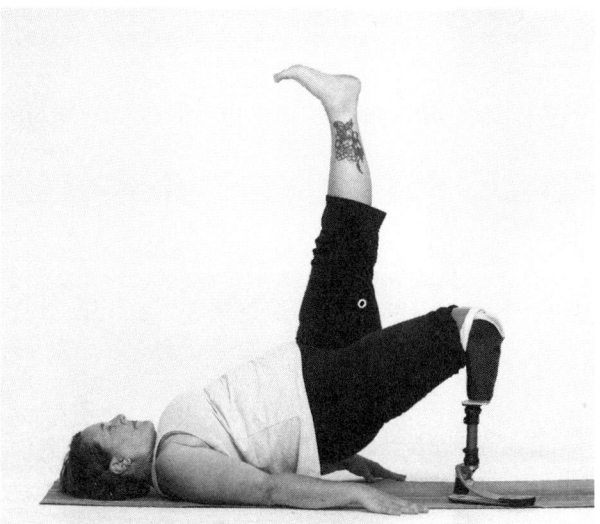

Bridge Pose (Setu Bandha Sarvangasana)

Fish Pose (Matsyasana)

Students can release the backbend and extend their legs out for Fish Pose. Their forearms press into the ground to lift their chest, creating just enough arch in their upper spine to place the crown of their head on the floor. They can place a block between their shoulder blades for support. This is a deep chest opener and a stretch most people are not used to, so remind students to be conscious to relax their breath and their mind. They should also soften their throat and the muscles of their face and send breath into any areas of discomfort. Insist they come down out of the pose at any time they feel discomfort, especially if there is any pain in their neck.

VARIATION: FISH POSE (MATSYASANA)
As a Fish Pose variation, students can hold palms pressed together over their head, fingers pointing to or on the floor. This opens the shoulders and the top of the back.

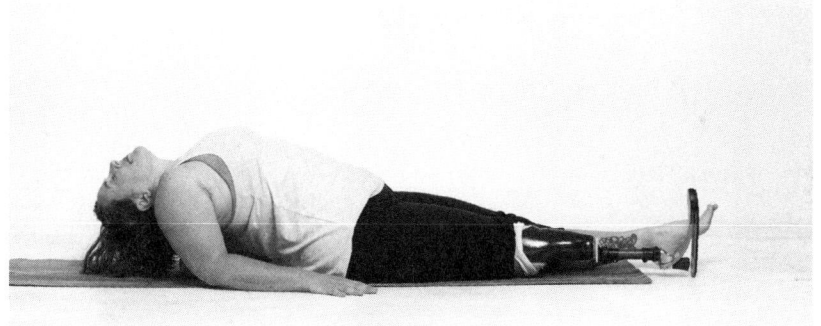

Fish Pose (Matsyasana)

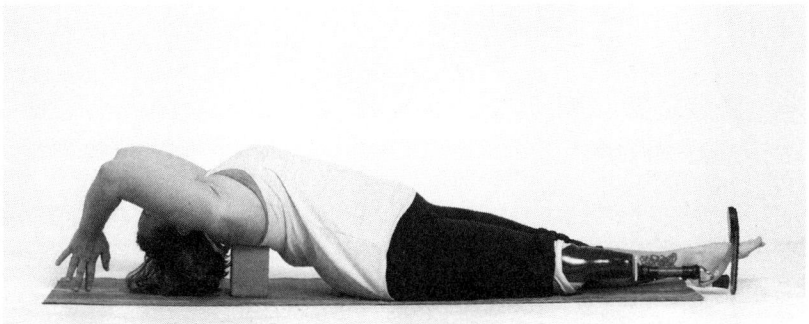

Fish Pose (Matsyasana) variation

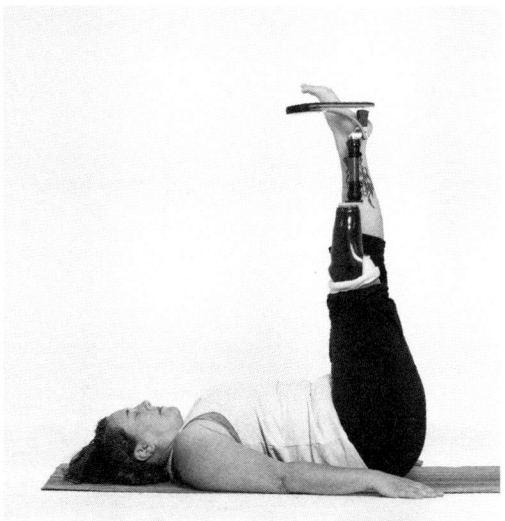

Legs Up the Wall (Viparita Karani)

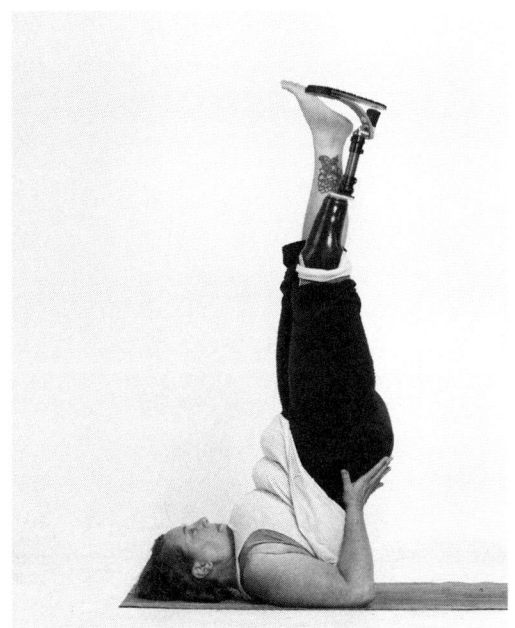

Shoulderstand (Salamba Sarvangasana)

Legs Up the Wall (Viparita Karani)

Long inversions are recommended after heart-opening postures. The easiest way to invert for a long time is by taking the Legs Up the Wall posture. This is one of the few yoga poses that can be taken at any time, independently throughout the day with no prep or warm-up. This version requires that students have unobstructed access to a wall. To get close to the wall and avoid back pain, recommend students enter the pose from their side, with their bottom against the wall, and flipping their legs upward to end up lying on their back. Their bottom and the backs of their legs are now extended up against the wall. Students can relax their arms at their sides or place their hands on their heart and belly. Both variations can be cued to bring variation into the posture during the longer hold. Cue twenty-five breaths in this posture.

If you have no free wall space or students prefer to stay where they are, this same pose can be done on the mat with the legs stretching up in the air unsupported. Alter the arm position to change the impact on the shoulders and chest area and to keep students interested in staying in the inversion during this longer hold.

Shoulderstand (Salamba Sarvangasana)

If Shoulderstand does not strain their neck or block their airway, students are welcome to take their lower back up and legs off the ground from Legs Up the Wall. A powerful inhale, their hands, and a clear intention help with the lift. Students should move their shoulders and elbows in toward each other under their upper back. Teach students to support their lower back with their hands. They should keep their gaze at their nose tip and take twenty-five slow deep breaths in this position. Insist they always come down (slowly) if there is any strain in the neck area.

Headstand (Sirsasana)

Like Shoulderstand, Headstand restores energy to the legs and slows down the body. Headstand is not necessary if you are offering a long Shoulderstand, but it can be fun, and when done properly, it can be more comfortable for the neck than Shoulderstand. Students should be able to do Headstand with no pressure on the neck, which means using their forearm strength and squeezing their legs up and together.

If you are teaching Headstand in a group class, always give the option for students to rest in Child's Pose or an alternate position. Prohibit jumping or kicking up to prevent accidents and injuries, and ensure students are using their strength and not momentum to come up into the posture.

Start by detailing the arm position. First, students kneel at the middle of their mat. Encourage students to place their elbows on the mat and then take opposite biceps with their hands to create a stable, triangular base for Headstand. Keeping their elbows glued to the ground, students release their biceps and swivel the forearms outward so their fingers can interlace. Then they open their palms to create a curved space to cup their head.

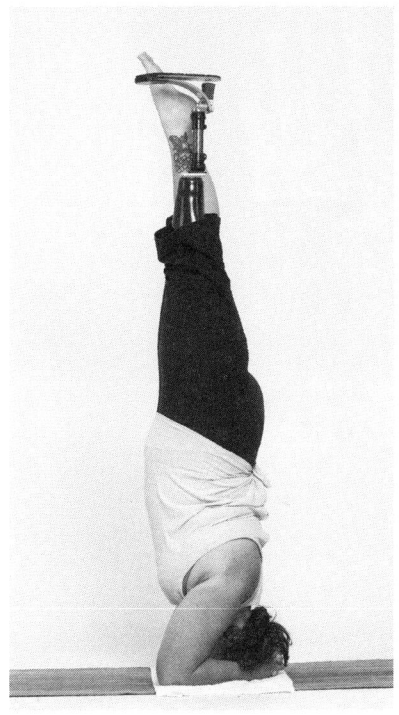

Headstand (Sirsasana)

Have students bring the crown of their head to the ground between their hands. Students lift their knees from the ground with toes pressing down and create a Downward Dog shape. Instruct them to squeeze their legs together and pull them forward, engaging from their hips, so they roll over onto the tops of their toes. Instruct them to continue pulling and squeezing their legs as they press their forearms down to keep pressure from their head. Over time, they may build enough strength, confidence, and body awareness to tip forward and squeeze in just the right amount that their toes will come up off the ground. Even if their toes never take flight, students will still enjoy the benefits of this posture, which include full-body strengthening, increased confidence, and body awareness. Count ten to fifteen breaths in this posture, encouraging folks to come out of it and rest whenever they feel called to.

After ten to fifteen breaths in Headstand, or when they are tired or finished, have students gently, slowly hinge at their waist, bringing their bent knees to the ground. Students then lower their body into Child's Pose and rest for one to two minutes. Make sure

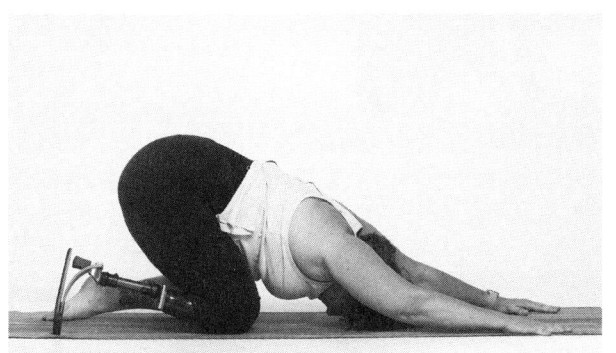

Child's Pose (Balasana)

One of the great benefits of this pose is the joy and confidence practitioners feel when they can get into it. It is often the pose that students directly relate to their ability to do daring things in life. It is for this reason that I recommend, when the student is ready, teaching this pose in the middle of the room and not up against a wall. In my experience, it is very hard to get students to transition from the support of the wall to a freestanding Headstand. It's much easier to learn to embody the confidence in this pose by starting in the middle of the room.

students never lift their head after Headstand or Headstand prep to prevent head rush and dizziness. Then they can step back into Chaturanga and take a vinyasa before moving into the final three closing postures.

BOUND LOTUS (BADDHA PADMASANA)

After the intensity of inversions, it is time to close and seal the practice. Invite students to take their legs into a comfortable cross-legged position or into Lotus if they prefer. They can cross their arms behind their back and take opposite elbows or reach around their hips to hold their big toes (yogic toe lock).

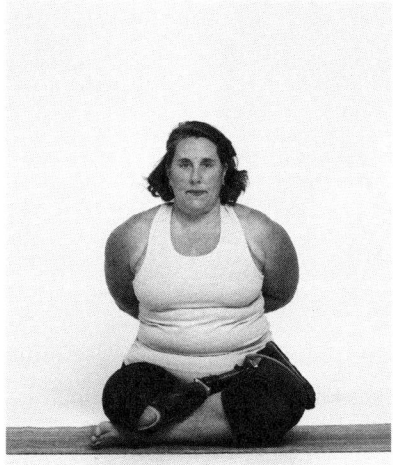

Bound Lotus (Baddha Padmasana)

Sealing the Practice (Yoga Mudra)

On an exhale, invite students to fold forward from Bound Lotus, bringing their forehead toward the ground. Instruct students to allow their spine to curve and gravity to help them take the most relaxed version of this shape. Encourage them to breathe their deepest ten breaths here.

Lotus (Padmasana)

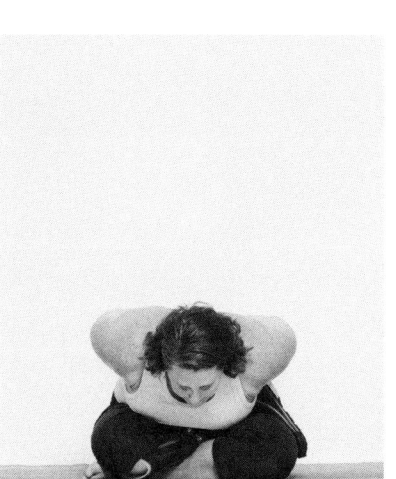

Sealing the practice (yoga mudra)

After ten breaths, cue students to inhale and sit up tall with their arms straight, the back of their hands resting on their knees, and their thumb and pointer fingertips touching. Invite them to lift their sternum slightly and drop their chin toward it. Their eyes can stay open with their gaze resting on the tip of their nose. Cue them to take ten full breaths, maintaining gentle awareness of their gaze, breathing pace, and body positioning.

Uprooting (Utpluthih)

Like a tense-and-release exercise, the final closing posture of this sequence is designed to squeeze out any last bits of stress and prepare
the body for rest. Ask students to remain in Lotus position and bring
their hands to the mat close to their body and slightly in front of their
hips. On an inhale, they can press down into the floor or on blocks, tuck
their crossed legs into their chest, and lift their body off the ground any
amount. If they are not taking Lotus, they remain in a cross-legged position and instead they can squeeze their knees tight into their body. If
their bottom or feet come down, encourage them to try again, engaging
again and pressing down with their hands and lifting up their bottom.
They should stay engaged for ten breaths, using all their energy even if
nothing lifts off the ground.

Final Rest (Savasana)

After this, your students can lie down and take rest. The body temperature will drop as the body rests, so a blanket over the body is often recommended. Remember to keep speaking to students through their rest,
encouraging them to stay present and focused on sensations that are
positive or neutral. They can continue to breathe through their nose and
allow the breath to return to its natural sound and rhythm.

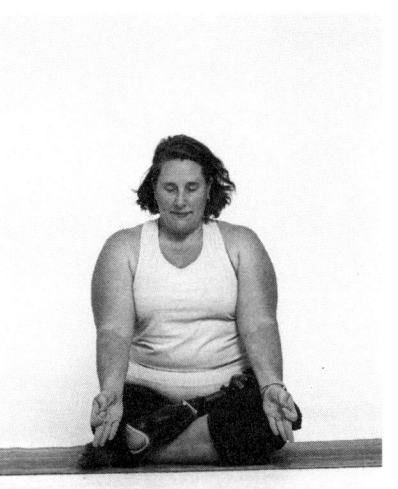

Lotus (Padmasana)

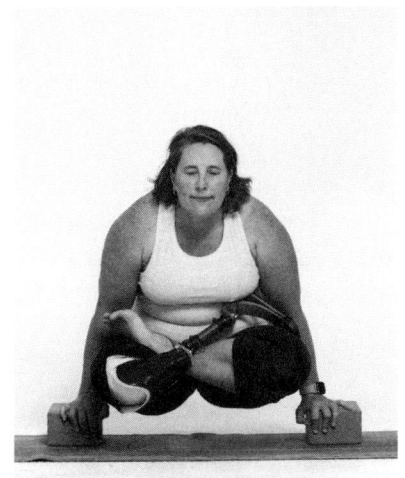

Uprooting (Utpluthih)

SLOW AND STEADY SEQUENCE: ADAPTABLE FLOW WITH ELSIE

Elsie's sequence is also inspired by the Ashtanga primary series; however, it offers fewer of the asanas and repeats others to allow for chair and standing instruction. This sequence focuses on flow; the body is meant to keep moving between postures to increase breath capacity and focus the mind. Her sequence features wider leg stances in the seated postures for knee safety and comfort. The extended closing series has a variety of Shoulderstand variations, but leave them out when teaching new students or for anyone with neck issues.

Consider ways to keep up the flow even as it is adapted for the chair or on the mat. I invite you to incorporate a simulated Chaturanga–Upward Dog flow from the Spacious and Opening Sequence with Nikki (page 137) between poses to stoke the heat while sparing the impact on shoulders and wrists. Remember, as the name of this sequence suggests, move slowly through the postures and vinyasas. Encourage students to feel into the difference moving forward with intention and not rushing. This sequence is especially good for groups who have the ability and desire to stand up and practice on the mat.

Accordion Breathing

Building breath capacity with your students is important, sensitive work. It's done mainly by helping them cultivate awareness of their breath and where it might be constricted. Many students conceive of breathing as something that happens in the chest or, at most, as a vertical process: the breath goes in and down, then up and out. I like to help them expand these notions through self-touch in an exercise called accordion breathing.

Ask students to place their hands on the sides of their body near or over their rib cage. Close to the armpits is preferable. Invite them to consciously send breath into their hands, trying to move their hands away from each other horizontally like the bellows of an accordion expanding. Breath should be through the nose if possible. Take ten to twenty breaths here.

Seated Equal Standing Pose (Samasthiti)

After their breathwork, bring students into stillness and give them a moment to feel the impacts of the breathing on their mind and body. Introduce the soft gaze and encourage awareness of the body in the seated position. Instruct these focal points as a grounding force and to bring their energy into the practice space.

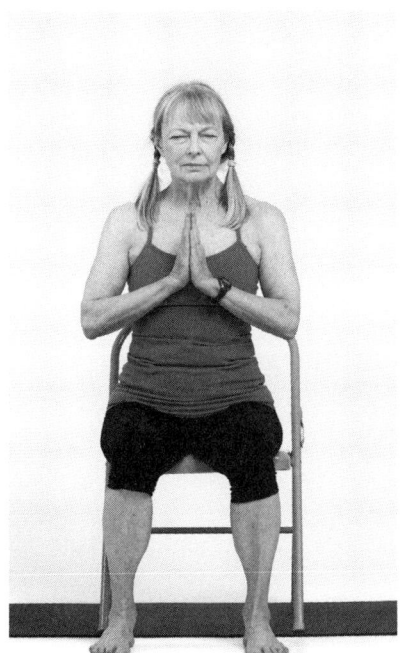 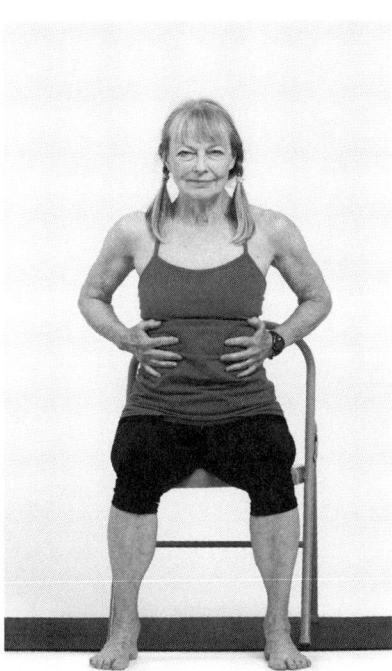

Seated Equal Standing Pose
(Samasthiti)

Accordion breathing

Arm Raises

Matching movement to breath awakens body awareness and presence and shows practitioners just how articulate their body can be. Special emphasis can be put on pairing the movement to the breath pace but also on exploring how to accomplish the intended movement with the most useful amount of activation and energy.

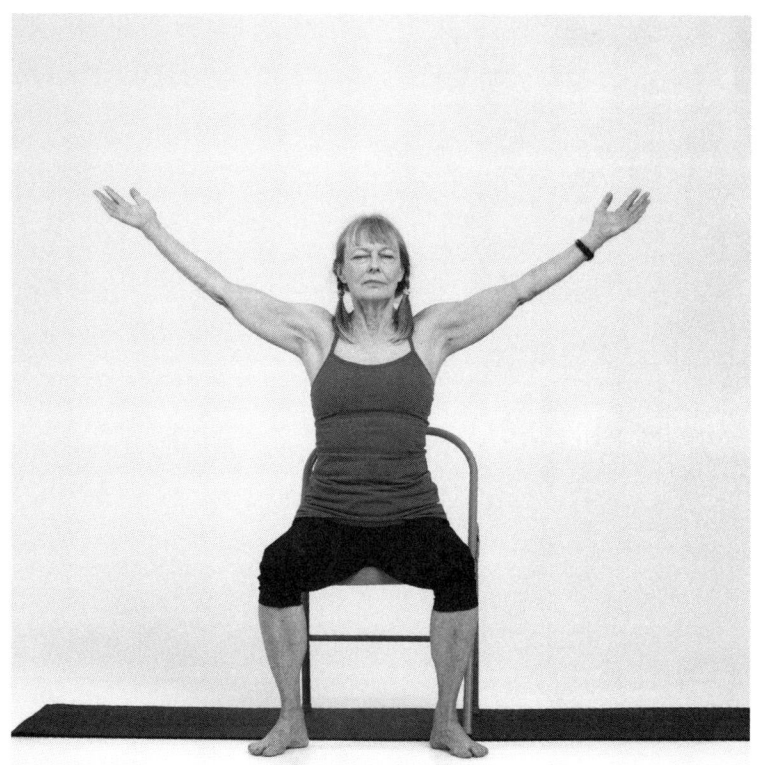 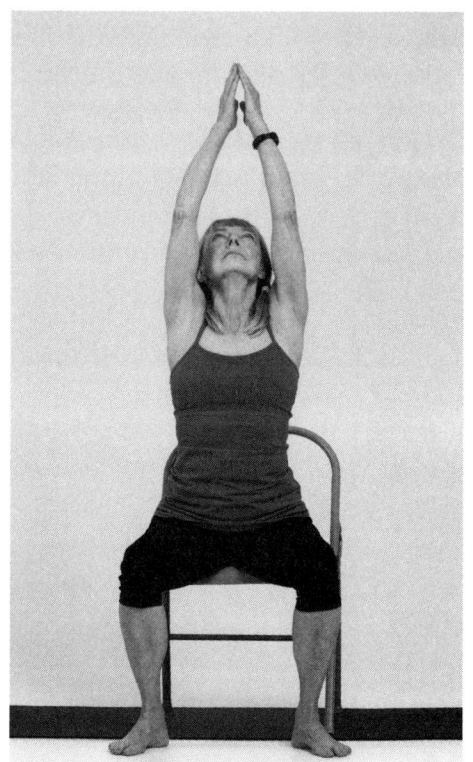

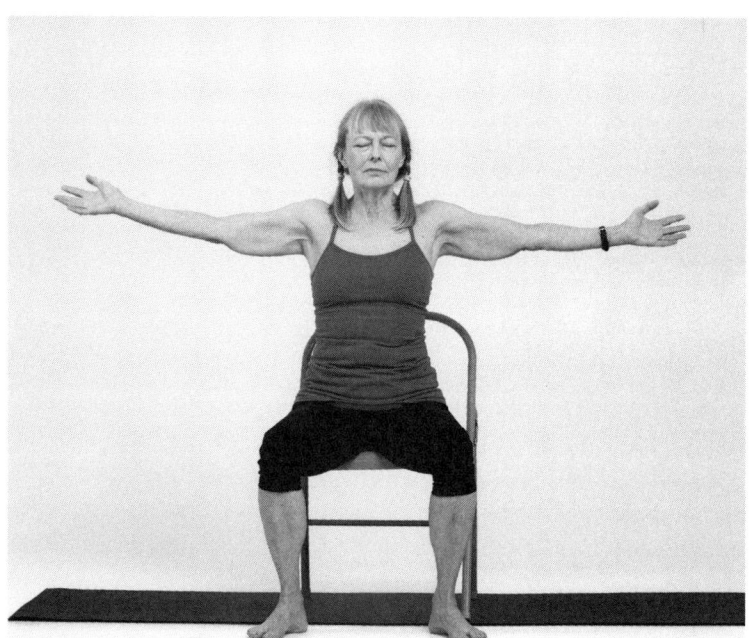 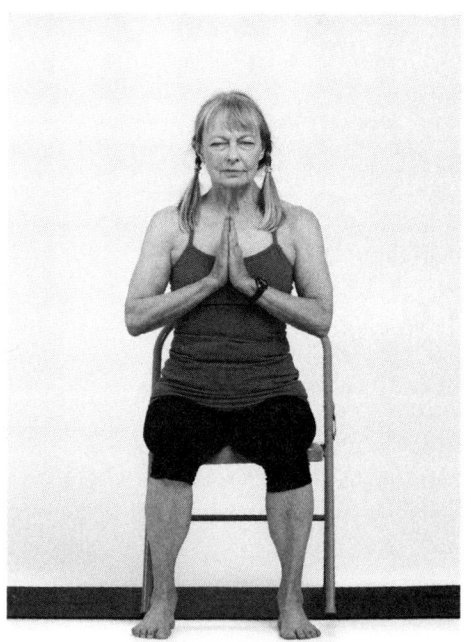

Arm raises

Invite students on their inhale to reach up their arms, allowing their gaze to follow if it doesn't hurt their neck to do so. They should complete the motion when they can inhale no more.

As their exhale begins, they can start to move their arms down, completing this motion at the exhale's end. They repeat this motion five to ten times, watching with curiosity as their breath and body work together and playing with breath and movement speed and effort.

Side Stretching

Next, invite students to stretch the sides of their body, creating more space for breath. On an inhale, have students arch one arm overhead, gently curving the side of the body. Exhaling, bring students back to center and the arm down to the side. Then on the next inhale, talk them through the opposite side stretch. Repeat this cycle five times. After the fifth repetition, invite students to stay in stillness on one side for five breaths. Transition the arm down and repeat on the opposite side, staying in stillness for five breaths again.

Gentle Seated Twist

Lead students to inhale and reach their arms up, then exhale into their seated twist. To do so, students move their left arm across their body and rest their hand on their right knee. They stretch their other arm behind their back to touch the chair, elongating their spine. They stretch their gaze behind them as they turn their head. On their next inhale, they can reach their arms up again and on the exhale, twist to the other side. Students can repeat this movement five times before settling into stillness, holding the stretch for five breaths on each side. During these longer holds they can work with the interaction of their hands on their chair and body to deepen the twist

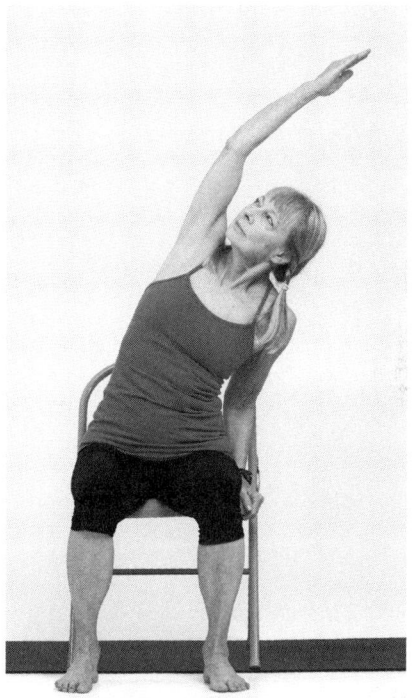

Side stretching

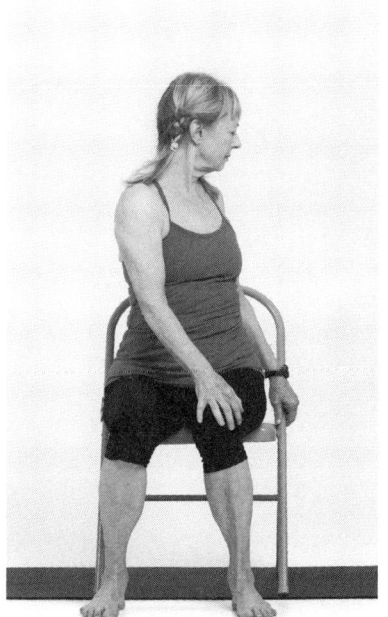

Gentle seated twist

further. Remind them not to strain but to soften their belly to deepen the posture and consciously continue to drop the opposite side down into the chair as they twist. Bring students back to stillness in seated Samasthiti.

Seated Sun Salutation (Surya Namaskar)

Sun Salutations are a key component of every sequence in this book. They are a valuable opportunity for practitioners to coordinate their breath and movement, get the body in flow, and learn about the self through repetition. In Seated Samasthiti, ask students to notice any changes that have occurred since sitting in stillness at the beginning of class. Remind them of their three-pointed focus.

When students feel settled and focused, cue students to, on the next inhale, lift their arms overhead. Then ask students to exhale and fold forward, with their hands on their knees. On their next inhale, they can lift

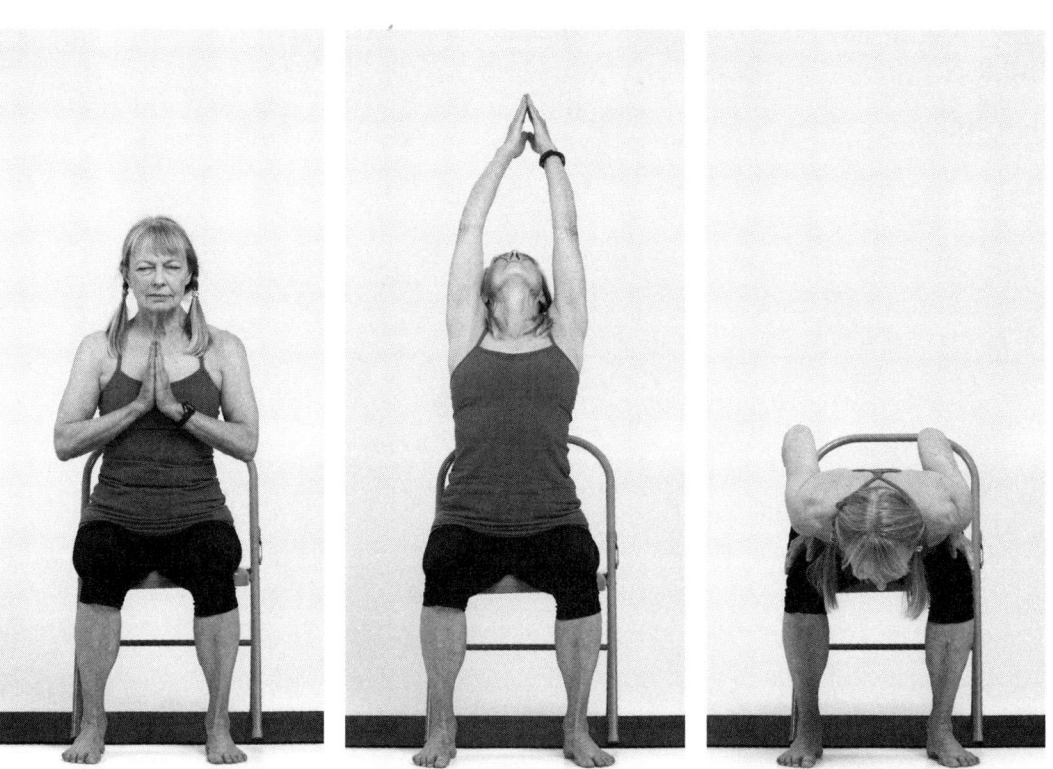

Seated Sun Salutation (Surya Namaskar)

halfway up with a gentle arch in the spine. On the exhale, fold forward more deeply, relaxing their head and neck.

On the next inhale, they rise all the way up with their arms overhead. End the sequence with an exhale to Seated Samasthiti. You can offer some resting breaths here or transition into repeating this sequence. Take three to five repetitions before finishing in Seated Samasthiti, inviting students to check in with any changes in their body, breath, or mind.

Seated Triangle Pose (Trikonasana)

Ask students to stretch their legs out in a wide seated straddle with their left toes pointing forward and their right toes pointing to the right. Encourage them to reach their arms out wide on their inhale. On the exhale, students reach farther to the right, then tilt their body to reach down their right leg for Triangle Pose. They can press the back of their

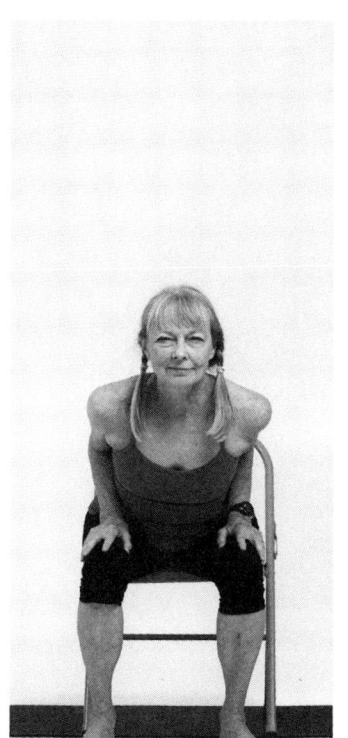
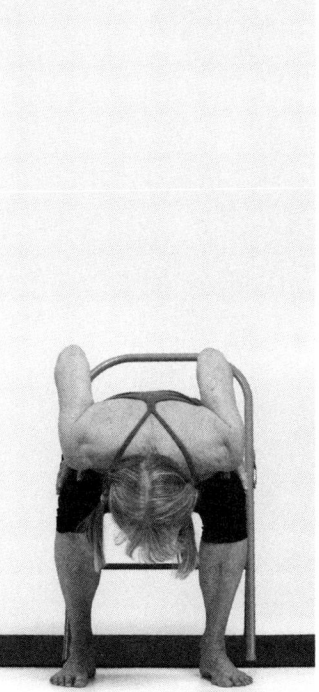
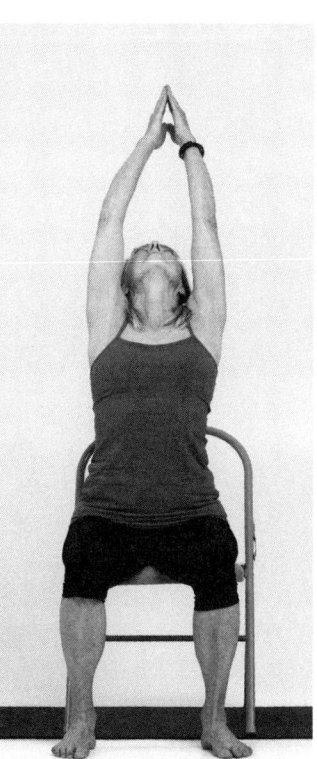
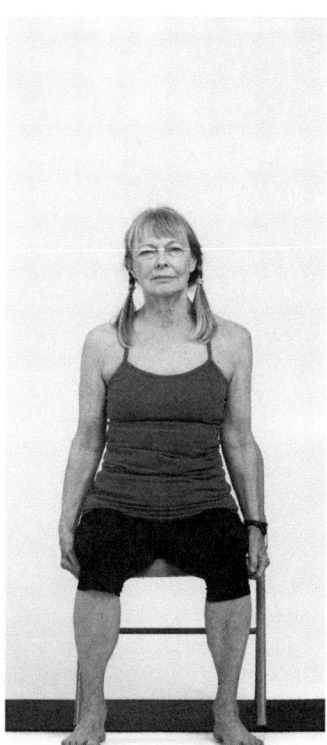

hand into their leg and use that pressure to lift up and out of their body, stretching in all directions. Lead five breaths here, continuing to cue for breath sounds and focus. Then use an inhale to bring the class up to center. On an exhale, guide everyone into the opposite side of the pose. Inquire after how the side of the body feels in this position after moving through the opening postures. Cue five breaths.

Seated Extended Side Angle A (Parsvakonasana A)

Invite students to rest their right forearm on their bent leg and extend their left arm over their ear at an angle instead of straight up. The gaze is up at their left hand or down at their right toe. Talk through five breaths here before inviting students to come up through center, straighten their legs, and rotate their feet for Extended Side Angle on the left side for five breaths each.

To vary the sequence, you could cue practitioners to stay on the right side of Triangle Pose and bend their knee deeply to set up for Extended Side Angle before taking Triangle on the left side. If you do so, the leg transition from this wide-legged Triangle to Extended Side Angle is just

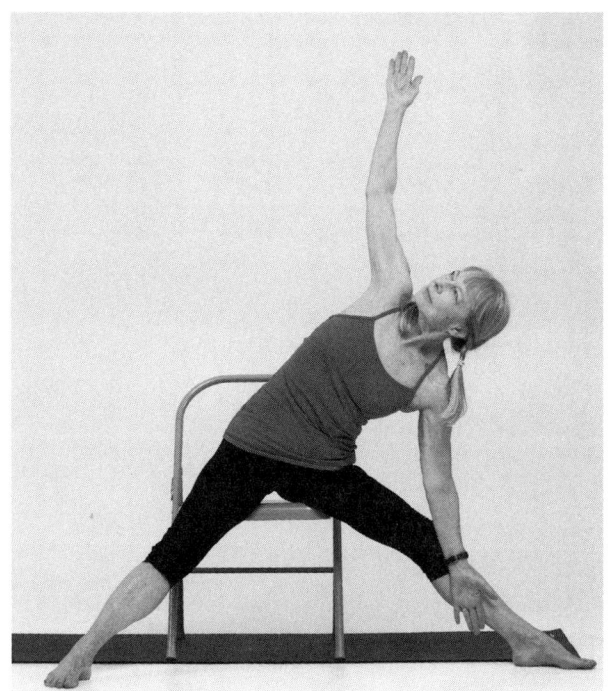

Seated Triangle Pose (Trikonasana)

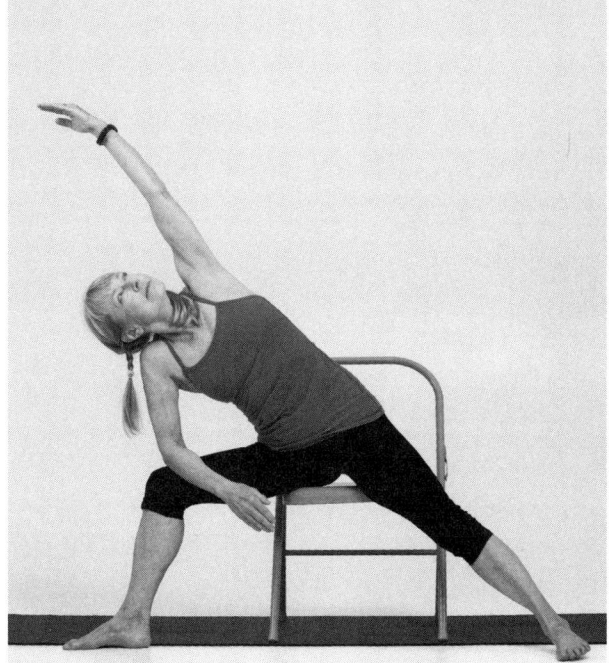

Seated Extended Side Angle A (Parsvakonasana A)

a bend of the right knee. Other than that, their legs don't need to shift. Repeat the sequence on the left side.

Wide-Legged Forward Fold A (Prasarita Padottanasana A)

On an inhale, invite students to straighten their bent leg, rising up to a seated posture and turning the toes of both feet out at an angle for a variation of Wide-Legged Forward Fold. If they are not at the front of their chair, they may want to scoot a bit forward and move there now. On an exhale, guide them to forward fold and bring their hands to the ground or as far down as they can reach.

On the next inhale, instruct students to lift halfway up and lengthen their spine. Exhaling, they can fold all the way forward and bring their head toward the ground, resting here for five breaths while gazing at their nose tip. Perhaps they can feel into the silliness of this childlike shape.

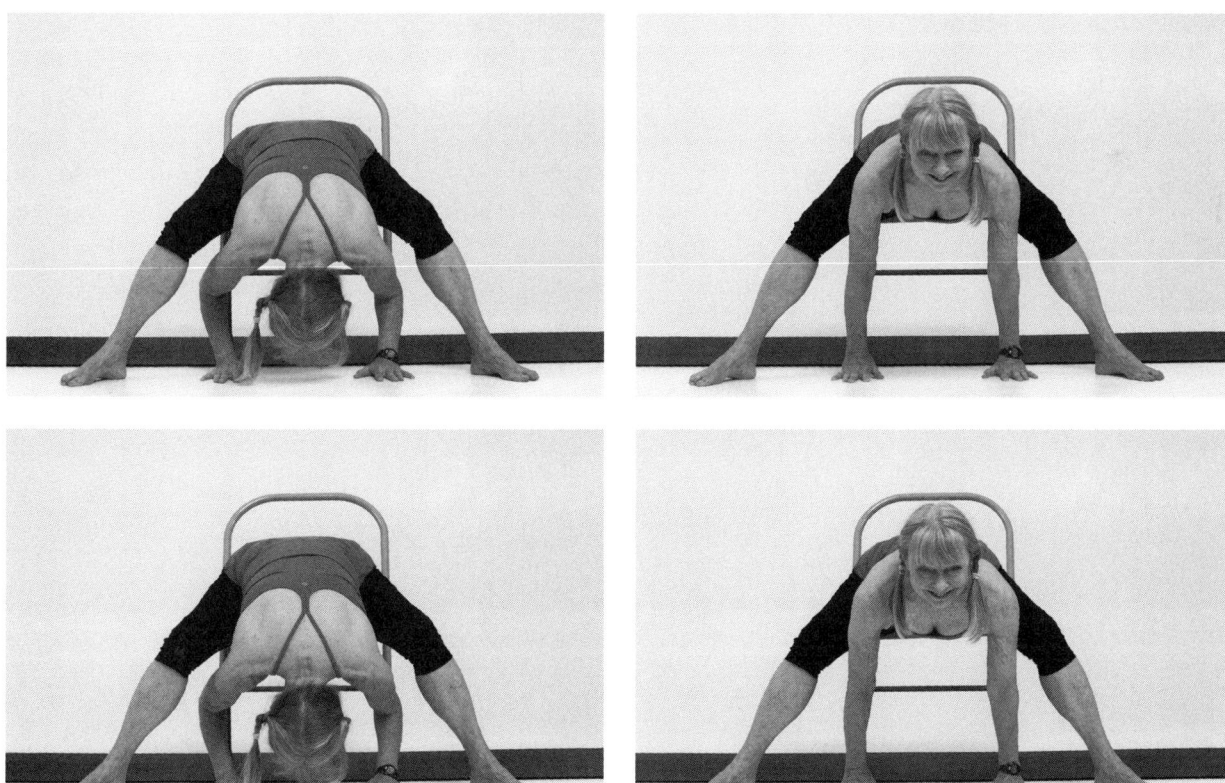

Wide-Legged Forward Fold A (Prasarita Padottanasana A)

After five breaths, have students inhale and hinge halfway up at the waist and stay there through the exhale before rising all the way up to seated, exhaling there.

Wide-Legged Forward Fold C (Prasarita Padottanasana C)

Invite practitioners to inhale and open their arms wide in a T. Exhaling, they clasp their hands behind their back, between their body and the chairback. They can take another inhale there.

On their next exhale, guide students to fold forward, bringing their head and arms toward the ground. Remind them to press back into their seat even as they fold forward to keep from falling and to further stretch their back in both directions. Count five breaths and then bring them all the way up to seated on an inhale.

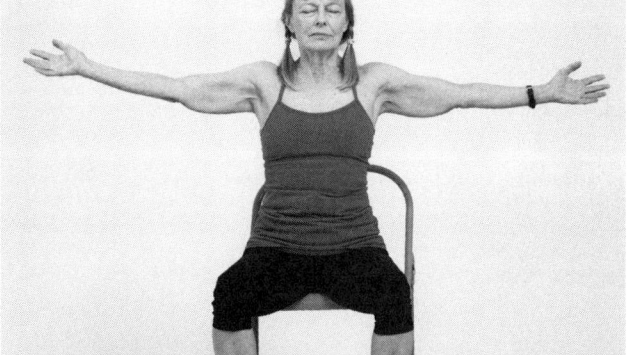

Intense Side Stretch Pose (Parsvottanasana)

Cue students to keep their hands clasped behind their back as you instruct them to pivot to the right side on an inhale, extend their back leg out long, and bend their right leg in front of them. Hips should be square over their right leg. Encourage students to keep activating their back foot to help with that rotation. Cue them to use their exhale to fold forward over their bent leg. They can work with the opposition of moving

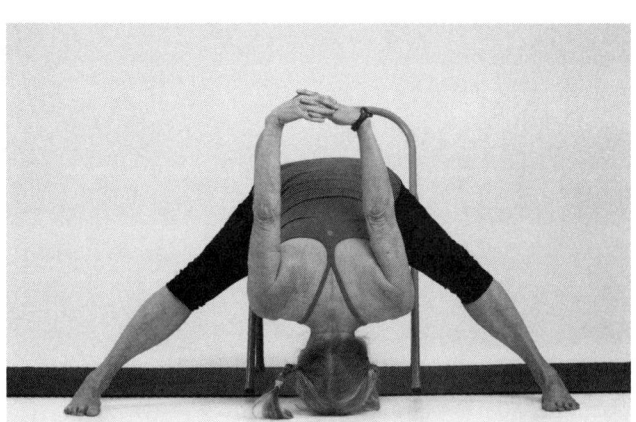

Wide-Legged Forward Fold C
(Prasarita Padottanasana C)

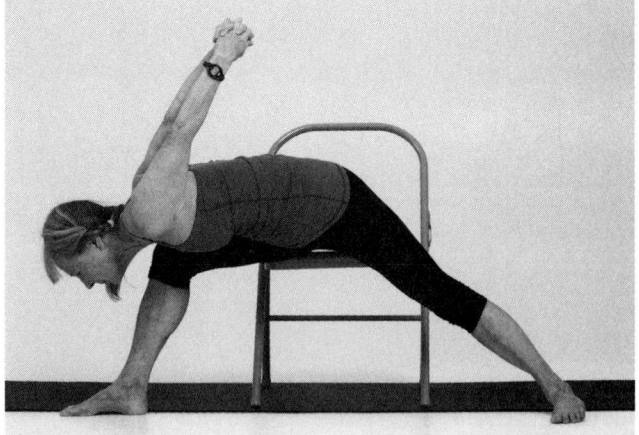

Intense Side Stretch Pose (Parsvottanasana)

forward with their chest as they reach back with their arms. What does this tension bring up for them energetically? For those who don't like the clasped hand position, taking opposite elbows is another option. Count five breaths as they stay there. On the next inhale, bring students upright and on the exhale, encourage them to pivot their feet and repeat the posture on the opposite side for five more breaths.

Tree Pose (Vrksasana)

Invite students to stand up and use their chair for support in Tree Pose. Work slowly with students through the many variations of this posture, exploring with them the subtle vacillations between being balanced and off-balance, in and out of control. Ask them to pay attention to how they react when they fall out of balance. What are the inner voices saying in those moments? Can those voices be controlled?

They can hold the top of the chair lightly with one hand as they press down into the leg closest to the chair. The downward motion invites the legs and spine to grow tall. They should turn their nonstanding foot out and take their toes to the ground and heel up to feel the shape of this pose. Have them bring one hand to their sternum and breathe here. If

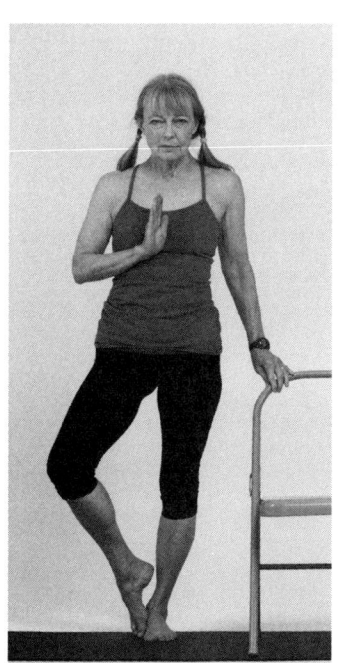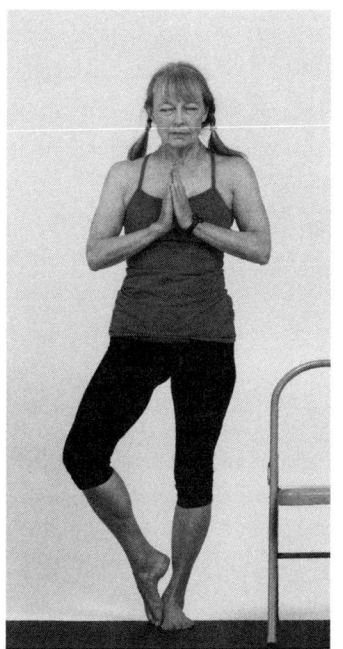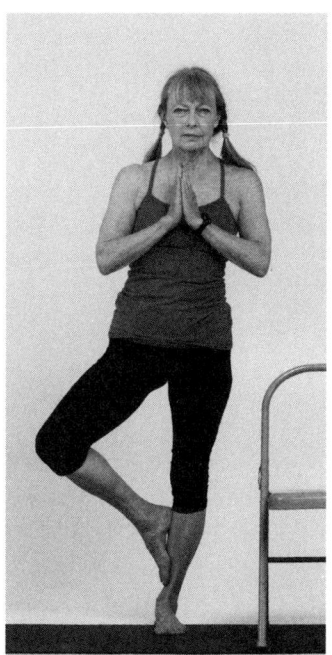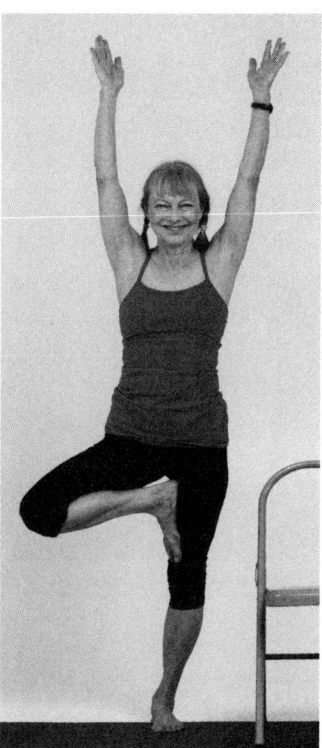

Tree Pose (Vrksasana)

Remind your students that, in general, it's best to go for a bit of a challenge while staying away from feeling overwhelmed. On physically and emotionally tough days, they should avoid challenging themselves at all and go for an expression of the asana that feels nurturing.

and when they feel ready, they can lift their other hand to meet the first in Anjali Mudra.

If this position feels easy, they may want to try placing their floating foot higher on their calf or on their thigh. Anywhere is fine as long as they avoid pressing on their knee. For more of a challenge, they can lift their arms overhead, followed by their gaze.

Straight-Leg Balance

Encourage students to take a straight-legged balancing asana. Students begin with both hands holding their waist and one leg lifted up as high as they can hold it. They can bring one hand to their chair and use it for support or just stand beside it. Challenge students to lift their leg higher and higher and test the limits of their balance, both mental and physical. This gives them a sense that you believe in their ability to do hard things. After five breaths, students lower their leg to the floor and repeat on the other side.

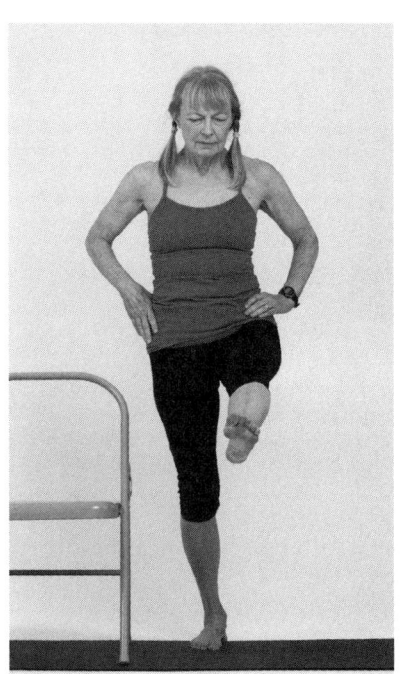

Straight-leg balance

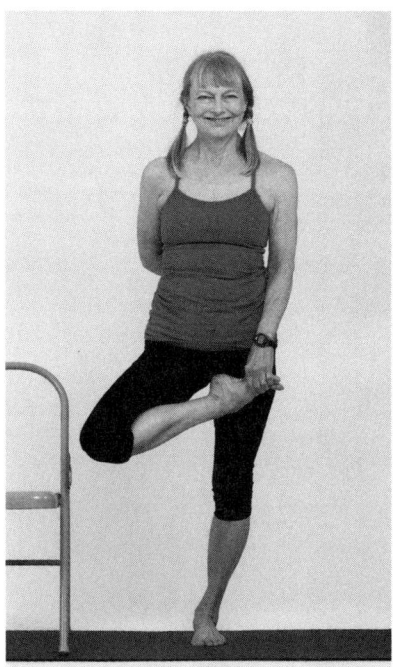

Half-Bound Lotus (Ardha Baddha Padmottanasana)

Half-Bound Lotus (Ardha Baddha Padmottanasana)

For Half-Bound Lotus, encourage practitioners to lift their right foot toward their navel, unfolding their leg so the outer edge of their foot presses against the thigh crease or thigh. They may need to hold their foot in place. Guide students to keep their foot in place without holding it by pressing their leg against their foot as they press back with their foot into their leg. Invite them to stay here for five breaths. If their foot slides down, students can turn the pose into an ankle-to-knee pose by flexing their foot, holding it above their knee, and balancing there. Students may also use the chair for support, resting their knee on the seat.

Half-Bound Lotus is a challenging balancing posture and should only be done when there is no problem with or injury in the knees. As an alternative, students may cross one foot over the other at the ankle, keeping that foot's toes on the ground. They can then fold forward from this position or take another round of Tree Pose. They may also sit in the chair and work on this asana as shown in previous sequences (see pages 103 and 151).

Seated Chair Pose (Utkatasana)

Guide students into their chair for a supported Chair Pose. Invite them to sit at the front edge of their seat with their feet and knees hip-width apart so they can be ready to stand up. Invite them to reach their arms up, letting the sternum rise. Encourage them to breathe into the sides of their body as they look up and take five breaths here.

Those who want to stand may now press into the floor, lean forward, and lift up out of the chair. Invite them to conjure a feeling of ease even as they work through the challenges of the pose. Count through five breaths, inviting folks to sit down any time they need to.

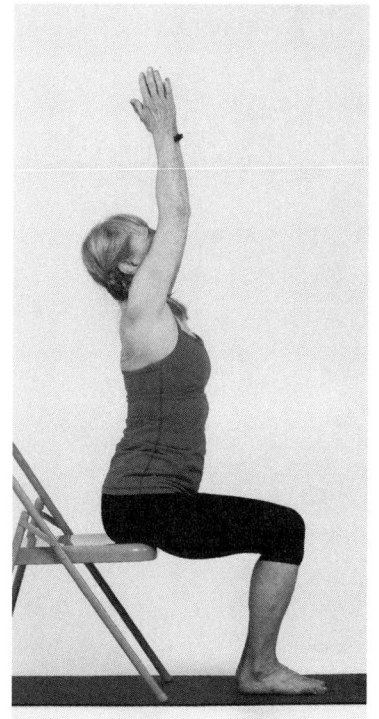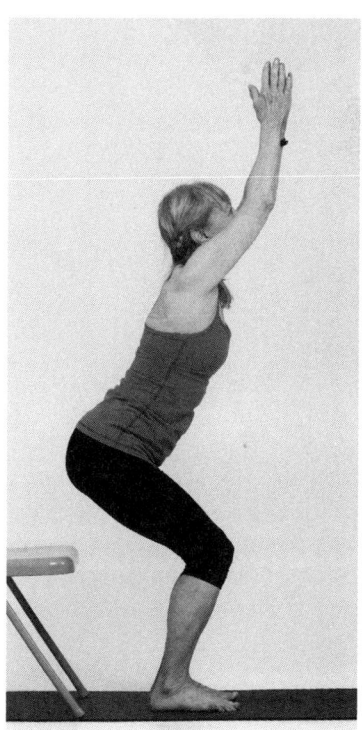

Seated Chair Pose (Utkatasana)

Seated Warrior 2 (Virabhadrasana 2)

Everyone can come to their chairs now for a Seated Warrior 2 posture. Instruct this version at the edge of the chair where the legs are forced to engage. Practitioners can align their feet in a wide straddle, then turn one foot out with their toes pointed sideways and their knee bent. The other leg is straight with the sole of the foot grounded. Invite students to open their arms out wide and gaze at the middle fingertip of the arm floating above their bent leg. At the end of five breaths, invite practitioners to pivot on their heels and transition into the other side.

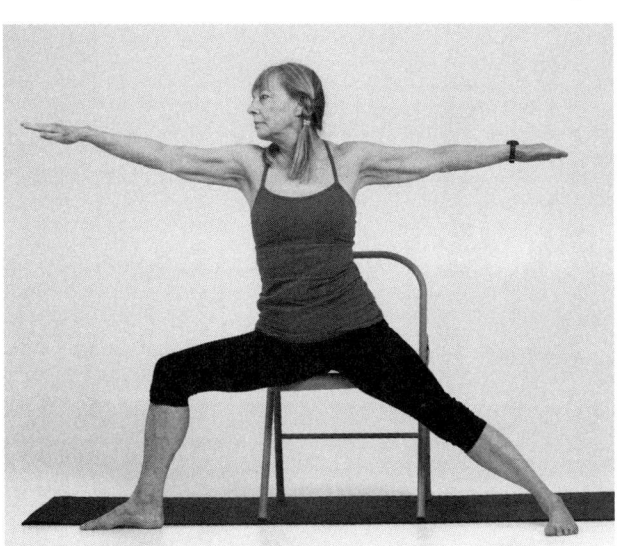

Seated Warrior 2 (Virabhadrasana 2)

Throughout this asana, draw students' attention to the feeling of their body in this shape as a whole. Then help them bring awareness into often neglected parts of the posture, such as the back arm and leg. Can they shift attention to those areas while holding their gaze steady? This movement of awareness and recognition of our ability to be aware is a key component of yoga. Can they work with 30 percent awareness in the front fingertip and 70 percent somewhere else? How can learning to bring some things into focus and let others be in the background support healing?

Standing Sun Salutation (Surya Namaskar)

Some of the sequence repeats now with the option to try the standing variations. Those who prefer to take a second round of Seated Sun Salutation are encouraged to do so.

Students who are standing can reach their arms up with an inhale. Then they exhale and fold forward. On the next inhale, they should lift their head up with a long spine. On the exhale, they can keep their head up and shoulders over their wrists as they hop or step back into a plank position, still exhaling as they bend their elbows and lower down, hovering two inches from the ground.

On the next inhale, they should let their hips move their body forward, coming onto the tops of their feet and lifting their chest for Upward Dog or Cobra, a gentler stomach-down backbend where the thighs remain on the ground as the chest lifts. Then, on the exhale, bring students into Downward Dog. Encourage them to spread their fingers and push down into their knuckles. Count five breaths here, inviting them

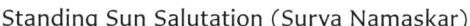

Standing Sun Salutation (Surya Namaskar)

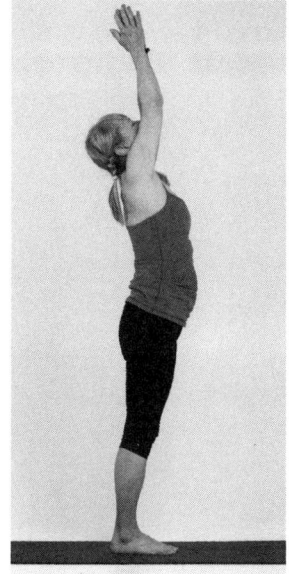
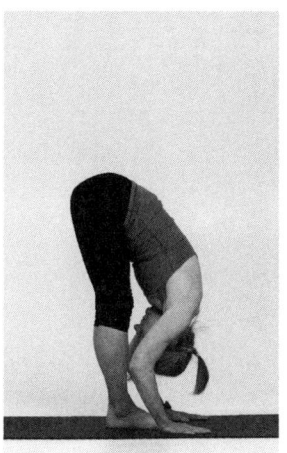
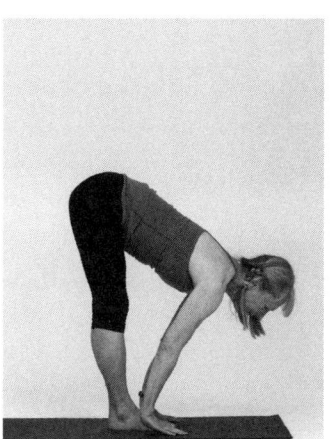
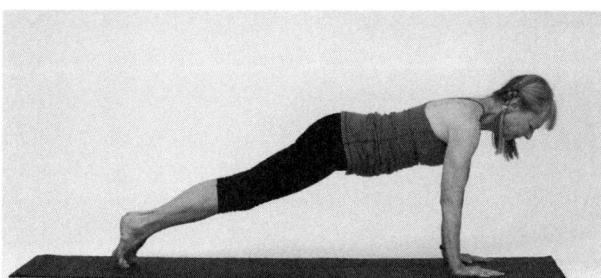
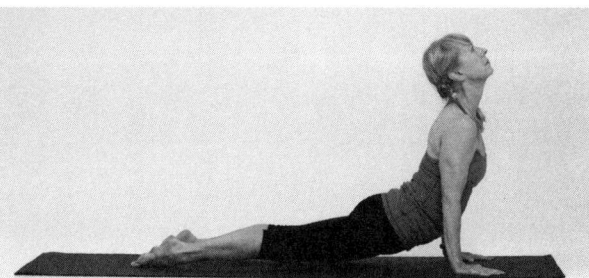
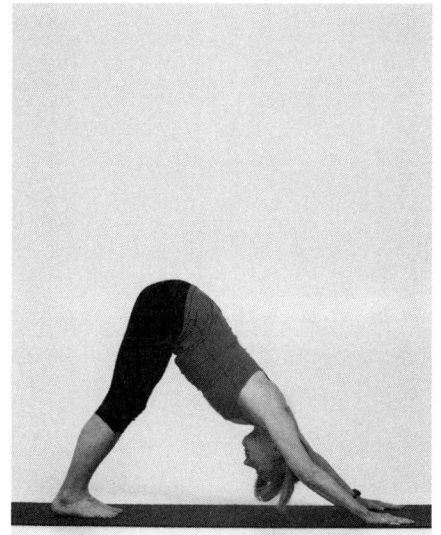
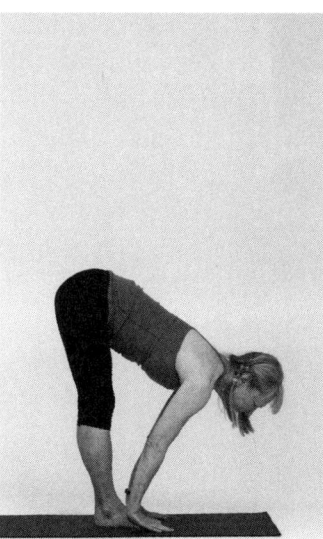
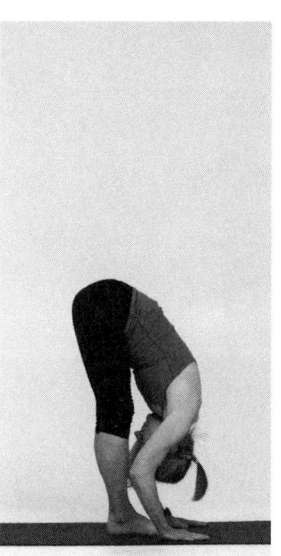
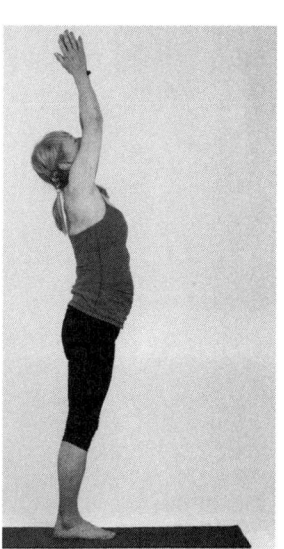

to breathe into the sides of their body as in accordion breathing. Give Child's Pose as an alternative.

After the fifth breath, students should step or jump forward, inhale, and lift their head. Then they can exhale and fold forward. Take them through a strong inhale to come all the way up with the arms up overhead. On their exhale, they can come to a starting position with their arms at their sides. Guide them to begin again when ready, repeating these salutations three to five times at their own pace.

Standing Triangle Pose A (Trikonasana A)

On an inhale, invite students to step out three feet to the side and open their arms wide. Exhaling, be with them as they turn one foot out and reach out and down toward their big toe. Encourage them to go as far as they can without straining, and then find stillness. They can press the back of their hand on their leg for support and to help them to reach up and out of their body instead of collapsing into the pose. Remind them to be sure their legs are doing the work, not their face, neck, and shoulders as they stay here for five breaths. Talk them through a strong inhale to come up before exhaling onto the other side.

Extended Side Angle A (Parsvakonasana A)

Invite students to take a five-foot step to the right on an inhale and reach their arms out wide. On their exhale, they can turn their right foot out, bend that knee, and reach their left arm over their ear at an angle. Invite them to turn their chest toward the ceiling and breathe into the sides of their body, perhaps even imagining that the breath is coming in and out from the armpit. What is the impact of breath being directed there? Count them through five breaths. Then invite them to use an inhale to come up through the center and pivot their feet to take the other side, coming into it as they exhale.

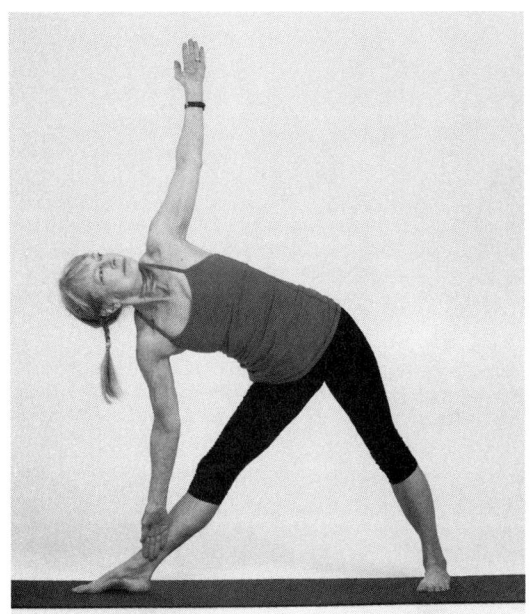

Standing Triangle Pose A (Trikonasana A)

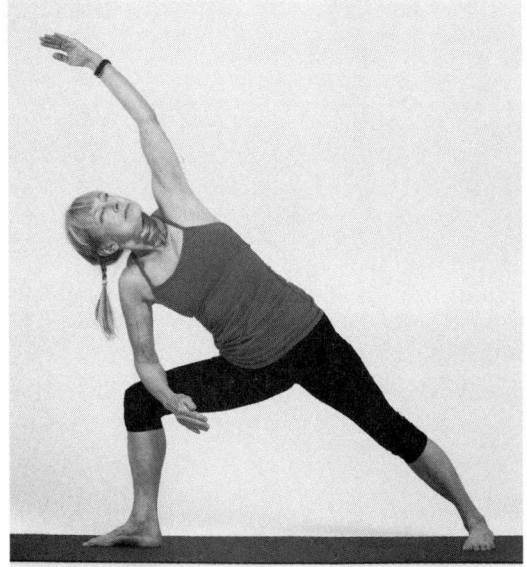

Extended Side Angle A (Parsvakonasana A)

Wide-Legged Standing Forward Fold Pose A
(Prasarita Padottanasana A)

Have students bring their hands to their waist as they face the center, feet slightly pigeon-toed, then inhale into their sides. On their exhale, invite them to fold forward, bringing their hands to the ground, shoulder-width apart, with fingertips in line with toe tips. They can inhale here, once more lifting their head.

Exhaling, students should bring their head toward the ground. Cue them to stay here for five breaths, gazing at their nose tip. Invite them to engage their legs as their head hangs heavy or touches the ground. Can they invite the idea of breathing into their back to color their experience in this position? What does it shift?

On the next inhale, instruct students to come halfway up. They should stay there for the exhale. Then on the inhale, students bring their hands

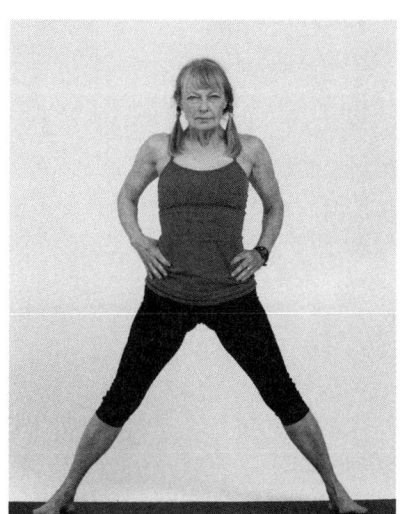
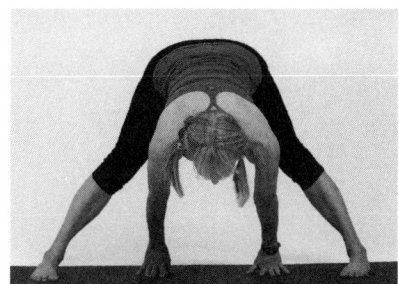
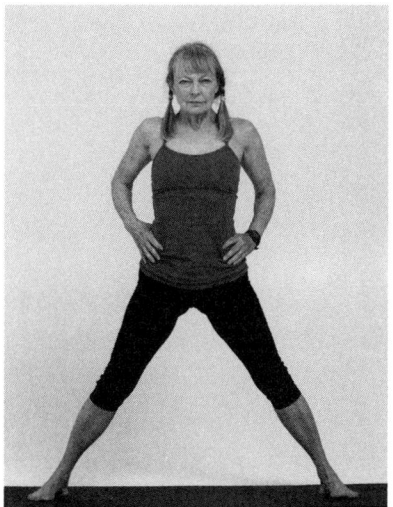

to their waist, come all the way up, then exhale in the standing position. Encourage them to tune in to any differences in their body since beginning the pose and note them as they ground through the feet.

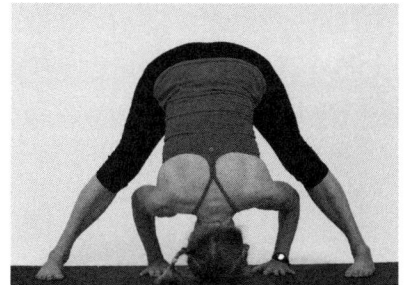
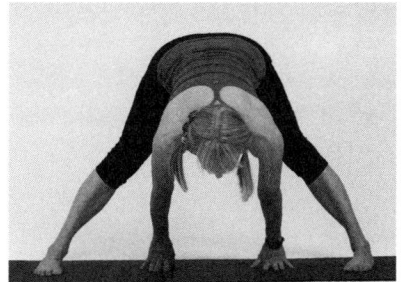

Wide-Legged Standing Forward Fold Pose A (Prasarita Padottanasana A)

Wide-Legged Standing Forward Fold Pose B
(Prasarita Padottanasana B)

For Wide-Legged Standing Forward Fold Pose B, invite students to inhale and open their arms into a T. They can take a moment to feel how spacious it is to be in this shape. On their exhale they should squeeze their waist with their hands, tuning in to their body's feelings in the pose. Next, invite them to inhale.

Exhaling, they can fold forward, bringing the crown of their head toward the ground as they continue to squeeze their waist. Encourage them to bring their chin toward their chest and reach down through the middle of their head toward the ground, firming up their legs as they do so. Stay here for five breaths. To come out of the pose, students inhale and rise all the way up to standing. Have them exhale there.

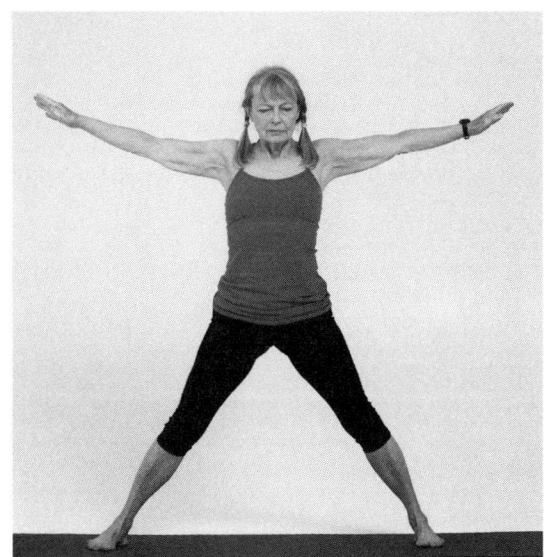

Wide-Legged Standing Forward Fold Pose C
(Prasarita Padottanasana C)

Students can start Standing Wide-Legged Forward Fold Pose C by inhaling and opening their arms wide. Encourage them again to take in the feeling of this shape in their body. Exhaling,

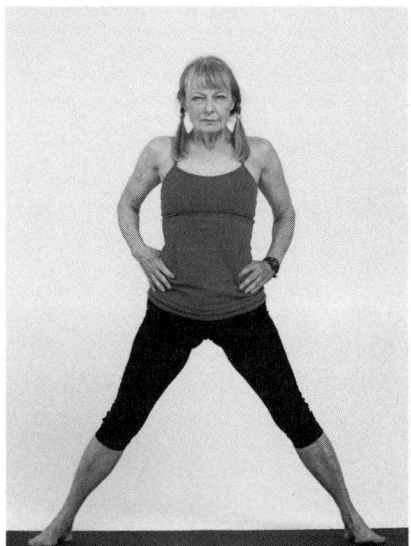 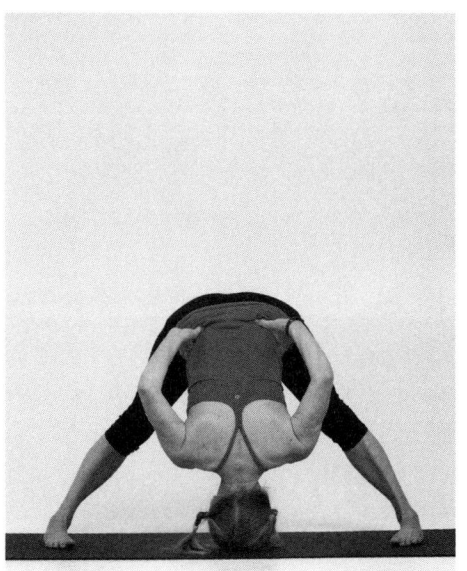 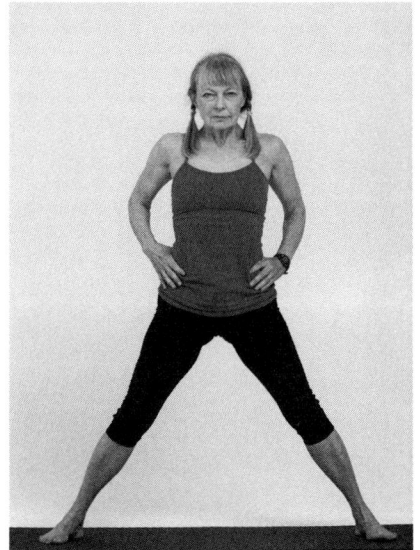

Wide-Legged Standing Forward Fold Pose B (Prasarita Padottanasana B)

they clasp their hands behind their back. Cue them to be aware of what this does to their body and their energetic sense. They can take an inhale here.

Exhaling, students can fold forward, bringing the crown of their head toward the ground and stretching their arms out and toward the ground as well. Remind them not to worry if that intention results in only a bit of movement from the shoulders. The arms will release as much as they are ready to do so and in time they may come forward. If there is any pain or pinching in the shoulders, encourage students to think about pressing their arms out instead of down. Invite students to stay here for five breaths. Cue them to keep their gaze on their nose tip as eyes tend to move around in this posture, which can make other students uncomfortable.

Students should meet tension they encounter by sending breath into their shoulder blades or other tight spots and actively releasing any holding or tension. They can let their arms fall more deeply toward the floor in their clasped position with each exhale. Stay here for five breaths. Ask students to inhale and come all the way up, then exhale there.

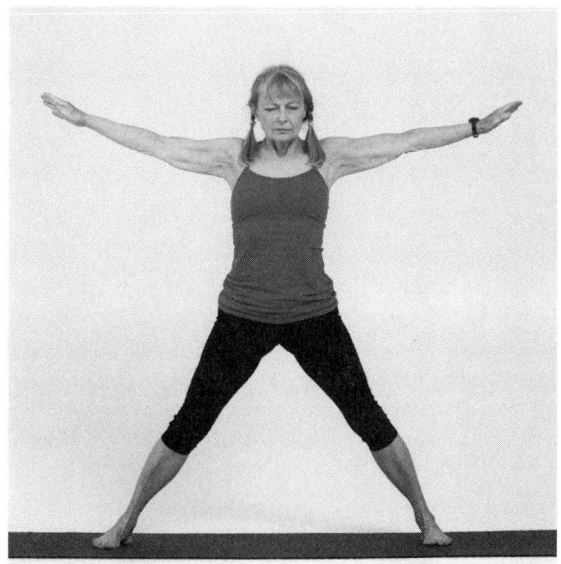 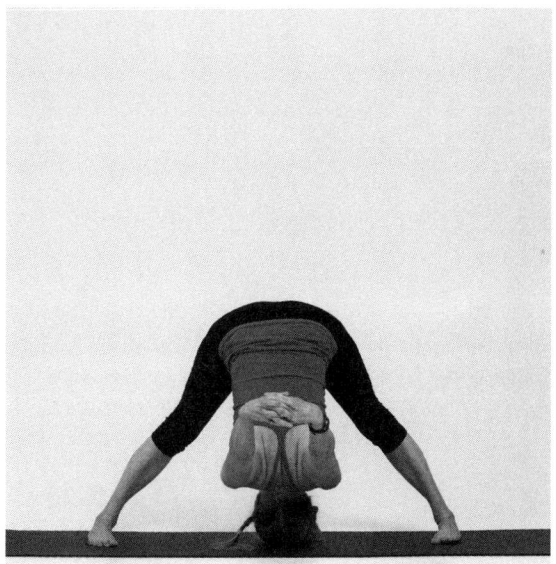

Wide-Legged Standing Forward Fold Pose C (Prasarita Padottanasana C)

Wide-Legged Standing Forward Fold Pose D (Prasarita Padottanasana D)

For Wide-Legged Standing Forward Fold Pose D, ask students to inhale and squeeze their waist with their hands. Then, exhaling, they can wrap their first two fingers around their big toes. Next, they can inhale and look up, keeping a hold on their toes and lengthening their spine. After that, invite students to exhale and pull their wrists and elbows up while reaching their head toward the ground. They can stay here for five breaths, gazing at their nose tip.

On the next inhale, invite students to look up, maintaining the toe hold and with a long spine. They can stay here for the exhale. On the next inhale, they can come all the way back up, exhaling when they are standing, with hands on their waist, before stepping forward to Samasthiti.

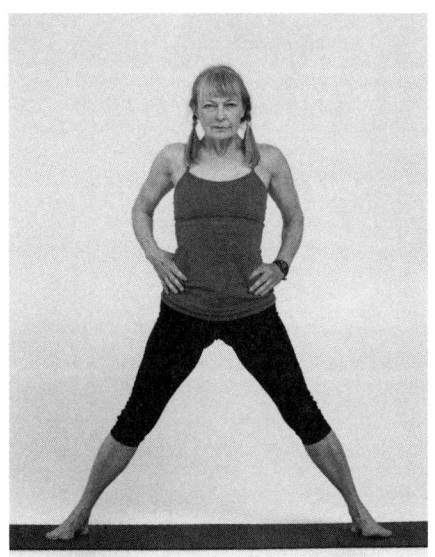
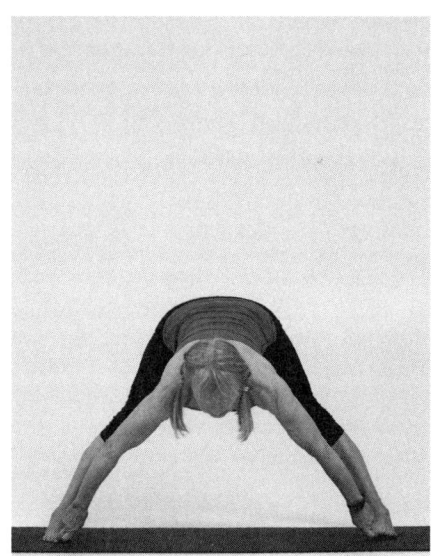
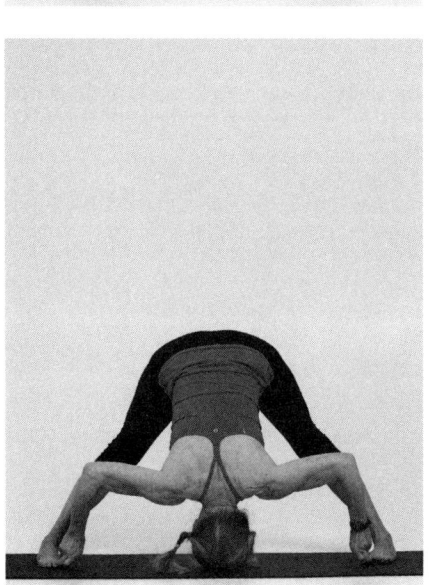
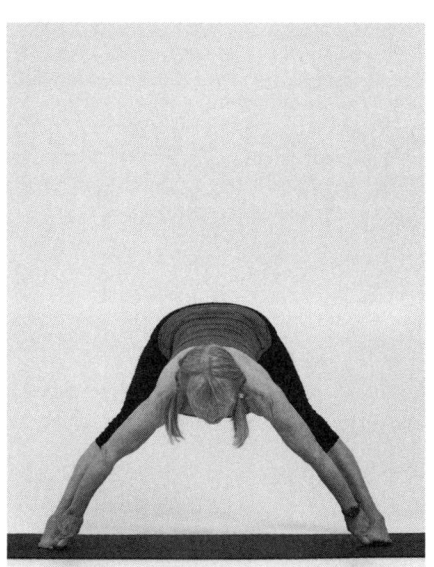
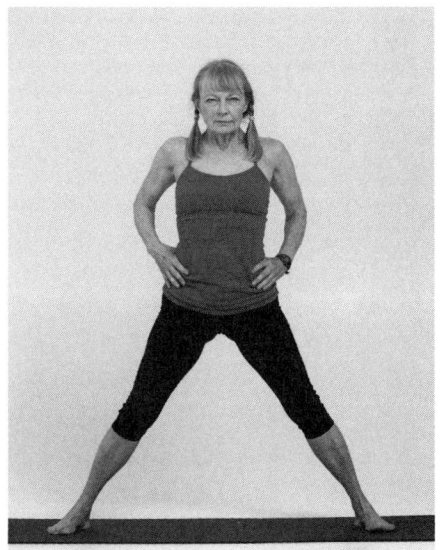

Wide-Legged Standing Forward Fold Pose D (Prasarita Padottanasana D)

Intense Side Stretch Pose (Parsvottanasana)

Ask students to pivot toward the back of their mat and step their right foot forward on an inhale. In this pose the feet are two and a half to three feet apart, the front foot is pointing forward, and the back foot is turned out slightly with heels aligned. Encourage students to square their hips over their extended leg. They can bring their arms behind their back either in Reverse Prayer Pose or to hold opposite elbows. As they exhale, invite students to fold over their extended leg. They can drop their head and gaze at their nose tip or, if their chest is resting on their leg, they can tilt their chin up to gaze at their big toe. Remind them to keep their knees soft to avoid hyperextension. Have them stay here for five breaths. Then bring them up through an inhale. Next, instruct them to exhale and pivot their feet, keeping the arms in their bind, and fold over the opposite leg.

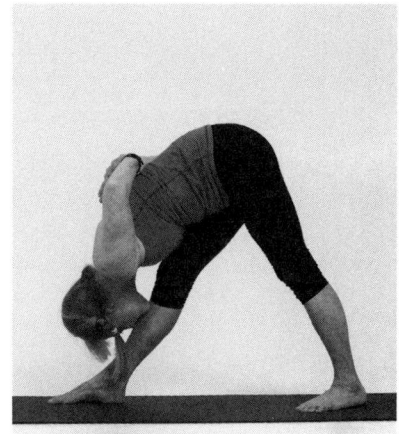

Intense Side Stretch Pose
(Parsvottanasana)

Extended Hand-to-Big-Toe Pose
(Utthita Hasta Padangusthasana)

Revisit Extended Hand-to-Big-Toe Pose, this time teaching a version without chair support, for those who want to try it. Ask students to see what, if anything, has shifted since taking this asana earlier in the sequence. This version offers the toe bind for those who want to increase the intensity of the pose.

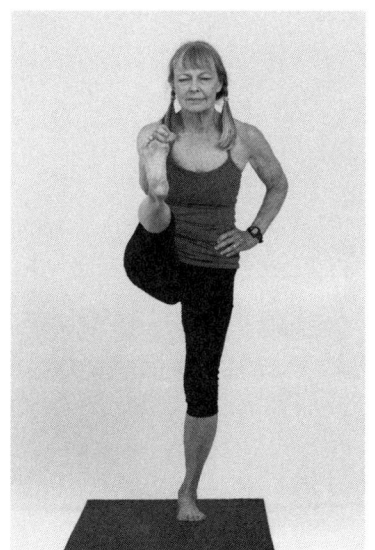 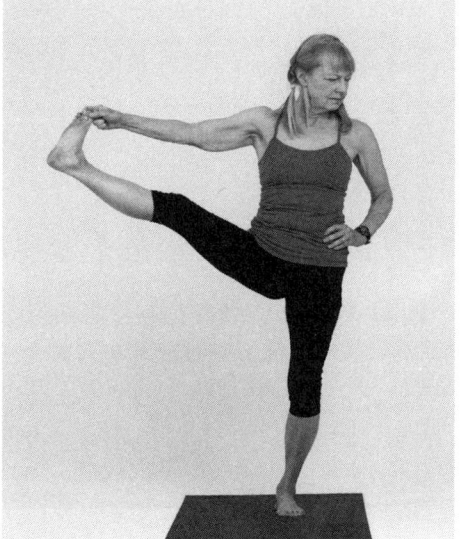 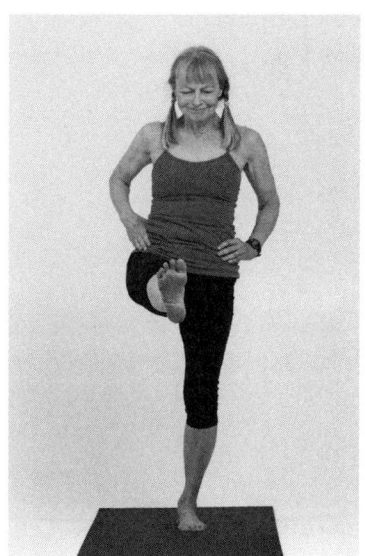

Extended Hand-to-Big-Toe Pose (Utthita Hasta Padangusthasana)

Students can ground down deeply through the left (standing) side of their body. Encourage them to press down so much through their left side that their right leg can't help but come up. If their toe is within reach, they can hook their big toe with their first two fingers. Ask students to lengthen their leg in front of them as much as they can while keeping their eyes resting on one still spot. Count five breaths here. On an inhale, invite them to stand up just a little bit taller.

On the exhale, ask students to bring their leg out to the side and encourage them to move their gaze to the opposite direction. Invite them to stay here for five breaths. They can always take their hand to the top of their knee if the leg extension is too intense or modify into Tree Pose.

Ask them to use an inhale to come back to center, and on the exhale, release the toe hold and bring their hand to their waist as they keep lifting their leg. They can gaze at their big toe for five breaths. Guide students to lower their leg to their mat on an exhale. Teach the posture on the other side.

Half-Bound Lotus (Ardha Baddha Padmottanasana)

Revisit Half-Bound Lotus now either with or without the chair. (Instructions and cues begin on page 197) Ask students what, if anything, has changed in their body since the first Half-Bound Lotus? Challenge them to find something new they can concentrate on or notice in this posture. How does shifting the awareness change the asana's expression? Invite students to fold forward, bringing their hands to the ground or to

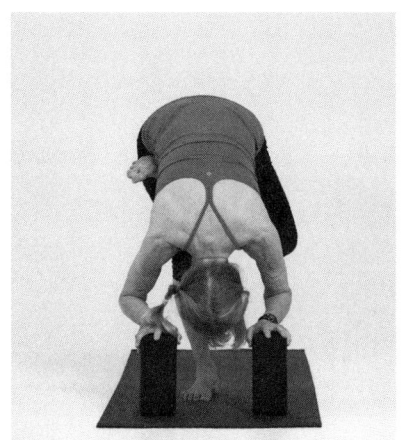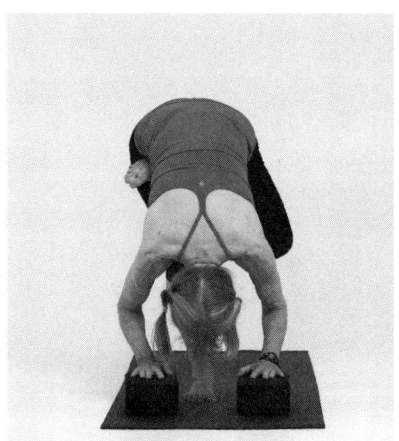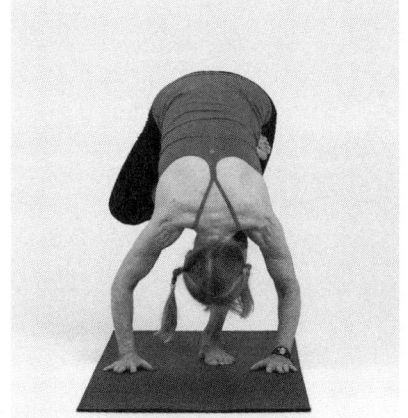

Half-Bound Lotus (Ardha Baddha Padmottanasana)

blocks and resting for five breaths. On an inhale, invite them to come up and switch sides.

Sun Salutation A (Surya Namaskar A)

A Sun Salutation gets the body in flow again and creates a transition from standing to the floor for seated postures. Compete instructions and cues for Standing Sun Salutation begin on page 198. When students are in Downward Dog, cue them to hop or step forward, folding their legs between their hands to sit.

Seated Forward Fold (Paschimottanasana)

Ask students to sit with their legs stretched out in front of them. On an inhale, they can use their first two fingers to hook their big toes, lengthening their spine as they lean forward. If they can't reach their big toes with straight legs, they can bend their knees.

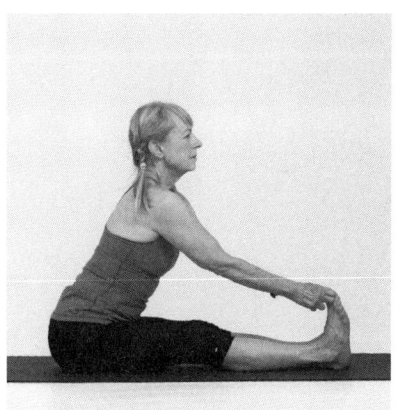

On an exhale, invite students to fold forward. This action could be uncomfortable in the lower back and hamstrings. Ask students to try to stay with uncomfortable sensations as they arise. This pose is good for this practice because it tends to burn for a short while and also because those sensations will often go away, move, and change. If that doesn't occur and pain is sharp or any numbness occurs, students should adjust or come out of the posture. A deceptively simple forward fold offers students an opportunity to explore the changing nature of sensations in a safe environment. Stay here for five breaths with the option for students to come out of the pose at any time.

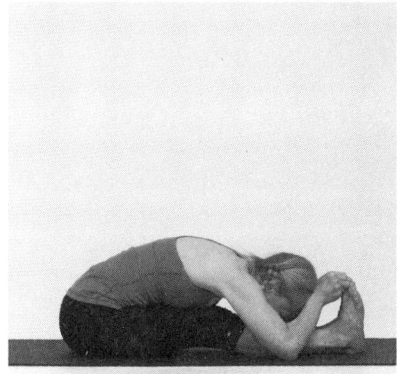 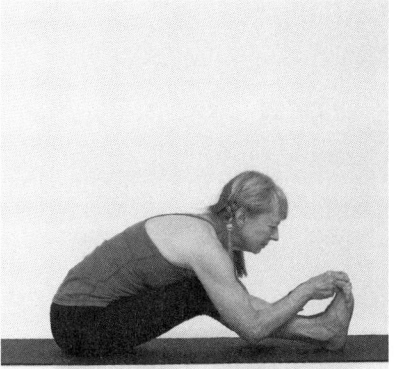 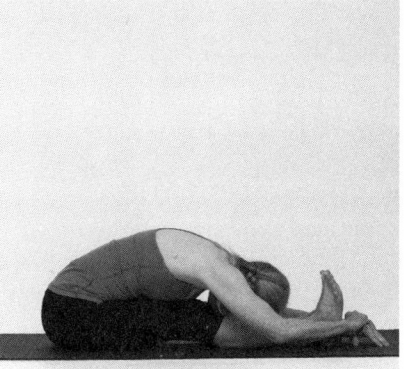

Seated Forward Fold (Paschimottanasana)

At the end of five breaths, ask students to lift their head on an inhale while still holding their toes. Next, invite them to wrap their hands around their feet for their deepest forward fold and exhale into it. They can stay there for another five breaths.

East-Facing Stretch/Upward Plank Pose (Purvottanasana)

Invite students to plant their hands about six inches behind their back with their fingers pointing forward. Encourage them to take some time in this position. They may even want to stay here for the full five breaths instead of moving into the following pose.

Those who want to feel more intensity can press down into their hands and lift their bottom and legs up as they point and press their feet toward the ground. Breathe here for five breaths. Be careful introducing this posture if students aren't ready for so much front body exposure. You'll know it's not time if poses such as Cat/Cow and Cobra are still triggering.

Ray of Light Pose/Sage Pose (Marichyasana A)

From East-Facing Stretch, invite students to lower their bottom and legs. From a seated position, students can bend one leg in toward their body as close as they can, foot planted toward their outside hip. They can extend their other leg out straight with the toes pointing upward. Make sure they leave space between the foot of their bent leg and their extended thigh. Invite students to inhale and stretch the arm (on the side of the bent leg) up and then out long. Then, exhaling, ask them

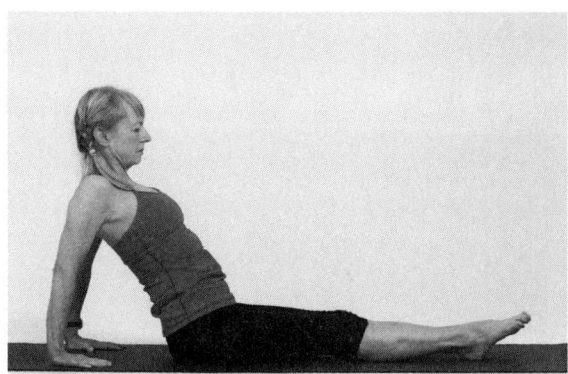 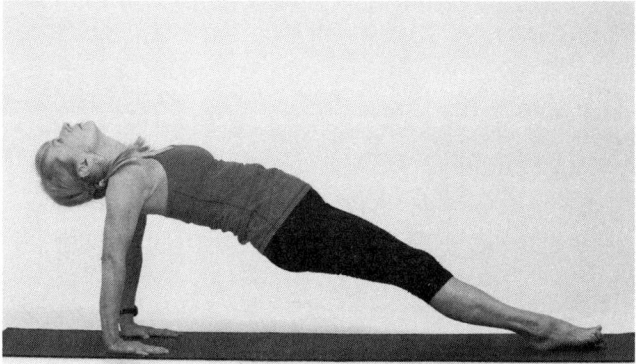

East-Facing Stretch/Upward Plank Pose (Purvottanasana)

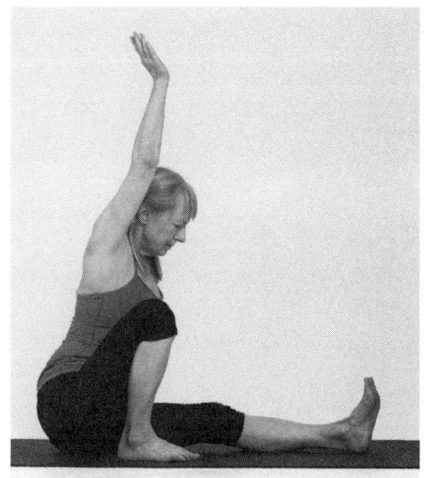

to wrap it around their leg. Guide them to inhale here, chest lifted and gaze forward, then exhale and fold forward, bringing their head to their extended leg. Breathe five times. Instead of switching sides, transition into Marichyasana C on the same side.

Ray of Light Pose/Sage Pose (Marichyasana A)

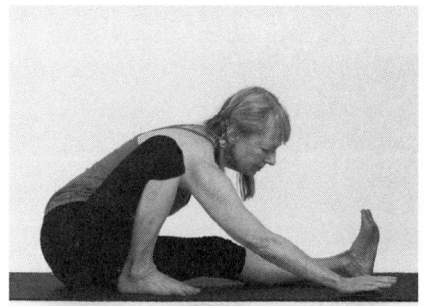
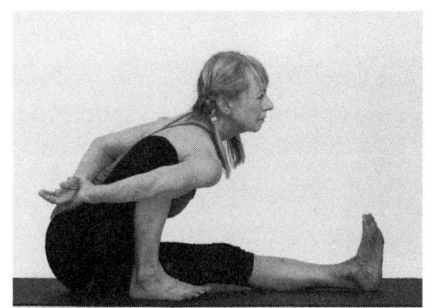
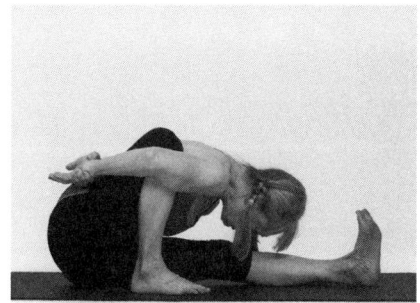

Ray of Light Pose/Sage Pose (Marichyasana C)

From Sage Pose, invite students to come back up to sit and release their arms. They can now reach across their body with the opposite elbow to press against the outside of their bent knee for a twist. They can stay here or try to get a deeper arm bind: students place their knee into their armpit, inwardly rotate their arm, bending their elbow, and reaching behind to find their other hand, which wraps around their waist. Remind them that it doesn't matter if they don't reach that other hand. The idea is about taking the

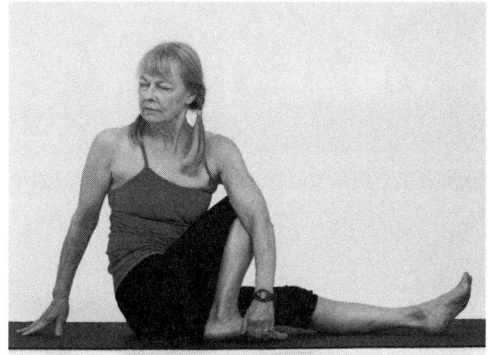
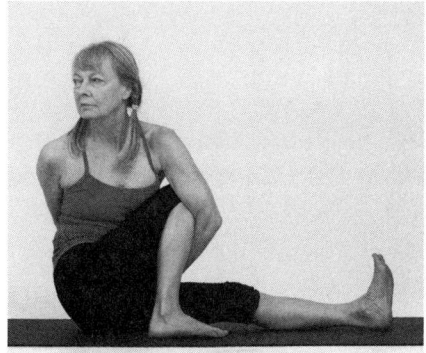

Ray of Light Pose/Sage Pose (Marichyasana C)

Poses with binds are potentially triggering for trauma survivors. Finding breath in a constricted position is challenging and can cause fear and all its related arousal to occur in the body. When the practitioner is ready to work with those feelings, it is an opportunity to practice calming the body in a time of crisis, which builds the practitioner's capacity for finding calm when their body is stressed.

Overwhelming a practitioner with challenging postures that trigger a fear response does not necessarily result in growth and can even cause harm. Introduce potentially stressful poses after a time if the student appears ready. Start with a shorter breath count, such as one to three breaths, to release them from feeling constricted.

deepest twist possible. Ask students to stretch their gaze back behind them and breathe five times in this position.

Invite students to release the bind or twist and switch legs for Marichyasana A and C on the other side.

Uprooting (Utpluthih)

Bring students back to center and invite them to bring their hands close to their body just in front of their bottom. Show them how to cross their legs at the shins and pull their knees in toward their chest. With an inhale, challenge them to press down into their hands and lift their bottom off the floor for one breath. Then ask them to come down on an exhale and immediately lift their legs up into Boat Pose.

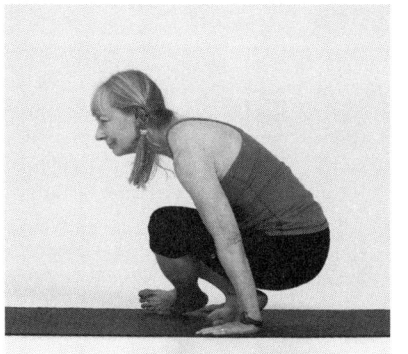

Uprooting (Utpluthih)

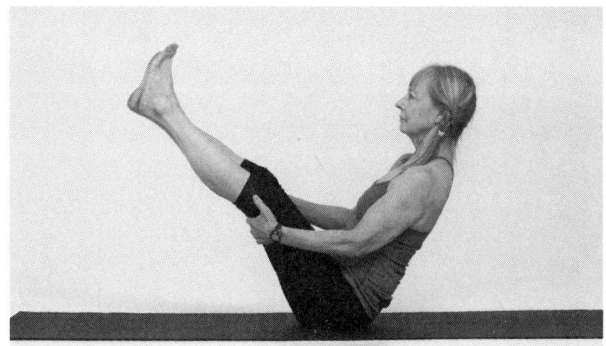
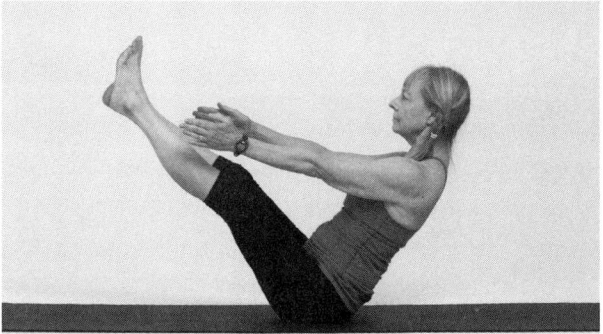

Boat Pose (Navasana)

Boat Pose (Navasana)

Encourage students to create a V shape with a straight spine and extended legs. They can either support their legs with their hands or let go and stretch their arms out. Ask them to gaze at their big toes and breathe five breaths. They can repeat this posture three to five times, coming to Utpluthih in between rounds.

Bridge Pose (Setu Bandha Sarvangasana)

Guide students to lie on their back with their knees bent and their feet placed on their mat hip-width apart or more. Ask them to keep their arms at their sides and stretch through their fingertips toward their heels. On an inhale, invite students to press down into their feet to lift up their bottom and back off the ground as high as they can. Invite them to bring their gaze to their chest where they can observe its rise and fall as they breathe five times before lowering down for one breath cycle.

VARIATION: BRIDGE POSE (SETU BANDHA SARVANGASANA)

Invite students to lift up again on an inhale, but this time roll their shoulders under, creating a deeper back arch and bring their hands together under their lower back for five more breaths. They can press down into their arms and clasped hands to lift up higher. After the fifth exhale, ask them to lower their bottom and back down to their mat.

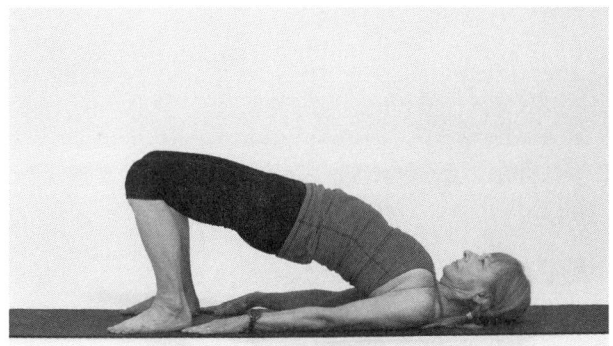

Bridge Pose (Setu Bandha Sarvangasana)

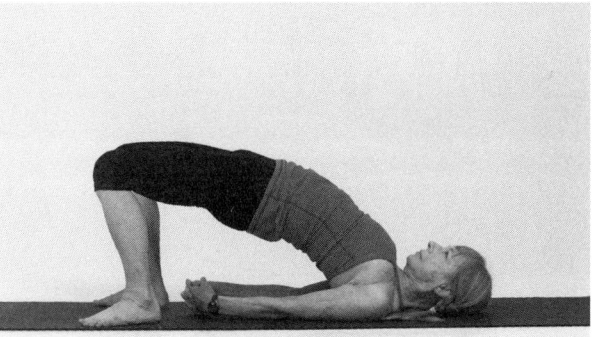

Bridge Pose (Setu Bandha Sarvangasana) variation

Wheel Pose (Urdhva Dhanurasana)

Invite students to choose one of the previous Bridge Poses or to prepare for Wheel Pose. To set up for Wheel Pose, students can bring their hands flat on their mat by their ears and bend their legs so their feet are in close to their body but hip-width apart or wider. Invite students to push into their hands and feet to lift their bottom, back, and shoulders off the ground, straightening their arms as much as possible.

This posture can be stimulating. Ask students to use their previous practice skills and knowledge of their body to try to relax and breathe here five times.

Wind-Relieving Pose (Pawanmuktasana)

After the intensity of the backbending sequence, it is time for counterposes. From Wheel Pose or Bridge Pose, bring students down to the mat on an exhale and invite them to hug their knees into their chest. Practitioners can move in any way that feels inviting to them: rolling, gentle rocking, or twisting, forward and back or side to side. If they are not sure what feels most inviting, encourage them to just move.

Shoulderstand (Sarvangasana)

When students seem ready, invite them to use their intention, inhale, and a little bit of a push to lift their back and legs into the air for Shoulderstand. They can support their lower back with their hands, inching their

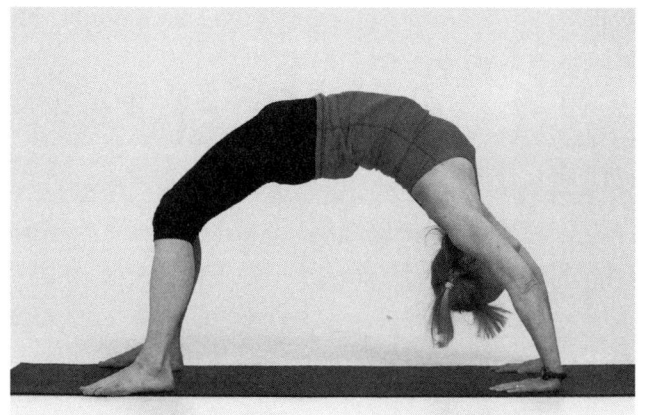

Wheel Pose (Urdhva Dhanurasana)

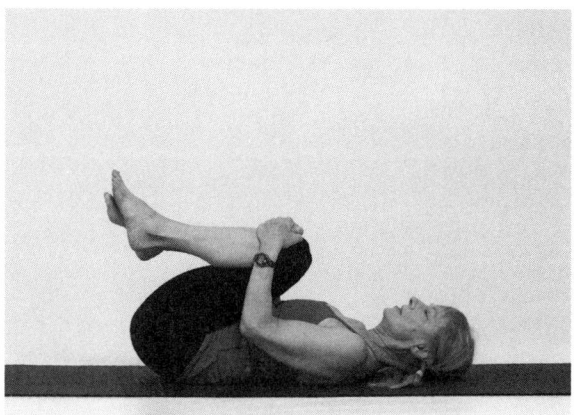

Wind-Relieving Pose (Pawanmuktasana)

elbows closer together as they do so. Legs up in the air or legs up a wall (if there's wall space) are alternatives (see page 182).

Shoulderstanding provides great relief for the legs, increases blood flow to the brain, and stimulates the thyroid. It stretches the spine and strengthens the legs. Folks give it credit for many health benefits including healing asthma, calming indigestion, and soothing menstruation. For these reasons, as long as there is no neck pain or other contraindications, it is great to stay in this pose for up to twenty-five breaths.

If the neck is open enough and the body is able, Shoulderstand variations can then be added to continue to stretch the body while also keeping it inverted. For many this feels strenuous for the neck. Encourage those students to come off the neck and take these poses reclined but not inverted. For instance, Ear-Pressure Pose (Karnapidasana) would now take the form of separating the legs and squeezing the knees in toward the shoulders; Embryo Pose (Pindasana) would take the form of crossed legs hugged in close to the chest.

Make sure to explain and demo the entire Shoulderstand sequence before your students are reclined so they can see and hear you. Remind them not to look around in Shoulderstand or Shoulderstand variations because it can injure the neck.

Plow Pose (Halasana)

After ten to twenty-five breaths in Shoulderstand, invite students to either stay there or drop their legs overhead toward the floor for Plow Pose. They should support their lower back with their hands unless their feet touch the floor. If toes are resting on the floor, they can remove their hands from their back, interlace their fingers, and extend

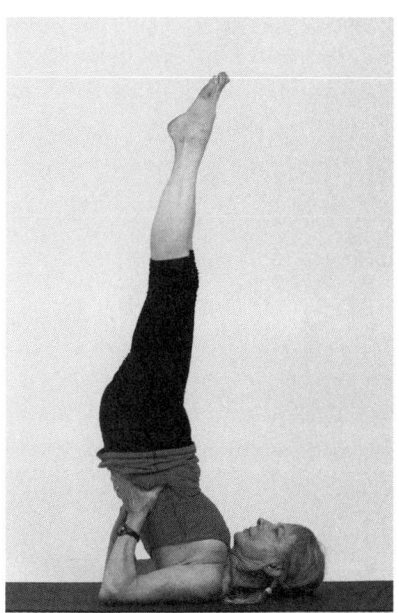

Shoulderstand (Sarvangasana)

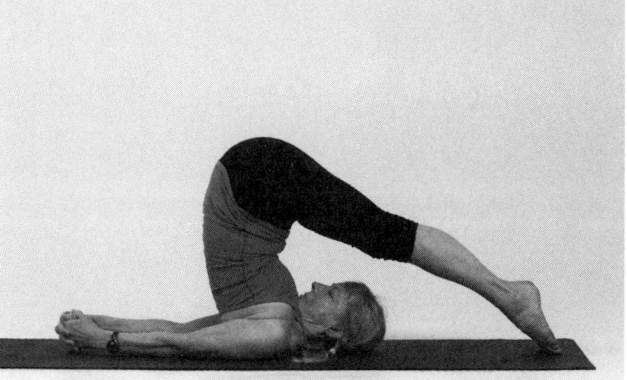

Plow Pose (Halasana)

their arms along the floor. Encourage them to keep toes and heels together and to gently lift their kneecaps. Count them through eight to ten breaths.

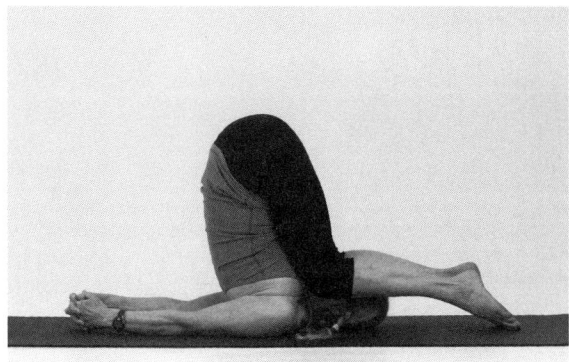

Ear-Pressure Pose (Karnapidasana) variation

VARIATION: EAR-PRESSURE POSE (KARNAPIDASANA)

Students who want to go deeper can bend their knees and squeeze their ears or the temples with their knees. Their toes and heels remain together, their hands clasped, and they press their arms into the ground. If they are regular practitioners, remind them to switch up their finger clasp every so often so the opposite thumb is on top! Remain in this pose for eight to ten breaths.

Upward Lotus (Urdhva Padmasana)

Invite students to support their lower back as they lift their legs into Shoulderstand position. From there, they can fold their legs into Lotus, or a cross-legged position. Newer students can begin to learn to balance on their shoulders by moving one hand to one kneecap while the other supports the lower back. Encourage them to breathe four breaths here and then switch hands. Remind everyone to position their hands like shelves beneath their knees and hold their Lotus legs so they are parallel to the ground.

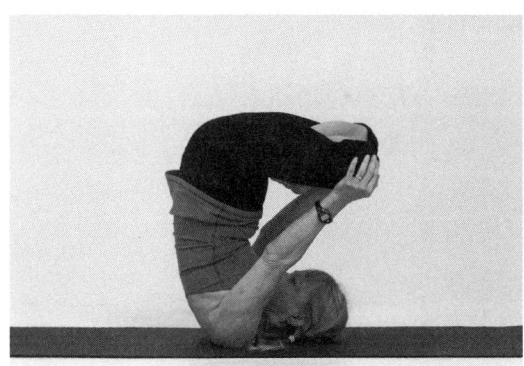

Upward Lotus (Urdhva Padmasana)

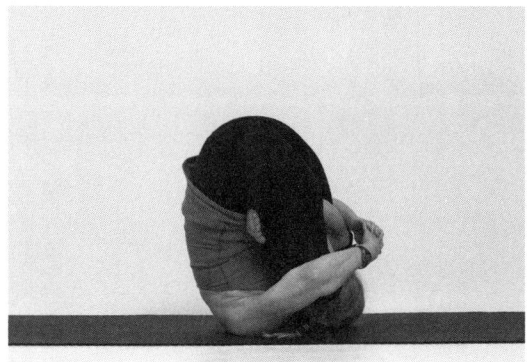

Embryo Pose (Pindasana)

Embryo Pose (Pindasana)

Next, invite students to fold their Lotus or crossed legs into their chest and hug their legs. If they can't balance like this, they can keep their hands on their lower back until they can balance on their shoulders. Caution them not to squeeze too hard in this position or they could pull a muscle. A gentle hug is what we are going for. Stay for eight to ten breaths.

Fish Pose (Matsyasana)

Invite students to release their arms to their mat and roll down their spine as slowly as they can, letting their knees drop. When their knees are as low as they can go, students can lift their chest and place the crown of their head on their mat. Then invite them to hold the outer edges of their feet or place their hands on their thighs. Their gaze is at their nose tip. Keep cuing for relaxing the body and mind. Count them through eight to ten breaths.

VARIATION: FISH POSE (MATSYASANA)
Invite students to extend their legs straight for a variation of Fish Pose, staying eight to ten breaths. Then ask them to release their head gently and slowly by engaging their hands and arms with the ground for support. Guide them to roll onto their side to sit up and onto their knees to prepare for Headstand.

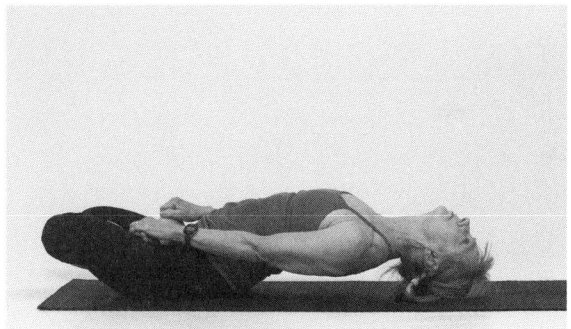

Fish Pose (Matsyasana)

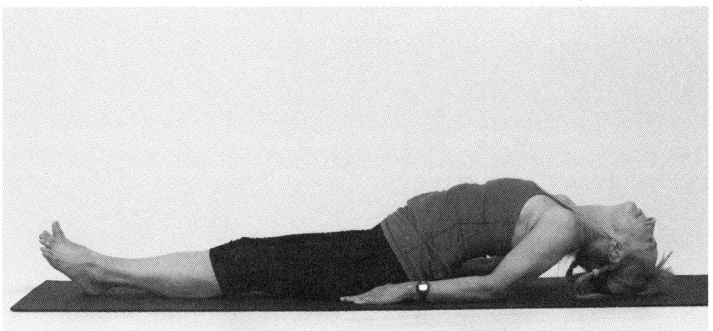

Fish Pose (Matsyasana) variation

Headstand (Sirsasana)

Ask students to bring their elbows in close as they cup their hands with threaded fingers, lift their knees up, and pull their legs forward trying to lift off the ground for Headstand. They should keep at this motion, pressing firmly into their forearms to keep pressure off their neck. Legs squeeze together, becoming like one big tail, and hips rock forward to get the right strength and alignment to eventually lift up. (For complete instructions and cues for Headstand, see page 183.)

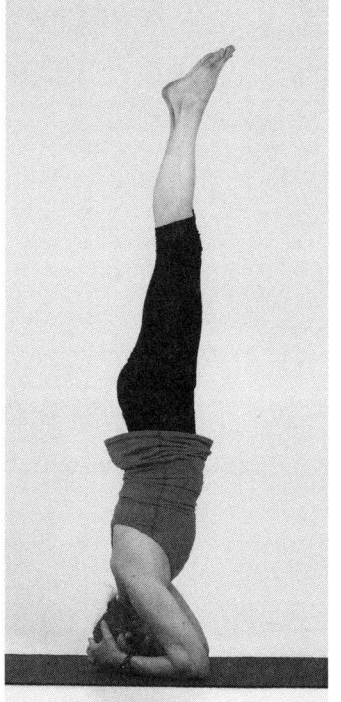

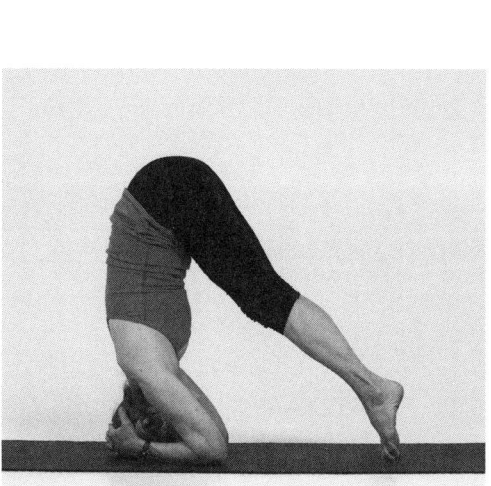

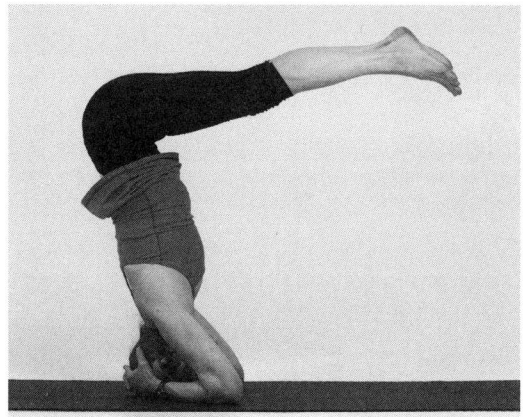

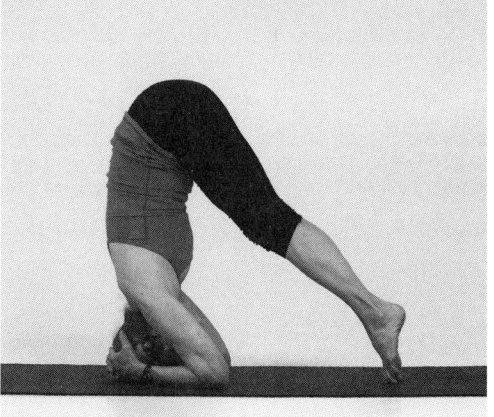

Headstand (Sirsasana)

Students can remain balanced in Headstand for up to fifteen breaths and then lower their legs halfway, parallel to floor, to build even more strength. Invite them to hold this L shape for ten breaths, with their gaze at their toes.

On an inhale, cue them to lift their legs upright again and, on an exhale, invite them to hinge at their waist, coming down very slowly. When their toes touch the ground, ask them to bend their knees, come to their mat, and rest in Child's Pose.

PREPARING FOR HEADSTAND

I prefer teaching the ascent into Headstand with straight legs because it builds the necessary strength. It also avoids the pop-up that one has to make from the crouched position into the straight legs. However, it's always good to have options for different students. Many like to explore balancing in a crouched position, and it can be fun to play in this shape. For those who want to try it, invite them to start as they would for a straight-legged Headstand. Instruct them to keep one leg straight and use it to push off the ground into a little hop as they pull the other leg in to a tucked position. If stable, they can then pull the jumping leg in at the top of the hop and squeeze their knees in tight to balance in a ball shape.

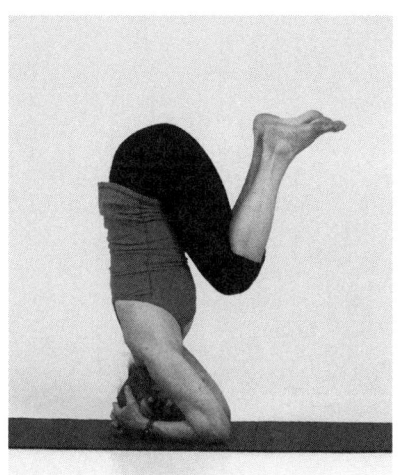

Preparing for Headstand

Child's Pose (Balasana)

Encourage students to stay in Child's Pose for a minute or two to rest their head and let the blood flow back in their body before sitting up.

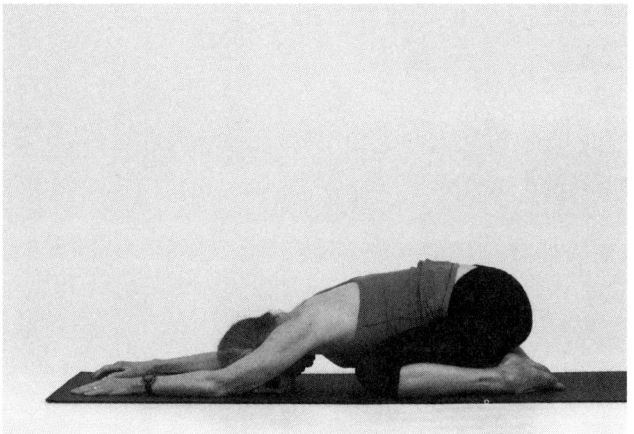

Child's Pose (Balasana)

Bound Lotus (Baddha Padmasana)

Finding a comfortable seat, students can take their legs into Lotus or any cross-legged position. Ask that they reach behind their back to hold opposite elbows or to take their big toes. They can work toward reaching the toes by practicing twisting and reaching in one direction at a time.

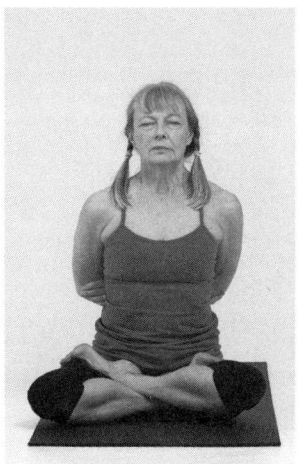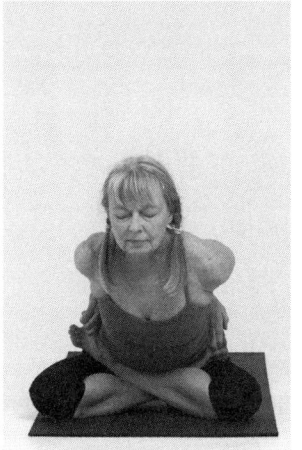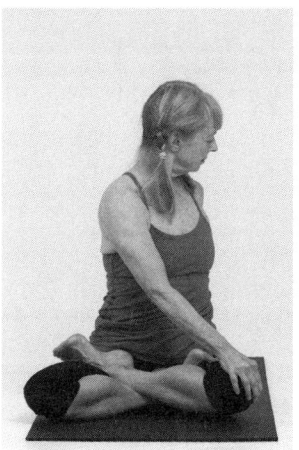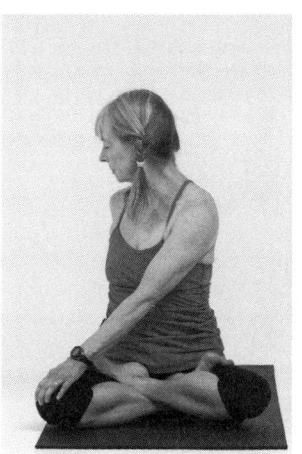

Bound Lotus (Baddha Padmasana)

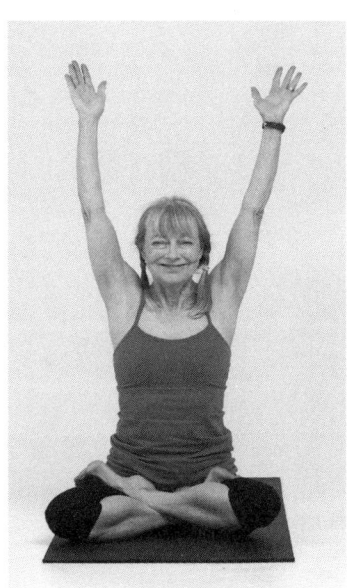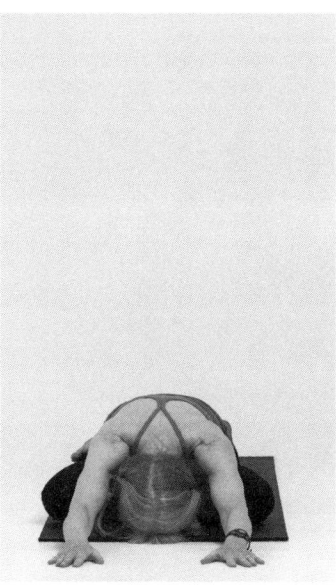

Sealing the Practice (Yoga Mudra)

Everyone can fold forward in this position. If they aren't holding their toes or elbows, invite them to reach their arms up and fold with outstretched arms. Count ten breaths in the forward fold. Challenge students to make these breaths fuller than any before them.

Lotus (Padmasana)

Bring them back up to sit and encourage them again to take the deepest ten breaths of their practice.

Sealing the practice (yoga mudra)

Uprooting (Utpluthih)

Finally, ask them to use the last pose to squeeze out any energy left in the body to get it ready to rest. Invite them into a crossed-legged or Lotus position with their hands close at their sides. Then lead them to press down and, with a big inhale, lift up their body. Keep challenging them to use all their focus and strength for ten breaths, even if they aren't lifting off the ground.

Final Rest (Savasana)

After ten breaths, bring everyone into rest. They can rest reclined or seated, with eyes open or closed. Invite them into stillness and presence, giving them the option to bring their attention to their breath or body as both relax. Remind them that if their mind wanders, they can bring it back to the present moment. If lying prone feels too intense, they can curl on their side or take any comfortable resting position with their eyes gently fixed on one spot.

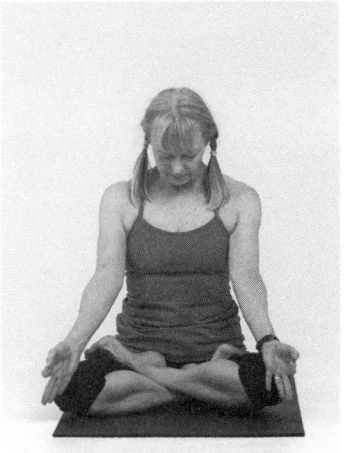

Lotus (Padmasana)

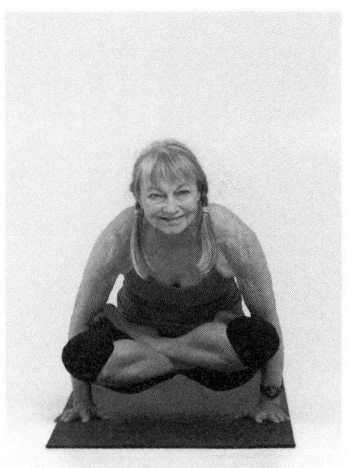

Uprooting (Utpluthih)

Closing Acknowledgments

Conclude by bringing the class up to sit and taking a moment to acknowledge their efforts and to feel the post-practice sensations. Give time for those who would like to share their experiences.

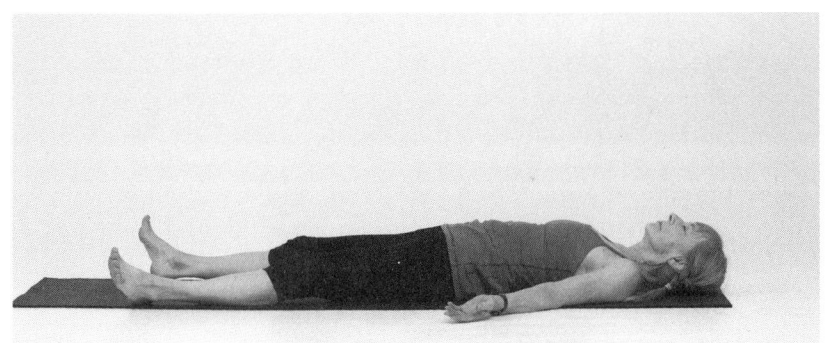

Rest (Savasana)

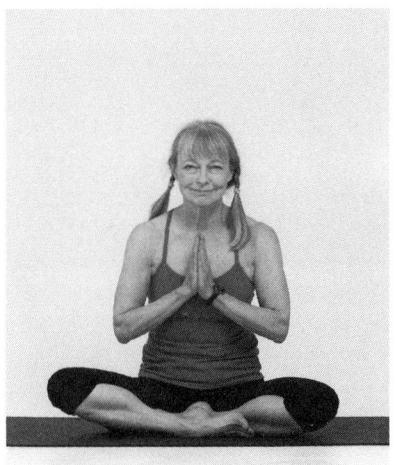

Closing acknowledgments

CONCLUSION:
YOGA AS SERVICE

CONGRATULATIONS! YOU'VE MADE IT TO THE FINAL CHAPTER of the book and the first chapter of your life as a trauma-informed yoga teacher. You may now be wondering, *What's next? What do I do with this knowledge? How do I know if I'm incorporating it correctly? Who are the others in my trauma sensitive yoga community?*

Orienting Yourself toward Healing

Yoga has always been trauma informed. It's rooted in self-healing, self-knowledge, personal expansion, and liberation. Yoga teachers from all traditions are now being called back to the original purpose and intentions of yoga study, for both personal sovereignty and world betterment. You are not alone. It's going to take a lot of us to break the spell the commercialization of yoga has sold us and to reeducate the world to what yoga really is. You are an ambassador of change and a corrector of misinformation. It's now on you to carry forth a definition of yoga that is true to its roots and honors its magnitude and power to heal. You can tell others about this mission, but you can be more effective by showing others through how you live, how you show up for life, and how you teach.

Continue your education. If you don't have a trauma-informed yoga certification, consider enrolling in a training, either from Three and a Half Acres or another of the wonderful organizations educating in this space (see the resources section in the conclusion). Train yourself in other areas such as yoga philosophy, chanting, somatics, conflict resolution, Alexander Technique, and so on. Continued education and self-betterment are your superpowers.

Practice teaching. One of the biggest pitfalls new teachers encounter is allowing fear of embarrassment to hold them back from making the mistakes necessary for growth. No one expects you to get it all right all the time, especially not in the beginning. Perfection is a false notion and impossible to reach; it does not exist. The idea of it keeps many potentially wonderful teachers from sharing their voices and talents, while people who have abundant confidence go wild sharing even though they may not be as well educated or informed, even spreading false information. We need more humble types willing to speak up. Pace yourself, teach what you know, and gradually add to your repertoire as you feel ready. Stay in a growth space, not becoming overwhelmed by trying too much too fast but daring to move out of your comfort zone. Stretch yourself and make sure to teach out loud. Too many new teachers make the mistake of practicing silently in their heads. Cerebral engagement will not do. We must say the words out loud to practice the movement from thought to sound, a transition that seems small but in fact makes all the difference. If you are too nervous to teach students in real time, record yourself teaching as a first step. Then teach a friend or family member, preferably someone without yoga experience, so you can see if your verbal explanations describe poses accurately enough.

Observe and assist experienced teachers. Who says mentorship and apprenticeship are over? In my opinion, they will always be the best ways to learn to teach yoga. Three and a Half Acres Yoga teacher trainee graduates are required to observe at least two classes, and they have the opportunity to mentor with senior teachers to improve their skills. Before deciding on one mentor, observe different teachers to see how they incorporate trauma-sensitive practices and alter sequences to work with their style and students. You can observe your mentor more regularly and perhaps assist and co-teach with and eventually fill in for them. There is nothing like being in the classroom to improve your skill sets. It places you in front of real challenges in real time that you could never simulate in a training session. You are forced to pull from all the resources inside of you while thinking on your feet, and you get immediate feedback via expressions, energy, and sometimes verbal responses as to how your facilitation has landed.

Preparing to Teach, Opportunities for Growth

Ready to teach trauma sensitive yoga but not sure how to get started or where to offer your classes? You have a few options to explore as you begin.

First, look inward. Practice on yourself and work on healing your own trauma. Whether it's a childhood experience, trauma from oppression, climate change or environmental trauma, or COVID-19 trauma, we are all working through different degrees of trauma. Healing from within is an ongoing process and essential to continue with so we don't transfer that trauma to others when we are in a position of leadership. Self-study and healing allow us to function and serve at our highest capacities and equip us for the problem-solving that life demands during challenging times.

Professionally, look at how you are putting yourself out there in your personal representation, website, newsletter marketing, and social media. Are your images representative of all and trauma sensitive? How can you better make your online spaces safer and to call in more folks? Write down one change you are ready to make now.

Look to the studios you teach at and the students you already have. Remember that trauma is in every room and folks do not wear signs that say "I am a trauma survivor." You can adjust your teaching immediately to make your "regular" classes more inclusive and trauma sensitive. What are three lessons you learned from this book? Pick three small changes you are ready to implement in your teaching style today. Write them down and hold yourself accountable.

You can begin to influence the studios you teach at and the culture of the classes offered by the way you teach. How can you bring more choice into the culture of the studios where you teach?

Beyond the Yoga Studio

Do you want to have an impact on the community beyond the yoga studio? I felt the same way when I began with trauma sensitive teaching. Teaching at a standard studio was not making enough of an impact for my vision and desire to serve. If this resonates, you can join us as a Three and a Half Acres Yoga teacher (see the resources section in the conclusion), or start your own program at a community organization or nonprofit in your area.

So many people ask me just how to go about this, as it may feel daunting. Here are some thoughts on getting started:

- Identify a community you feel drawn toward supporting, such as folks in recovery, LGBTQIA+ people, domestic abuse survivors, or the elderly.

- Get to know what organizations are out there supporting that community and what services are already being offered. There are large nonprofits such as Children's Aid Society, United Way, and Boys & Girls Clubs of America, but there are many small- and medium-sized local nonprofits as well.

- What is your offering? A weekly class? Monthly workshop? Make sure you are clear on what you'd like to share and for how long. One month? Three? I highly suggest a trial period of two to three months and an evaluation afterward to see if you and the students and organization feel the program is working and, if not, what could be tweaked to make it better.

- Will you offer a trial? Free ongoing classes or a fee-based structure?

- What will you do if you are sick or traveling, move, or decide to end classes so that you don't abandon a community with whom you have an established relationship and risk further traumatization to the students you wish to help?

- If you choose to offer your services for free, have you considered how much time you will be donating? Have you accounted for travel time and time spent planning your class? How will you manage burnout? Low attendance? It's important to consider all these factors in advance so you are prepared to take on the pragmatics of the class, not just the ideals.

- Identify the person or persons in charge of programming and reach out via email and phone. Share your skill sets and your personal reasons for wanting to get involved. You'll probably need to follow up more than once and at more than one organization before you make a promising connection.

- Respond quickly and thoughtfully to any interest. Ask to meet in person so you can see the space and get a sense of the needs specific to that space. This will also give you a sense of your travel time.

- Ask how they will promote your offering. Is there a flyer they could circulate or a newsletter they use to get information around their community? What times and days do they see the most participation? Could you come to an established, well-attended group and offer a short sample class? Is there a trusted person or persons on-site who could attend and support getting the word out?

- Show up! After you've done your background work, you are ready to do the real work of showing up each moment of your commitment prepared, curious, compassionate, in a beginner mindset, ready to share and learn!

You are needed. With political polarization, climate change, and many social systems in disarray, the times we are living in and the times coming are guaranteed to produce trauma across communities and populations. The only way through this requires calling on more of us to boost our own capacities for growth and that of others to stand strong and centered and to create safe spaces to love and to heal.

Sequence Worksheets

Download the Essential Guide to Trauma Sensitive Yoga Class Lesson Plan templates at www.shambhala.com/traumasensitiveyoga/. Two additional yoga sequences are available at https://laraland.us/wp-content/uploads/2022/11/Lara-Land-Bonus-Sequences.pdf.

Resources

BOOKS

Barkataki, Susanna. *Embrace Yoga's Roots: Courageous Ways to Deepen Your Yoga Practice*. Orlando, FL: Ignite Yoga & Wellness Institute, 2020.

Ballard, Jacob. *A Queer Dharma: Yoga and Meditations for Liberation*. Berkeley, CA: North Atlantic Books, 2021.

Cohen, Elizabeth. *Light on the Other Side of Divorce: Discovering the New You*. Miami: Mango, 2021.

Germer, Christopher K. *The Mindful Path to Self-Compassion: Freeing Yourself from Destructive Thoughts and Emotions*. New York: Guilford Press, 2009.

Goldstein, Joseph. *Mindfulness: A Practical Guide to Awakening*. Boulder: Sounds True, 2016.

Heyman, Jivana. *Yoga Revolution: Building a Practice of Courage and Compassion*. Boulder: Shambhala Publications, 2021.

———. *Accessible Yoga: Poses and Practices for Every Body*. Boulder: Shambhala Publications, 2019.

Johnson, Michelle Cassandra. *Finding Refuge: Heart Work for Healing Collective Grief*. Boulder: Shambhala Publications, 2021.

————. *Skill in Action: Radicalizing Your Yoga Practice to Create a Just World*. Boulder: Shambhala Publications, 2017.

Kabat-Zinn, Jon. *Full Catastrophe Living: Using the Wisdom of Your Body and Mind to Face Stress, Pain, and Illness*. New York: Bantam Books, 2013.

Khouri, Hala. *Peace from Anxiety: Get Grounded, Build Resilience, and Stay Connected Amidst Chaos*. Boulder: Shambhala Publications, 2021.

Levine, Peter. *Waking the Tiger—Healing Trauma: The Innate Capacity to Transform Overwhelming Experiences*. Berkeley, CA: North Atlantic Books, 1997.

Linklater, Kristin. *Freeing the Natural Voice: Imagery and Art in the Practice of Voice and Language*. London, Nick Hern Books, 2006.

Magee, Rhonda V. *The Inner Work of Racial Justice: Healing Ourselves and Transforming Our Communities through Mindfulness*. New York: Tarcher Perigee, 2019.

Menakem, Resmaa. *My Grandmother's Hands: Racialized Trauma and the Pathway to Mending Our Hearts and Bodies*. Las Vegas: Central Recovery Press, 2017.

Mortali, Micah. *Rewilding: Meditations, Practices, and Skills for Awakening in Nature*. Boulder, CO: Sounds True, 2019.

Murthy, Vivek. *Together: The Healing Power of Human Connection in a Sometimes Lonely World*. New York: Harper Wave, 2020.

Owens, Lama Rod. *Love and Rage: The Path of Liberation through Anger*. Berkeley, CA: North Atlantic Books, 2020.

Parker, Gail. *Restorative Yoga for Ethnic and Race-Based Stress and Trauma*. London: Singing Dragon, 2020.

Porges, Stephen. *The Polyvagal Theory: Neurophysiological Foundations of Emotions, Attachment, Communication, and Self-Regulation*. New York: W. W. Norton, 20211.

Salzberg, Sharon. *Real Love: The Art of Mindful Connection*. London: Bluebird, 2017.

Sanford, Matthew. *Waking: A Memoir of Trauma and Transcendence*. Emmaus, PA: Rodale, 2006.

Sapolsky, Robert. *Why Zebras Don't Get Ulcers*. New York: Henry Holt, 2004.

Selassie, Sebene. *You Belong: A Call for Connection*. New York: HarperOne, 2020.

Siegel, David. *The Developing Mind: How Relationships and the Brain Interact to Shape Who We Are*. 3rd ed. New York: Guilford Press, 2020.

Treleaven, David. *Trauma-Sensitive Mindfulness: Practices for Safe and Transformative Healing*. New York: W. W. Norton, 2018.

Van der Kolk, Bessel. *The Body Keeps the Score: Brain, Mind, and Body in the Healing of Trauma*. New York: Penguin, 2014.

Walker, Matthew. *Why We Sleep: Unlocking the Power of Sleep and Dreams*. New York: Scribner, 2017.

Yang, Larry. *Awakening Together: The Spiritual Practice of Inclusivity and Community*. Somerville, MA: Wisdom Publications, 2017.

PODCASTS

Accessible Yoga, https://www.accessibleyogaschool.com/podcast

Beyond Trauma Podcast, https://beyondtraumapodcast.com/

Ear Hustle, https://www.earhustlesq.com/

Emerge: Making Sense of What's Next, https://www.whatisemerging.com/emergepodcast

Ten Percent Happier with Dan Harris, https://www.tenpercent.com/podcast

The Trauma-Sensitive Mindfulness Podcast, https://davidtreleaven.com/podcast/

Yoga Is Dead, https://www.yogaisdeadpodcast.com/home

WEBSITES

Land Yoga School, https://landyogaschool.teachable.com/p/intro-to-ashtanga-yoga

Three and a Half Acres, www.threeandahalfacres.org

Yoga Philosophy, https://yogaphilosophy.com/

ACKNOWLEDGMENTS

AMPLIFYING ONE'S INDEPENDENCE CAN REVEAL AGENCY, energy, and action, but understanding our interdependence unlocks awe, humbleness, and a truth that, if we embody it, is capable of making change. I will never be able to thank all the people who have gotten to my soul, formed connections in my mind, and influenced this body of work. I'll do my best to name a few.

Thank you to my husband, Thimo Wittich, who is always bringing me the works of great teachers and opening the depths of my understanding. You are a thought partner, a supporter, and an anchor for me. I appreciate all the early mornings and evenings you watched Hannah so I could write.

Big thanks to my parents, David and Sheryl, who are the most parenty parents one could ask for. I am so lucky to have them so close and still caring for me and my family—a deep, deep privilege.

Gratitude to the many teachers who have sparked curiosity in me and helped me to see the narratives that aren't always so obvious. Especially I want to thank Elaine Vaan Hogue, who taught me about using my body to hold and express meaning and whose introduction to and stories of civil disobedience still resonate with me today. Thank you also to Betsy Polatin, who brought the Alexander Technique into my life, which forced me to own choices in life-changing ways.

Thank you to Andrea Matura, one of my earliest yoga teachers, who saw my passion and was generous enough to send me to other teachers who would influence my path. What a rare and honorable gift.

I'm forever grateful to Christopher Hildebrandt, my first Mysore-style Ashtanga teacher. Thank you for believing in me and for taking me on my first trip to India, a decision that changed the next twenty years of my life.

ACKNOWLEDGMENTS

To my teachers in India, Sharath Jois and Hema Venkatesh: you changed my vibration, you taught me dedication, and you gave me the deepest respect for the subtle lessons of the early morning hours. Thank you for sharing your lineages and your culture with me for over a decade.

I also give thanks to the other teachers who have come to my path, especially in more recent years, many of whom are referenced in this book. Thank you Jivana Heyman, Suzanna Barkataki, Dr. Shyam Rangatham, David Treleaven, and my teachers at The Embody Lab: Dr. Maureen Gallagher, Karine Bell, Dr. Peter Levine, Kai Cheng Thom, Dr. Scott Lyons, Euphrasia "Efu" Nyaki, Dr. Dan Siegel, Bonnie Bainbridge Cohen, Jessica Montgomery, Dr. Albert Wong, and Dr. Diane Poole Heller.

Big thanks to Michelle Cassandra Johnson for not only her teaching but also her influence, energy, and kindness in writing the foreword for this book.

Thanks to all the many partnerships that have helped me grow in ways working solo never can. I'm in deep gratitude to present and former Three and a Half Acres Yoga board members Kristin Krantz, Caitlin Condy, Maria Lupardo, Jennifer Scullion, Karen Murray-Archer, and Jessica Swenson. Working with these women has been one of the greatest gifts of my life. To Iana Velez, my partner on SOULFest: thank you for remaining by my side as life has been filled with this book-writing work.

Thank you to my editor Beth Frankl for believing in me and this project in its earliest stages and to everyone at Shambhala for consistently taking extra time to show kindness and support for me and this body of work.

Special thank you to my editor Rochelle Bourgault, whose clear, precise, and gentle nature was exactly what I needed at the stage she arrived. I appreciate you and the energy you brought with you through our final edits. I also want to send these same sentiments to the book's photographer, Simon Keough, who has showed up so generously and wholeheartedly for me through this entire process and made the models look and feel so good.

Big sturdy hugs to the models in this book who shared so transparently their images and their unique and personal stories that have made this book all the more real and compelling. Timothy Lewis, Samantha Lucas, Elsie Scimecca, Nikki Walker, and Pratiba Premkumar: I am in awe of each one of you. Thank you for your time, your insights, and your friendship.

Finally and most importantly are the true teachers: the students. Each time I train another class of yoga teachers in trauma sensitivity, I always impart to them that the real training happens in the classroom. This is no cliché. The students are the teachers. To each student who has trusted me with your precious mind-body-spirit system, I send you a continuous flow of gratitude. This book is for and because of you.

NOTES

Introduction

1. Dalai Lama, *Worlds in Harmony: Dialogues on Compassionate Action* (Berkeley, CA: Parallax Press, 1992), 95.
2. Adrienne Maree Brown, *Emergent Strategy: Shaping Change, Changing Worlds* (Chico, CA: AK Press, 2017), 68.
3. Lama Rodd Owens, interview by Dan Harris, "What Is a Meditation Anchor?" May 27, 2020, *Ten Percent Happier*, podcast, 00:20:22, https://www.tenpercent.com/tph-live/52-lama-rod-owens.

1. Defining Trauma

1. A 2015 study on Holocaust survivors that showed hints at trauma inheritance brought intense attention to this field of research, though it is still very early for broad claims.
2. Gail Parker, *Restorative Yoga for Ethnic and Race-Based Stress and Trauma* (Philadelphia: Singing Dragon, 2020), 25.
3. Kristin Neff, *Fierce Self-Compassion: How Women Can Harness Kindness to Speak Up, Claim Their Power, and Thrive* (New York: HarperCollins, 2021), 190.
4. William J. Hall, Mimi V. Chapman, Kent M. Lee, Yesenia M. Merino, Tainayah W. Thomas, B. Keith Payne, Eugenia Eng, Steven H. Day, and Tamera Coyne-Beasley, "Implicit Racial/Ethnic Bias Among Health Care Professionals and Its Influence on Health Care Outcomes: A Systematic Review," *American Journal of Public Health* 105, no. 12 (December 2015): e60–76. https://doi.org/10.2105/AJPH.2015.302903.
5. Dr. Vivek Murthy, former surgeon general and author of *Together*, explains it's not how many relationships but having ones in which you can bring "the entirety of yourself to the table" that protects against loneliness. Furthermore, it is a connection to one's own self, particularly

one's self-worth, that allows this kind of deep connection with others. Research shows loneliness is as lethal as smoking fifteen cigarettes per day, and lonely people are 50 percent more likely to die prematurely than those with strong social connections. Murthy, *Together: The Healing Power of Human Connection in a Sometimes Lonely World* (New York: HarperCollins, 2020), 61.

6. Larry Yang, *Awakening Together: The Spiritual Practice of Inclusivity and Community* (Somerville, MA: Wisdom Publications, 2017), 130.

7. Jivana Heyman coined the term *accessible yoga*, and his book *Accessible Yoga: Poses and Practices for Every Body* (Boulder, CO: Shambhala Publications, 2019) is a great resource to delve more deeply into this topic.

8. Peter Levine, *Waking the Tiger—Healing Trauma: The Innate Capacity to Transform Overwhelming Experiences* (Berkeley, CA: North Atlantic Books, 1997), 156.

9. "With chronic sleep restriction over months or years, an individual will actually acclimate to their impaired performance, lower alertness, and reduced energy levels. That low-level exhaustion becomes their accepted norm, or baseline. Individuals fail to recognize how their perennial state of sleep deficiency has come to compromise their mental aptitude and physical vitality, including the slow accumulation of ill health." Matthew Walker, *Why We Sleep: Unlocking the Power of Sleep and Dreams* (New York: Scribner, 2017), 137.

10. Pamela Stokes Eggelston, "How One Yoga Teacher Found Strength After Her Husband's War Injury," *Yoga Journal*, May 15, 2020, https://www.yogajournal.com/yoga-101/yoga-advice-for-finding-strength-post-war-trauma/.

11. Robert Sapolsky, *Why Zebras Don't Get Ulcers* (New York: Henry Holt, 2004).

2. Softening the Trauma Response through Yoga

1. Presentation by Shyam Ranganathan based on *Patañjali's Yoga Sūtra*, trans. Shyam Ranganathan (Delhi: Penguin India, 2008).

2. Bessel van der Kolk, *The Body Keeps the Score: Brain, Mind, and Body in the Healing of Trauma* (New York: Penguin, 2014), 21.

3. The esteemed yoga teacher Matthew Sanford who was paralyzed at age thirteen said in a 2010 interview with *Gulf News* that it did not take long for the effects of yoga to begin showing in his body and mind. "For the first time after [my accident], I could feel the energy flow through my whole body. Through yoga, I encountered a richness and texture within part of me that I never thought possible. It helped me feel whole again. My paralyzed body pulses with life and sensation and has much to teach me about the experience of living." Suchitra Bajpai Chaudhary, "Making the Connection," *Gulf News*, March 2020, https://www.matthewsanford.com/sites/default/files/media/gulf-news-march-2010.pdf?phpMyAdmin=4qrRaMSfaJdSKnrro9UtvUEcrT1.

4. The term *window of tolerance* was coined by Dan Siegel, a clinical profes- sor of psychiatry, to describe the landscape of stimulation a person can function within. When outside this "window," either through over- or understimulation, the person's ability to function will be diminished. This window is unique to each individual and can be expanded through capac- ity-building practices.

5. David Treleaven, *Trauma-Sensitive Mindfulness: Practices for Safe and Transformative Healing* (New York: W. W. Norton, 2018), 113.

6. Winthrop Sargeant, trans., *Bhagavad Gita* (Albany: State University of New York Press, 1994), 132.

7. Michelle Casandra Johnson, *Skill in Action: Radicalizing Your Yoga Practice to Create a Just World* (Boulder, CO: Shambhala Publications, 2017), 19.

8. Kristin Linklater, *Freeing the Natural Voice* (Los Angeles, CA: Drama Pub- lications, 1976), 184.

9. Jivana Heyman, *Yoga Revolution: Building a Practice of Courage and Com- passion* (Boulder, CO: Shambhala Publications, 2021), 113.

10. Joseph Goldstein, *Mindfulness: A Practical Guide to Awakening* (Louis- ville, CO: Sounds True, 2016), 313.

11. Resmaa Menakem, *My Grandmother's Hands: Radicalized Trauma and the Pathway to Mending Our Hearts and Bodies* (New York: Penguin, 2021), 93–94.

3. Becoming a Skilled Trauma-Informed Yoga Teacher

1. There are no perfectly safe spaces, and sometimes in group classes, attend- ing to one person's safety compromises another's. For instance, one per- son in your class may feel safest walking around and another may feel un- comfortable when there is lots of movement around them. This highlights the complexity of teaching trauma-informed yoga to groups as opposed to the therapeutic individualized way it's often been described. Our goal is to make our spaces as safe as possible, which involves shifting acceptable prac- tices group to group. It requires agility. It may never be perfect, but it can be safe enough.

2. Stephen Porges, *The Polyvagal Theory: Neurophysical Foundations of Emotions, Attachment, Communication, and Self-Regulation* (New York: W. W. Norton, 2011), 13.

3. While there are studies that indicate certain poses have calming effects, those same poses could be triggering for someone whose trauma is associated with that position, even if it is deemed restful. It's also essential to note that it is not the pose but how we bring breath and awareness into the experience of being in the posture that determines its impact.

4. Building a Safe Trauma-Informed Yoga Class

1. Hala Khouri, *Peace from Anxiety: Get Grounded, Build Resistance, and Stay Connected Amidst the Chaos* (Boulder, CO: Shambhala Publications, 2021), 9.

2. See my *Huffington Post* article "The Positivity Problem: Why Yoga Imaging Must Go Deeper," last updated February 3, 2017, https://www.huffpost.com/entry/the-positivity-problem-wh_b_9138968.

3. Tristan Katz, "Creating Trans Affirming Yoga Spaces," Tristan Katz Creative (website), https://www.katz-creative.com/trans-affirming-yoga-spaces.

ABOUT THE AUTHOR

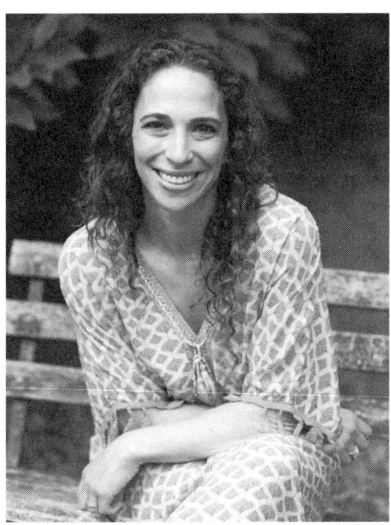

LARA LAND (she/her) is a deeply compassionate somatic therapist, life coach, consultant, and yoga-teacher trainer specializing in trauma sensitivity. Her work is directed in helping to heal trauma, both subtle and significant, and to train others to do the same using yoga, meditation, mindfulness, and breathing practices. Lara has spent the last twenty-five years studying and sharing yoga asana, chanting, meditation, and philosophy directly from her teachers in India. Her commitment is to honor the traditions of yoga by responding to the needs of each individual using a unique combination of practices and techniques that are appropriate for their personal growth. Lara is the owner of Land Yoga, coproducer of SOULFest, and executive director of Three and a Half Acres Yoga. Her self-published life-purpose planner, *My Bliss Book*, was released in 2018. She has been featured in *Yoga Journal*, *New York Magazine*, the *Huffington Post*, and on NY1, Fox5, CBS, and Pix11.